Treatment and Management of Melanoma

Treatment and Management of Melanoma

Edited by **Frederick Nash**

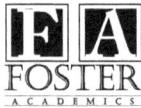

FOSTER
ACADEMICS

New Jersey

Published by Foster Academics,
61 Van Reypen Street,
Jersey City, NJ 07306, USA
www.fosteracademics.com

Treatment and Management of Melanoma
Edited by Frederick Nash

International Standard Book Number: 978-1-63242-408-2 (Hardback)

Printed in the United States of America.

Contents

Preface

This book intends to present data and knowledge from most experienced experts in the field. The book encompasses important topics on multiple approaches in melanoma treatment as well as related features. It provides a global perspective concerning one of the most frequent types of cancer, which a large number of people come across at some point of time in their life. This book is an invaluable source of reference for those interested in the research and treatment of melanoma.

Significant researches are present in this book. Intensive efforts have been employed by authors to make this book an outstanding discourse. This book contains the enlightening chapters which have been written on the basis of significant researches done by the experts.

Finally, I would also like to thank all the members involved in this book for being a team and meeting all the deadlines for the submission of their respective works. I would also like to thank my friends and family for being supportive in my efforts.

Editor

Melanoma Treatment Approaches

Management of Brain Metastasis in Melanoma Patients

Sherif S. Morgan*, Joanne M. Jeter, Evan M. Hersh,
Sun K. Yi and Lee D. Cranmer*

Additional information is available at the end of the chapter

1. Introduction

The American Cancer Society estimates that 76,250 Americans will be diagnosed with malignant melanoma and 9,180 will die from the disease in 2012 [1]. The incidence is increasing both in the United States and worldwide [2]. Brain metastasis is a common problem in this population with 45-60% of those with metastatic melanoma developing brain metastases during the course of their illness [3]. Post-mortem studies demonstrate that brain lesions are present in 70-90% of patients who die of melanoma [3]. Development of brain metastases may have adverse impact both on a patient's prognosis and, if symptomatic, severe effects on quality-of-life (QOL) [4]. If left untreated, symptomatic brain lesions may be fatal within several weeks [3].

The literature pertaining to the treatment of brain metastasis from melanoma is scant when compared to brain metastases from more common solid tumors. In particular, brain metastases from non-small cell lung cancer (NSCLC) and breast cancer have been the subject of a larger number of investigative efforts. This chapter will extrapolate relevant results from other common solid tumors to the treatment of melanoma. In addition, systemic treatment approaches that may be useful in managing intracranial disease will be presented. Leptomeningeal involvement of the central nervous system, a less common form of central nervous system (CNS) invasion by melanoma, will not be discussed.

2. Treatment modalities

2.1. Surgery

Three randomized trials have investigated treatment of a single brain metastasis with whole brain radiation therapy (WBRT) alone or combined with surgical resection (Table 1) [5-7]. In all three, overall survival (OS) was the primary endpoint. In one study, the addition of surgery to WBRT achieved better control at the target lesion site than did WBRT alone [7]. Two of the trials indicated a survival benefit conferred by surgical treatment when added to WBRT, compared to WBRT alone. Differences in the proportion of patients with NSCLC, percentages of patients with extracranial disease, treatment of patients with non-metastatic intracranial disease, and cross-over from one treatment arm to the other may explain why the study of Mintz and co-workers did not indicate a survival benefit [6]. Extent of extracranial disease status was a consistent predictor of survival.

Study	Centers (#)	Patients (#)	Disease Types # (%)	Median Survival	Recurrence/ Progression in CNS		Comments
					Treated Site	Distant	
Patchell et al., 1990 [7]	1	48 25-S 23-R	37 NSCLC (77%) 3 Mel. (6%)	40 w-S 15 w-R P<0.01	20%-S 52%-R P<0.02	20%-S 13%-R P=0.52	37% of enrolled patients with metastatic disease at enrollment. Extracranial disease and older age predicted decreased survival in multivariate analysis.
Noordijk et al., 1994 [5]	5	63 32-S 31-R	33 NSCLC (52%) 6 Mel. (10%)	10 m-S 6 m-R P=0.04	NR	NR	Survival benefit in those with stable extra-cranial disease (12 m-S vs. 7 m-R, p=0.02) and patients younger than 61 y (19 m-S vs. 9 m-R, p=0.003). No survival benefit for surgery in patients with progressive extracranial disease or age"/>60.
Mintz et al., 1996 [6]	8	84 41-S 43-R	45 NSCLC (53%)	5.6 m-S 6.3 m-R P=0.24	NR	NR	45% of enrolled patients with metastatic disease at enrollment. Only extracranial disease status predicted survival in multivariate analysis.

KPS: Karnofsky performance status; Mel: Melanoma patients; NR: Not reported; NSCLC: Non-small cell lung cancer; OS: Overall survival; QOL: Quality of life; R: Refers to treatment arm receiving WBRT alone; S: Refers to treatment arm combining surgery and WBRT

Table 1. Randomized trials of surgical resection of a single brain metastasis combined with WBRT versus WBRT alone

Since these studies primarily enrolled patients with primary NSCLC or breast cancer, their applicability to melanoma is uncertain. No prospective trials of surgery for melanoma patients with brain metastases have been published to date. However, a number of large retrospective studies have been reported (Table 2) [8-13]. Surgical treatment is consistently reported as a factor strongly associated with prolonged survival over those treated with WBRT alone. Selection biases are inherent in retrospective studies. Indeed, two of the studies specifically identified factors predicting patient selection for more or less aggressive treatment and follow-up based on the presumed severity of CNS involvement [10, 12]. Given that these retrospective reports in melanoma concur with the randomized trials of surgical therapy in non-melanoma brain metastases, similar randomized trials of surgery for melanoma brain metastases are probably unnecessary.

Traditionally, surgical management of brain metastases was restricted to individuals with a single accessible lesion. Bindal and co-workers found that individuals with a variety of primary solid tumors (n=56; melanoma=25/45%) undergoing resection of 2-3 brain metastases had survival rates equivalent to those undergoing resection of a single lesion [14]. In patients with complete resection of all known lesions, median survival was 14 months, equivalent to that for patients treated surgically for a single CNS lesion. Patients who could not undergo complete resection of CNS disease demonstrated inferior median overall survival of 6 months. Thus, presence of multiple CNS metastases is not a contra-indication to surgical treatment, although the advent of stereotactic radiosurgery (SRS) has made this approach less common.

2.2. Stereotactic Radiosurgery (SRS)

Stereotactic radiosurgery (SRS) has become a major modality in the local treatment of brain metastases. When compared to conventional techniques, SRS allows for safe and effective dose escalation. This is achieved through use of multiple modulated beamlets from a variety of angles, allowing optimized conformality and avoidance of normal tissues. SRS is minimally or non-invasive and allows targeting multiple CNS lesions including those that may be surgically accessible. Treatment is often performed on an outpatient basis and over a short time duration. Retreatment of the same or of new lesions is possible.

The Radiation Therapy Oncology Group (RTOG) conducted a large randomized study of SRS combined with WBRT (n=164) versus WBRT alone (n=167) (Table 3) [15]. The study enrolled patients with a variety of tumor types, although NSCLC patients comprised the largest proportion. The addition of SRS to WBRT resulted in a survival benefit for patients with a single brain lesion (6.5 months for combination therapy versus 4.9 months for WBRT alone, p=0.0393), but not for patients with multiple lesions (5.8 months for combination therapy versus 6.7 months for WBRT alone, p=0.9776) or all patients combined (6.5 months for the combination versus 5.7 months for WBRT alone, p=0.1356). At 6 months, SRS-treated patients required lower doses of corticosteroids and were more likely to discontinue steroid use altogether (52% in SRS+WBRT decreased their dose compared to 33% in the WBRT only group, p<0.0158). Patients receiving SRS also were more likely to improve their performance status (13% improved vs. 4% improved in WBRT group, p=0.0331). Local control of targeted tumors was better with SRS. Disease control at distant sites within the brain was equivalent.

Study	Dates, Patient Source Population, Institution	Melanoma Patients Studied and Treatment	Median Survival	CNS Recurrence Rates Based on Therapy Received	QOL
Raizer et al., 2008 [13]	1991-2001 All metastatic melanoma patients (n=1114) at a single center	355 total 12 S/R +SRS 20 S + SRS 58 S/R 20 R + SRS 36 S 26 SRS 100 R 83 Supp.	Surgery (9 m) vs. no surgery (4 m), p<0.0001 R 4.0 m Supp. 2.0 m	NR	NR
Fife et al., 2004 [12]	1985-2000 All patients with brain metastasis from melanoma (n=1137) at a single center	686 total 158 S/R 47 S 236 R 210 Supp.	All pts. 4.1 m S/R 8.9 m S 8.7 m R 3.4 m Supp. 2.1 m S= S/R, p=0.21 S or S/R >R > Supp., p<0.001	NR	NR
Buchsbaum et al., 2002 [10]	1984-1998 All brain metastasis patients (n=1154) at a single center	74 total 14 S/R 19 R + SRS 3 S/R + SRS 10 S or SRS 25 R 3 Supp.	All pts. 5.5m (S or SRS) + R 8.8 m S or SRS 4.8 m R 2.3 m Supp. 1.1 m (S or SRS) + R vs. other groups, p<0.0001 S/R =R + SRS, p=0.5128	49% Local + R 17% R 20% S or SRS	NR
Zacest et al., 2002 [11]	1979-1999 All surgically treated melanoma patients with brain metastasis at a single center	147 total 9 S 102 S/R 33 S/R/C 3 S/C	All pts. 8.5 m	50% overall recurrence rate	Neurological symptoms after treatment: Resolved 52% Improved 26% Unchanged 9% N/A 13%
Wronski and Arbit, 2000 [9]	1974-1994	91 total 49 S/R	All pts. 6.7 m	56% S/R vs. 46% S, p=NR	NR

Study	Dates, Patient Source Population, Institution	Melanoma Patients Studied and Treatment	Median Survival	CNS Recurrence Rates Based on Therapy Received	QOL
	All surgically treated brain metastasis patients (n=702) at a single center	29 S 13 died within 62 d of surgery	S/R (9.5 m) vs. S (8.3 m), p=0.67		
Sampson et al., 1998 [8]	~1978-1998 All melanoma patients (n=6953) treated at a single center	524 total 87 S/R 52 S 180 R 205 C	Surgical therapy (NR) vs. R (120 d), p<0.0001 S/R (268 d) vs. S (195 d), p=0.9998 R (120 d) vs. C (39 d), p<0.0006	NR	No sig. difference in symptomatic results between patients treated with surgery and those treated with radiation (p=0.138)
Skibber et al., 1996 [53]	1979-1991 All surgically treated melanoma patients with a single brain metastasis at two centers. No active non-CNS metastases present.	34 total 22 S/R 12 S	S/R (18 m) vs. S(6 m), p=0.002	Overall CNS relapse rate: 30% S/R vs. 90% S, p=0.02	NR
Hagen et al., 1990 [54]	1972-1987 All surgically treated melanoma patients with a single brain metastasis at a single center	35 total 16 S 19 S/R	S (8.3 m) vs. S/R (6.4 m), p=NS	Median time to CNS relapse: S/R (26.6 m) vs. S (5.7 m), p<0.05	NR

C: Chemotherapy; Local Therapy: Treatment of CNS lesions with either surgery or stereotactic radiosurgery; KPS: Karnofsky performance status; NR: Not reported; NS: not significant; OS: Overall survival; QOL: Quality of life; R: Whole brain radiotherapy; S: Refers to treatment arm using surgery alone; Sig: Statistically significant; S/R: Surgery combined with whole brain radiotherapy; SRS: Stereotactic radiosurgery; Supp: Supportive care;

Table 2. Retrospective case series of surgery as treatment for brain metastasis in melanoma

A smaller study used the same design, but its primary endpoint was local disease control in patients with 2-4 brain lesions (Table 3) [16]. The study was halted at 60% of planned accrual due to meeting its primary endpoint (27 patients; 5 with melanoma). SRS-treated patients had significantly improved local disease control (p=0.0016). Median time-to-progression at SRS-treated sites was 6 months in patients treated with WBRT alone, versus 36 months in those treated with SRS and WBRT (p=0.0005). Extracranial disease status was the major survival determinant in a *post hoc* analysis.

Only two relatively small, single-arm prospective studies of SRS in melanoma have been published. One of these studies enrolled 31 patients, including 14 (45%) with melanoma (Table 3) [17]. Patients received only SRS as CNS therapy. Overall intracranial failure rate was 50% at 6 months. About one-third of patients failed within the SRS-treated tumor volume. The second study enrolled 45 melanoma patients receiving SRS at one of two treatment centers (Table 3) [18]. Up to 6 metastases were treated. Use of WBRT in conjunction with this therapy was not reported. Median survival of all patients was 4.2 months. The local control rate with SRS was 86%, although the follow-up period was not defined. Follow-up imaging was available for only 71 out of 86 treated lesions.

Numerous retrospective studies have reported the results of SRS therapy in melanoma (Table 4) [19-41]. These are quite variable in design. While some studied melanoma patients exclusively, others enrolled patients with other tumor types. Several studies appear to include the same set of patients treated at a given institution during overlapping time periods (noted in Table 4). Treatment and follow-up plans were not pre-specified or standardized. Although all patients received SRS, they often received a wide array of other therapies, including immediate or delayed WBRT, concurrent or delayed surgery, and partial brain irradiation. Patients received SRS both as primary brain metastasis therapy and as salvage therapy after failure of prior treatment. Some patients received therapy for a single metastasis, while others were treated for multiple brain metastases. Several studies specifically identify selection bias in the treated population, with more aggressive therapy being reserved for patients with more severe CNS disease [37, 38]. Collectively, the study heterogeneity limits the conclusions that can be reached from these retrospective analyses.

Reported median survival of melanoma patients in these series ranged from 4.4 to 11.1 months. These values approximate ranges reported in patients with brain metastases from other primary tumor types, in which median survival is estimated to be 6.5 to 10.5 months [10, 42, 43]. Several factors predicted shorter survival in multiple studies: decreased performance status or its surrogate indicators, multiple CNS lesions, greater intracranial tumor volume, infratentorial lesion location, and active extracranial disease.

Some studies did not find that the initial number of lesions predicted survival [28, 29, 34, 37, 39]. This contradicts the results of the only randomized trial of SRS with survival as the primary endpoint, in which a survival benefit was observed only in patients with a single CNS lesion (OS was 6.5 months in patients with SRS+WRBT compared to 4.9 months in the WBRT group alone; p=0.0393) [15]. This may be due to inadequate statistical power in the retrospective studies, given the heterogeneity of the populations under study.

CNS disease control was reported in most of these retrospective studies as 1-year actuarial control rates. At SRS-treated sites, reported in most of the studies, this was 47-87%. One-year control at non-SRS treated sites was 24-57%. The overall CNS control at one year was only 24-38%.

Study	Study Design	Patient Numbers & Tumor Types	Treatment	Median Survival	CNS Recurrence
Andrews et al., 2004 [15]	Randomized Multi-institution, cooperative group study 1996-2001 Primary endpoint: median survival	331 total 64% Lung 10% Breast 5% Melanoma 21% Other 1-3 CNS metastases	164 SRS+R 167 R	Overall 6.5 m S+R vs. 5.7 m R, p=0.14 Single met. 6.5 m SRS+R vs. 4.9 m R, p=0.39 Multiple met. 5.8 m SRS+R vs. 6.7 m R, p=0.98	Time to intra-cranial progression SRS+R=R, p=0.13 Local control at 1 yr 82% SRS+R vs. 71% R, p=0.01
Kondziolka et al., 1999 [16]	Randomized Single institution Primary endpoint: local control at SRS-treated site	27 total: 44% Lung 19% Melanoma 15% Renal 15% Breast 7% Other 2-4 CNS metastases	13 SRS+R 14 R	11 m SRS+R vs. 7.5 m R, p=0.22.	Median time to CNS failure: Local: 36 m SRS+R vs. 6 m R, p=0.0005 Any: 34 m SRS+R vs. 5 m R, p=0.002
Manon et al., 2005 [17]	Single-arm Multi-institution, cooperative group study 1998-2003 Primary endpoint: 3m and 6m intracranial progression rate	31 total 45% Melanoma 45% Renal 10% Sarcoma 1-3 CNS metastases	31 SRS	8.3 m	Intra-cranial Failure Rates 3 m: Any 25.8% SRS-treated 19.3% Outside SRS 16.2% 6 m: Any 48.3% SRS-treated 32.2% Outside SRS field32.2%
Friehs et al., 1998 [18]	Single-arm Multi-institution 1998-2003 Primary endpoint: Overall survival	45 total 100% Mel. 1-6 CNS metastases	45 SRS	4.2 m	86% of SRS-treated tumors controlled at follow-up. 13 (29%) with known distant failure in CNS.

KPS: Karnofsky performance status; Mel: Melanoma; Met: Metastasis/metastases; MMSE: Mini-Mental Status Examination; NR: Not reported; QOL: Quality of life; R: Whole brain radiotherapy; SRS+R: Stereotactic radiosurgery combined with whole brain radiotherapy; SRS: Stereotactic radiosurgery

Table 3. Prospective trials of stereotactic radiosurgery as treatment for brain metastases in melanoma

Study	Study Design	Patient Numbers & Tumor Types	Treatment	Median Survival	CNS Control Rates (1-yr actuarial unless otherwise stated)	Comments (Prognostic factors multivariate unless otherwise noted)
Liew et al., 2011 [31]	1987-2008 Single institution All patients with mel. receiving GK	344 total 100% mel.	163 SRS 118 SRS+R 63 SRS + other	5.6 m after SRS 8.3 m from diagnosis of brain met	SRS treated sites 63% Distant 33%	R not sig. for survival or recurrence. Population may overlap with that of Mori et al., 1998 and Somoza et al., 1993.
Hara et al., 2009 [27]	1999-2005 Single institution All pts. receiving Cyberknife therapy for mel. or renal cancer	62 total 44 mel. 18 renal	33 SRS 17 SRS sal. 5 SRS+R 7 SRS + Surg.	8.3 m 5.6 m for mel.	SRS-treated sites 87% Local and distant 38%	
Powell et al., 2008 [34]	1998-2007 Single institution All patients receiving GK	76 total 50 mel. 23 renal 3 sarcoma	39 SRS 37 SRS+R	5.1 m Histology does not predict outcome	SRS-treated sites 78% Distant 37% Local and distant 26%	Local control higher for renal than mel . (94% vs. 63%, p=0.001)
Redmond et al., 2008 [36]	1998-2006 Single institution All mel. pts. receiving GK	59 total 100% mel.	32 SRS 27 SRS+R	4.4 m	NR	Timing between SRS and R undefined.
Samlowski et al., 2007 [37]	1999-2004 Single institution All mel. patients receiving LA-SRS	44 total 100% mel.	19 SRS 4 SRS +partial R 14 SRS+R 16% SRS with salvage R	11.1 m from brain metastasis diagnosis 48% 1-yr survival 18% 2-yr survival	SRS-treated sites 47%	Patients receiving SRS+R had a higher mean number of presented metastases (3.8) than those receiving salvage R after SRS failure (1.6). 22 (50%) treated with surgery at some point. Multiple lesions treated in 22 (50%).
Christopoulou et al., 2006 [22]	1998-2004 Single institution All mel. patients receiving GK	29 total 100% mel.	All SRS 4 with prior R 2 with prior surg.	5.7 m	NR	
Gaudy-Marqueste et al., 2006 [23]	1997-2003 Single institution All mel. patients receiving GK	106 total 100% mel.	106 SRS	5.1 m 13% 1-yr survival	SRS-treated sites 69%	No patients received planned R
Chang et al., 2005 [20]	1991-2002 Single Institution	189 total 103 mel. 77 renal	130 SRS 16 SRS + R 43 SRS sal.	7.5 m	For mel. SRS-treated sites 47%	Inadequate patients treated with R to assess effects.

Study	Study Design	Patient Numbers & Tumor Types	Treatment	Median Survival	CNS Control Rates (1-yr actuarial unless otherwise stated)	Comments (Prognostic factors multivariate unless otherwise noted)
	All patients with mel., renal cancer or sarcoma receiving SRS as therapy	9 sarcoma		24% 1-y survival for mel.	Distant 24%	
Koc et al., 2005 [29]	1999-2003 Single institution All mel. patients receiving GK as initial therapy	26 total 100% mel.	12 SRS 14 SRS+R	6 m 25% 1-yr survival	NR	
Radbill et al., 2004 [35]	1996-2001 Single institution All mel. patients receiving GK	64 total 100% mel.	32 SRS 13 SRS sal. 8 SRS+R 8 SRS+surg. 2 SRS + R + surg. 1 NR	26 wk Single CNS met. (77 wk) vs. multiple (20 wk), p=0.003	SRS-treated sites 56% Distant 25%	Adjuvant R did not decrease distant failure, although small population receiving it.
Selek et al., 2004 [38]	1991-2001 Single institution All mel. patients receiving LA-SRS	103 total 100% mel.	61 SRS 12 SRS + R 30 SRS sal.	Overall 6.7 m SRS 7.5 m SRS+R 3.7 m SRS sal. 5.4 m 25% 1-y survival	SRS-treated sites 48% SRS alone 60% SRS+R 0% SRS sal. 5% Distant 24% SRS alone 18% SRS+R 0% SRS sal. 51%	Patients with more aggressive disease were more likely to receive R after SRS.
Herfarth et al., 2003 [28]	1986-2000 Two institutions All mel. patients treated with LA-SRS	64 total 100% mel.	All SRS	10.6 m	SRS-treated sites 81% Lesions ≥2 cm (64%) vs. <2 cm (88%), p=0.05 Distant CNS control NR	
Brown et al., 2002 [19]	1990-2000 Single institution All patients with mel., renal cancer or sarcoma receiving SRS.	41 total 23 mel. 16 renal 2 sarcoma	20 SRS 4 R with SRS sal. 8 Surg. with SRS sal. 9 SRS + surg.	14.2 m No difference in survival SRS+R vs. SRS, p=0.54	6 m CNS control SRS-treated sites: SRS+R (100%) vs. SRS (85%), p=0.02 Distant: SRS+R (91%) vs. SRS (35%), p=0.004	
Gonzalez-Martinez et al., 2002 [25]	1996-2002 Single institution All mel. patients receiving GK	24 total 100% mel.	10 SRS 14 SRS+R	5.5 m	NR	

Study	Study Design	Patient Numbers & Tumor Types	Treatment	Median Survival	CNS Control Rates (1-yr actuarial unless otherwise stated)	Comments (Prognostic factors multivariate unless otherwise noted)
Mingione et al., 2002 [32]	1989-1999 Single institution All mel. patients receiving GK	45 total 100% mel.	29 SRS 16 SRS+R	10.4 m 31% 1-yr survival	NR	Adjuvant R had no impact on survival or CNS recurrence rate.
Yu et al., 2002 [41]	1994-1999 Single institution All mel. patients receiving GK	122 total 100% mel.	83 SRS 12 SRS + R 10 SRS/R >1.5 m before SRS 17 SRS/R >1.5 m after SRS	7 m 26% 1-yr survival	SRS-treated sites 84% Distant 57%	Population may overlap with that of Lavine et al., 1999 and Chen et al., 1999.
Chen et al., 1999 [21]	1994-1999 Single institution All patients receiving GK	199 total 88 mel. 40 NSCLC 5 SCLC 12 Renal 12 Breast 9 Colon 24 Other	199 SRS	8.5 m 7 m for mel.	89% of lesions with follow-up "controlled for the lifetime of the patient"	Use of R reported, but not defined. Population may overlap with that of Yu et al., 2002 and Lavine et al., 1999. Follow-up available for only 69% of lesions.
Lavine et al., 1999 [30]	1994-1997 Single institution All mel. patients receiving GK	45 total 100% mel.	43 SRS. 2 SRS + R	8 m	3 m CNS control SRS-treated sites 97% Distant 81%	Population may overlap with that of Yu et al., 1999 and Chen et al., 1999. Other therapies in addition to SRS depending on clinical condition. Only 2 (4%) received SRS+R
Grob et al., 1998 [26]	1993-1996 Single institution All mel. patients receiving GK	35 total 100% mel.	35 SRS	7 m	Actuarial control rate of evaluable, treated lesions: 3 m 98% 6 m 100% 9 m 95% 12 m 87% Distant CNS control not reported	
Mori et al., 1998 [33]	1988-1996 Single institution All mel. patients receiving GK	60 total 100% mel.	12 SRS 36 SRS+R 12 SRS sal.	7 m median survival 21% 1-yr survival	Control in 46 pts. receiving SRS +/-R: SRS-treated sites: Overall 85%	Population may overlap with that of Mathieu et al., 2007 and Somoza et al., 1993.

Study	Study Design	Patient Numbers & Tumor Types	Treatment	Median Survival	CNS Control Rates (1-yr actuarial unless otherwise stated)	Comments (Prognostic factors multivariate unless otherwise noted)
					SRS+R 80% SRS 100% SRS sal. 86% Distant: Overall 70% SRS+R 77% SRS 56% SRS sal. 57%	
Seung et al., 1998 [39]	1991-1995 Single institution (UCSF) All melanoma patients receiving GK	55 total 100% melanoma	28 SRS 11 SRS+ R 16 SRS sal.	35 wk	SRS-treated sites 77% Distant 36% Entire CNS 24%	
Gieger et al., 1997 [24]	1992-1994 Single institution All mel. patients receiving LA-SRS	12 total 100% mel.	1 SRS 10 SRS+R 1 SRS sal.	8 m 36% 1-y survival	At least 6 patients with at least one SRS-treated lesions progressing. At least 3 (25%) developing new distant CNS lesions	Imaging follow-up not consistent.
Somoza et al., 1993 [40]	1988-1992 Single institution All mel. patients receiving GK	23 total 100% mel.	19 SRS + R 4 SRS with R 3-12 m later	7 m 26% 1-y survival	NR	Population may overlap with that of Mathieu et al., 2007 and Mori et al., 1998.

CNS: Central nervous system; GK: Gamma knife-based stereotactic radiosurgery; KPS: Karnofsky performance status; LA-SRS: Linear accelerator-based stereotactic radiosurgery; Mel: Melanoma; Met: Metastasis/metastases; NR: Not reported; QOL: Quality of life; Partial R: Partial brain irradiation; R: Whole brain radiotherapy; RPA: Recursive Partitioning Analysis; Sig: Statistically significant; SIR: Score Index for Radiosurgery; SRS: Stereotactic radiosurgery; SRS+R: Stereotactic radiosurgery combined with whole brain radiotherapy; SRS sal: Stereotactic radiosurgery salvage after failure of prior therapy; SRS+Surg: Combination therapy of stereotactic radiosurgery and conventional surgical resection; Surg: Surgical resection

Table 4. Retrospective studies of stereotactic radiosurgery for brain metastasis in melanoma

2.3. Comparative benefit of SRS versus surgery

The relative benefit of SRS versus surgery has not been tested in randomized clinical trials to date. One small randomized trial indirectly addressed this question, although not specifically for melanoma (Table 5) [44]. Sixty-four subjects with a single, surgically accessible brain lesion were randomly assigned to surgical excision and adjuvant WBRT or to SRS alone. A direct comparison of surgery and SRS is not possible due to the inclusion of adjuvant WBRT for all surgical patients and its omission in SRS-treated patients. Nine (14%) of the subjects had melanoma. No difference in overall survival was observed (9.5 months for surgery versus 10.3 months for SRS, p=0.8). A statistically non-significant improvement in local tumor control favored SRS (82% for surgery plus WBRT versus 97% for SRS, p=0.06). The one-year recurrence rate at distant CNS sites was significantly higher in the group receiving SRS alone (3% for surgery plus WBRT versus 26% for SRS alone, p<0.05). Thus, this study perhaps served to highlight the risks of omitting adjuvant treatment, rather than the relative merits of SRS versus surgery.

Two retrospective studies compared SRS to surgery [45, 46]. Melanoma patients were in the minority in both studies. O'Neill and co-workers analyzed patients seen from 1991-1999 at the Mayo Clinic who underwent either SRS or surgery for a solitary brain metastasis [45]. Eligible patients were candidates for either procedure: all had solitary lesions measuring less than 35 mm (maximum size conventionally treated with SRS), none of the lesions were surgically inaccessible, and none required immediate surgical decompression. Ninety-seven patients met these criteria, of whom only seven were melanoma patients. Seventy-four were treated surgically and twenty-three were treated with SRS. Although not achieving statistical significance, more SRS-treated patients received WBRT (96% SRS vs. 82% surgery, p=0.172). The treatment groups differed at baseline in performance status (worse in the SRS group, p=0.0016). Overall survival was similar between the two groups and was predicted by age, performance status, and systemic extracranial disease status rather than the type of brain metastasis treatment. Similar proportions of patients had CNS recurrence (29% SRS versus 30% surgery), but patients receiving surgery were more likely to have local recurrence at treated sites (58% of recurrences in 19 patients vs. 0% out of 6 recurrences in SRS-treated patients, p=0.02). Although this study suggests that local recurrences are more common after surgery, the retrospective nature of the study and the small number of patients limits its applicability.

In contrast, another single institution, retrospective study from a similar time period (1991-1994) suggested that SRS led to higher local recurrence rates than surgery [46]. Thirty-one patients were treated with SRS and sixty-two with surgery for brain metastases. Twenty-one patients (23%) had melanoma. Patients were matched with regard to histology, extracranial disease status, performance status, time from initial diagnosis to CNS metastasis, number of CNS metastases, age, and gender. Patients in the two groups were equally likely to have received WBRT. Patients receiving surgical treatment survived significantly longer than those treated with SRS (16.4 months surgery vs. 7.5 months SRS, p=0.0018). This improvement in survival was attributable to decreased rates of death from neurological causes in the surgical group (19% surgery vs. 50% SRS, p=0.037); deaths due to systemic disease were equivalent (p=0.28). Surgery yielded lower local tumor recurrence rates than SRS (8.1% surgery vs. 38.7% SRS). There was no statistically significant different in distant CNS recurrence rates between the two groups.

This retrospective study is subject to the biases inherent in such an undertaking. The authors matched patients for a variety of known relevant parameters, but the differences in local control may reflect the use of older SRS technology, high quality neurosurgical treatment at the referral center where the study was undertaken, or a combination of both. These discrepancies might explain the differences in results when contrasted with the results of the two other studies described [44, 45].

Collectively these studies do not indicate whether surgery or SRS is superior. There are no easily detectable differences in local control rates. Logistic differences therefore are important in selecting therapy. Unless a clinical situation arises in which surgery provides clear superiority (e.g. rapid control of symptomatic lesions; histological diagnosis), SRS will likely be the predominant modality employed to treat macroscopic melanoma lesions in the CNS.

2.4. Adjuvant Whole Brain Radiotherapy (WBRT)

Adjuvant therapy of the CNS is that which is administered in conjunction with definitive local therapy (surgery or SRS) of radiologically evident tumors to treat co-existing micrometastatic disease. This is distinguished from prophylactic cranial irradiation (PCI). PCI is administered in patients with systemic cancer after responses to systemic therapy, and has proven benefit in several conditions, such as small cell lung cancer (SCLC) [47, 48]. In melanoma, PCI has not been adequately assessed to recommend. Adjuvant CNS therapy has traditionally relied on WBRT. Although new systemic agents with proven anti-melanoma activity and CNS penetration may come to be used for this purpose as well, such use is experimental at present. Adjuvant WBRT is a controversial topic in metastatic brain tumor management, primarily due to questions of efficacy and of neurocognitive toxicity.

Three factors must be considered in determining whether or not to use adjuvant WBRT: (a) the effectiveness of WBRT in preventing emergence of new brain tumors; (b) the adverse effects of WBRT; and (c) the competing adverse effect of foregoing WBRT, namely an increased rate of CNS tumor progression. As new systemic therapies are proposed for this purpose, the same considerations apply. The relevant adverse effects relate to deterioration of neurocognitive function (NCF) and QOL, which could result from either WBRT itself or from progressive brain tumors. It is in balancing these factors that a rational decision regarding the use, or non-use, of adjuvant WBRT can be made.

2.4.1. Randomized trials of adjuvant WBRT in solid tumor patients

Despite the frequency of brain metastasis in melanoma patients, no prospective trials have been conducted to assess adjuvant WBRT in this population. Data from the treatment of brain metastases focusing on other tumor types must be reviewed to come to any conclusions (Table 5). Five randomized trials of adjuvant WBRT have been reported. Four of these are multi-institutional efforts, reflecting the difficulty in conducting this type of study [49-52]. A fifth study, discussed earlier, compared outcome in patients with a single brain metastasis treated with surgery and WBRT or with SRS alone [44]. The majority of patients in all of the studies were those with NSCLC primary tumors. Relatively few melanoma patients were enrolled.

Only one study used intracranial recurrence rate as the planned primary endpoint [52]. Ninety-five patients were enrolled after surgical resection of an isolated brain metastasis. Sixty percent had NSCLC. Forty-nine patients were randomized to receive adjuvant WBRT (50.4 Gy administered as 28-1.8 Gy fractions). The remaining forty-six patients were observed. Only

Study	Evaluable Patients (#)	Disease types #	Primary Endpoint	Median Survival	Recurrence/Progression in CNS		Comments
					S/SRS-site	Distant	
Patchell et al., 1998 [52]	95 total 49 S+R 46 S	57 NSCLC 9 Breast 29 Other	CNS recurrence rate	S+R (48 wk) vs. S (43 wk), p=0.39	10% S+R 46% S P<0.001	14% S+R 37% S P<0.01	Single brain metastasis. Overall CNS recurrence rate (primary endpoint) significantly less in R-treated patients (18% S+R vs. 70% S, p<0.001). Decreased rate of neurological cause of death in group receiving R (14% S +R vs. 44% S, p=0.003)
Aoyama et al., 2006 [49]	132 total 65 SRS+R 67 SRS	88 NSCLC 9 Breast 11 GI 10 Renal 14 Other	OS	SRS+R (7.5m) vs. SRS (8 .0 m), p=0.42	1-y rate 11% SRS +R 38% SRS P=0.002	1-y rate 42% SRS+R 64% SRS P=0.003	1-4 brain metastases. Overall CNS recurrence rate at 1-y: 47% SRS+R 76% SRS P<0.001 Salvage treatment required: 15% SRS+R 43% SRS P<0.001
Muacevic et al., 2008 [44]	64 total 31 SRS 33 S+R	22 NSCLC 10 GU 11 Breast 9 Mel. 4 GI 8 Other	OS	9.5 m S+R 10.3 m SRS P=0.8	1-y rate 3% SRS 18% S+R P=0.06	1-y rate 26% SRS 3% S+R P=0.04	Single, surgically accessible brain metastasis. Study stopped early due to poor accrual.
Chang EL et al., 2009 [50]	58 28 SRS+R 30 SRS	32 NSCLC 8 Breast 7 Mel. 4 Renal 7 Other	HVLT at 4 m vs. baseline	SRS+R (5.7 m) vs. SRS (15.2m), p=0.003	1-y rate 0% SRS+R 33% SRS P=0.01	1-y rate 27% SRS+R 55% SRS P=0.02	Up to 3 brain metastases. Decline in function at 4 m (primary endpoint): 48% SRS+R 24% SRS P=0.04 Study accrual stopped early due to achieving primary endpoint.
Kocher et al., 2011 [51]	359 total SRS 100 SRS+R 99 S 79 S+R 81	190 NSCLC 29 Renal 42 Breast 18 Mel. 30 Colon 50 Other	Duration of functional independenc e (measured as deterioration of WHO PS to >2)	WBRT (10.7 m) vs. No WBRT (10.9 m), p=0.89	2-y rate S – 59% S+R – 27% (p < 0.001) SRS – 31% SRS+R – 19% (p = 0.040)	2-y rate S – 42% S+R – 23% (p = 0.008) SRS – 48% SRS+R – 33% (p = 0.023)	1-3 brain metastasis eligible. Either stable extracranial disease for 3 months or no extracranial metastases. Median Survival with WHO PS ≤2 (primary endpoint) 9.5m WBRT vs. 10.0 m no WBRT, p=0.709 Overall rate of CNS progression at 6 and 24 m: 15.2% and 31.4% WBRT vs. 39.7 and 54% no WBRT, p<0.0001 Neurological cause of death 25% WBRT vs. 43% no WBRT, p=NR

Table 5. Randomized trials of adjuvant WBRT with surgery or stereotactic radiosurgery for brain metastases

one patient in each group had melanoma. The CNS recurrence rate was 18% (9/49) in those receiving adjuvant WBRT. This contrasted sharply with a 70% (32/46) CNS recurrence rate in the observation group (p<0.001). The median time-to-CNS recurrence was markedly prolonged in those receiving adjuvant WBRT (220 weeks versus 26 weeks observation, p<0.001) due to decreased recurrence rates both at resection sites (10% WBRT versus 46% observation, p<0.001) and at distant sites within the brain (14% WBRT versus 37% observation, p<0.01). There was no difference in median survival (49 weeks WBRT versus 43 weeks observation, p=0.39) or in maintenance of independent function (maintenance of KPS >60%). A decreased rate of neurologic cause of death was evident in the WBRT-treated group (14% WBRT versus 44% observation, p=0.003), although the determination of this was less objective than determination of intracranial recurrence by imaging.

Another randomized trial tested adjuvant WBRT (30 Gy in 10 fractions) in conjunction with SRS [49]. The study enrolled 132 patients with one-to-four metastases measuring less than 3 cm in maximal dimension. Sixty-five patients received SRS and WBRT; sixty-seven received SRS alone. Two-thirds of those enrolled had NSCLC. The majority of the remainder had breast, colon or renal primary sites. The primary endpoint was overall survival. The researchers initially estimated that 89 evaluable patients per group would be required to detect a 30% difference in median survival time. A planned interim analysis, performed after 122 patients enrolled, led to early study termination. Four-to-five-fold more patients would have been required to detect a significant difference in the primary endpoint.

Although underpowered to detect a survival advantage, a number of secondary endpoints yielded significant results. CNS progression at 1 year was 47% in the combination therapy group and 76% in the SRS monotherapy group (p<0.001). WBRT improved control at one year for both SRS-treated sites (89% WBRT versus 72% without, p=0.002) and distant CNS sites (58% WBRT versus 36% without, p=0.003). No differences were observed in median survival, neurological cause of death, and acute or late neurological toxicity. Rates of systemic functional preservation (assessed by KPS), neurological preservation, and neurocognitive preservation (assessed by the Mini-Mental Status Examination, MMSE) were also not different.

A third trial randomized patients with 1-3 brain metastases to either SRS or SRS combined with adjuvant WBRT (30 Gy in 12 fractions) [50]. A novel endpoint for the study was chosen: change in performance on the Hopkins Verbal Learning Test-Revised (HVLT) at 4 months after primary therapy. The majority of enrolled patients were those with NSCLC primary tumors (55%), with melanoma in the minority (12%). The study was stopped early after accrual of 58 patients (28 SRS+WBRT, 30 SRS) due to its achieving the primary endpoint. Patients treated with the combination demonstrated a 52% decline in HVLT score at 4 months, versus a 24% decline in those receiving SRS only (p=0.04). This difference persisted at 6 months. Significant differences in performance on a panel of other neurocognitive tests were not detected. The study was stopped early and may have therefore been underpowered to detect other important differences in outcome. Decreased HVLT performance occurred despite decreased rates of CNS progression at one year in the combination therapy group (SRS-treated sites: 0% SRS +WBRT vs. 33% SRS, p=0.01; distant CNS: 27% vs. 55%, p=0.02). The authors also reported improved survival in the group treated with SRS alone (5.7 months SRS+WBRT vs. 15.2 months SRS, p=0.003).

Patients who were treated only with SRS required salvage therapy for intracranial progression in 87% of cases. Ten (33%) of the patients treated with SRS alone required craniotomy, ten (33%) received salvage WBRT and six (20%) received salvage SRS. In the group treated with SRS and adjuvant WBRT, two patients (7%) received salvage WBRT, and three (11%) progressed intracranially, but received no salvage therapy.

This study provides convincing evidence that the addition of adjuvant WBRT to SRS therapy for brain metastases impairs HVLT performance. This occurs despite a decreased rate of intracranial progression in those receiving WBRT. Salvage therapy for intracranial progression was required in the majority of patients treated with SRS alone, including salvage craniotomy in one-third of the patients. The clinical significance of HVLT deterioration due to adjuvant WBRT, vis a vis that of frequently needed salvage therapy for CNS disease was not addressed.

A fourth randomized trial assessing adjuvant WBRT enrolled patients with 1-3 brain metastases and stable or absent extracranial disease [51]. The majority of patients had NSCLC (53%); only 5% were melanoma patients. Patients received SRS or surgery as primary therapy and were then randomized to receive adjuvant WBRT (30 Gy in 10 fractions) or no additional therapy. The composite primary endpoint was median overall survival in patients with KPS of 0-2. In the intent-to-treat analysis, 180 patients were assigned to receive WBRT and 179 to observation. At the end of the study, per protocol, 164 patients received WBRT and 166 patients were on observation. Analysis was by intention-to-treat.

No differences were detected in the primary endpoint of survival with functional independence (9.5 months WBRT versus 10.0 months observation, p=0.709) or median overall survival (10.7 months WBRT versus 10.9 months observation, p=0.891). Intracranial recurrence rates were markedly suppressed by adjuvant WBRT. Overall intracranial progression occurred in 48% of WBRT-treated patients and in 78% of the observation group (p<0.001). This translated to improved progression-free survival (PFS) in the WBRT-treated group (4.6 months vs. 3.4 months observation, p=0.002). Two years after surgery, WBRT reduced the probability of relapse at intial site from 59% (observation) to 27% (p<0.001) and at distant CNS sites from 42% (observation) to 23% (p=0.008). Similarly, after SRS, WBRT reduced the probability of relapse at SRS-treated site from 31% (observation) to 19% (p=0.040) and at distant CNS sites from 48% (observation) to 33% (p=0.023). Neurological cause of death was suppressed by adjuvant WBRT (28% WBRT versus 44% observation; p<0.002). Extracranial disease progression rates at 24 months were identical (65% WBRT and 63% observation, p=0.73).

All four randomized trials showed decreased intracranial recurrence rates when adjuvant WBRT was administered, both at the site of treatment and at distant sites within the brain. Similar effects from adjuvant WBRT on distant CNS recurrence were reported by the trial of Muacevic and co-workers, in which patients were randomized to surgery with adjuvant WBRT versus SRS alone, discussed above [44]. The impact on the reduction in distant CNS recurrence with the use of adjuvant WBRT is likely from the eradication of subclinical microscopic disease present at the time of brain metastasis diagnosis. The effect of WBRT on CNS seeding from uncontrolled extracranial disease is unclear, but likely has a lesser effect. If seeding from extracranial disease was a dominant mechanism leading to CNS failure, adjuvant WBRT would not be predicted to decrease its occurrence.

No trial to date evaluating the omission of adjuvant WBRT after local therapy has demonstrated a survival benefit to WBRT. The study by Chang and co-workers indicated that the use of adjuvant WBRT after local therapy might be associated with a decrement in survival. It is difficult to draw firm conclusions about these data, as the study was stopped early, was not powered to detect a survival benefit, and contradicted the survival results of the other four larger randomized studies presented above. This includes the study by Aoyama and co-workers [50], which evaluated overall survival as its primary endpoint and was unable to detect a survival difference between its treatment arms, without a marked increase in sample size to over 800. The study by Kocher and co-workers demonstrated an improvement in PFS associated with adjuvant WBRT [51]. This study excluded patients with uncontrolled or progressive primary disease, mitigating extracranial disease burden as a competing risk for death

The studies presented here represent the best assessment of the efficacy of adjuvant WBRT therapy in treatment of solid tumor brain metastases. This therapy is clearly able to decrease intracranial recurrence rates, both at locally treated and distant sites within the CNS. The effect of this therapy on survival and the relative benefits versus the cognitive effects of the therapy are less clear. Melanoma patients formed a small fraction of the patients enrolled in these trials and one might therefore question whether these results even apply in the melanoma setting. To do so requires examination of the rather imperfect retrospective dataset regarding adjuvant WBRT specifically in melanoma.

2.4.2. Adjuvant WBRT in melanoma patients

The randomized studies discussed above primarily enrolled patients diagnosed with NSCLC. There have been no prospective studies evaluating the role of adjuvant WBRT specifically in the melanoma patient population. Many retrospective studies have been reported; unsurprisingly, these have indicated that adjuvant WBRT confers no survival benefit (see Tables 2, 4) [8-10, 12, 19, 29, 31, 32, 34, 35, 38, 39, 41, 53]. Since most melanoma patients with brain lesions present with active extracranial disease, any potential survival benefit due to adjuvant WBRT after local CNS therapy is probably undermined: extracranial disease serves as a competing cause of death, diluting any study's statistical power.

It is difficult to make firm conclusions based on the numerous melanoma case series on whether adjuvant WBRT actually decreases the rate of intracranial recurrence after local therapy. Selection and ascertainment biases are major concerns. Patients with clinically advanced disease are often selected for more aggressive therapy. Groups receiving aggressive therapy are likely to undergo more frequent and detailed surveillance for recurrence.

Several retrospective studies identify such biases. In the study of Buchsbaum and co-workers a paradoxically *higher* rate of CNS recurrence (49%) was identified in patients having received combined local CNS lesion therapy and adjuvant WBRT versus local therapy alone (20%) [10].

Follow-up scans were more frequent in the combined therapy group, possibly explaining the increased detection of progression and therefore higher documented recurrence rates. Samlowski and co-workers indicated that patients having received combined SRS and adjuvant WBRT had a higher mean number of CNS lesions at presentation than those selected for SRS alone [37]. Not surprisingly, more aggressive upfront therapy is apparently administered to patients with a greater initial disease burden.

Another study reported that patients receiving SRS with WBRT had 0% 1-year actuarial control within the CNS versus 60% for those treated with SRS alone (p=0.0005), strongly suggesting selection bias [38]. Those patients with initially more advanced disease were more likely to be treated with the combined modality technique. Advanced disease was found as a strong predictor for poorer outcomes. Therefore local control rates were likely confounded by the level of disease burden at presentation and not necessarily by the choice of treatment modality.

Other studies indicate similar paradoxical results in patients treated with adjuvant WBRT. Wronski and Arbit reported an increased risk of CNS recurrence (56%) in patients treated with surgery and WBRT versus 46% in those treated with surgery alone [9]. Another study reported a 20% failure rate at SRS-treated sites in patients receiving adjuvant WBRT versus 0% in those treated with SRS alone [33]. Perhaps indicative of a possible beneficial effect from adjuvant WBRT, failure at distant sites within the CNS was only 23% in the combination therapy group versus 44% in those treated with SRS alone. Those failing at the local site after combined modality treatment had larger initial volumes of disease compared with those treated with SRS alone. The additional fractionated dose contributed from WBRT at the site of failure may not have adequately addressed the increased tumor burden initially present. This was likely a significant confounder in local control outcomes.

Several studies concluded that WBRT does not significantly impact CNS recurrence rates. In one study of 333 melanoma patients, WBRT before or after SRS did not alter the intracranial recurrence rates [31]. The same study also showed that patient survival was significantly shorter with WBRT (4.5 months) compared to SRS alone (6.4 months, p=0.05). Again, selection bias for patients with more lesions or more aggressive disease could explain this result. Radbill et al. reported that adjuvant WBRT did not decrease the rate of failure at non-SRS-treated sites in the CNS (p=0.13) [35]. However, the number of patients treated with adjuvant WBRT (13%) was potentially too small to detect a benefit. Mingione et al., studying 45 melanoma patients, of whom 16 received adjuvant WBRT, concluded that WBRT had no impact on outcomes [32]. Yu et al. also found that adjuvant WBRT did not decrease distant CNS recurrence; this conclusion was again limited by the small proportion of WBRT-treated patients (32/122 patients; 32%) [41].

Three studies have suggested a benefit from WBRT in preventing CNS recurrence in the melanoma population. One retrospective study of 35 melanoma patients undergoing resection of a single brain metastasis at a single institution from 1972 to 1987 documented a CNS recurrence rate of 37% in those treated with adjuvant WBRT, versus 69% in those not receiving this therapy (Table 2) [53]. Median time to CNS relapse was 26.6 months in the group receiving adjuvant WBRT, as compared to 5.7 months in those not receiving such therapy (p<0.05). Survival was predicted by the extracranial disease status, rather than receipt of adjuvant

WBRT. Death due to neurological causes was more common in the group that did not receive WBRT (24% WBRT versus 85% observation, p<0.01).

Another study during approximately the same time period (1979-1991) examined adjuvant WBRT after surgery in patients with a solitary CNS metastasis from melanoma (Table 2) [54]. Patients had no active extracranial disease and underwent resection of a single metastasis. Of the 34 subjects, 22 received WBRT. Median survival was improved in the combination therapy group (18 months versus 6 months with surgery alone, p=0.002), but CNS relapse rates were similar (30% surgery+WBRT vs. 22% surgery only; p=0.65). This study evaluated a highly selected patient group. This study and that of Hagen also suffer from being older studies, with more limited CNS imaging capabilities [53]. Nevertheless, the results tend to echo those of Patchell's randomized trial, suggesting a decreased CNS recurrence rate in CNS melanoma patients treated with adjuvant WBRT after local therapy [52].

Another report reviewed a single institution's experience with SRS in the treatment of 41 patients with radioresistant tumors, including 23 with melanoma [19]. Adjuvant WBRT improved local control (100% control with SRS and WBRT versus 85% with SRS alone at 6 months) and distant brain failure rates (17% failure with SRS and WBRT versus 64% failure with SRS alone). As might be predicted, adjuvant WBRT did not affect overall survival.

In summary, retrospective case series in melanoma indicate that adjuvant WBRT does not convey an overall survival benefit. This is consistent with the results of the randomized trials of WBRT primarily conducted in non-melanoma brain metastases. It is therefore reasonable to conclude that the addition of adjuvant WBRT does not improve the overall survival of the majority of melanoma patients with brain metastases.

As regards the effect of adjuvant WBRT on the prevention of CNS recurrence in melanoma, this collection of retrospective studies provides conflicting data. Some have shown no effect, others have shown decreased intracranial recurrence rates with the addition of WBRT, and still others have indicated that WBRT is associated with increased recurrence rates. Biases in treatment selection and ascertainment are strong confounders in many of the studies.

An ongoing randomized phase 3 trial is currently accruing for the comparison of distant intracranial control with the addition of adjuvant WBRT to observation following surgery and/ or SRS in melanoma patients with 1-3 brain lesions (NCT01503827) [55]. Secondary endpoints will include the effects on OS, QOL, and NCF. This prospective, randomized, melanoma-specific trial will hopefully reconcile the contradictory observations reported in the retrospective studies discussed above. With improving systemic therapy, including agents able to penetrate the CNS at clinically relevant concentrations, even this randomized trial may not be able to answer its major questions about adjuvant WBRT in melanoma patient.

Salvage SRS: An alternative to WBRT?

An alternative strategy to managing CNS metastases involves the use of "salvage" SRS. After patients receive initial local therapy with SRS alone, WBRT is omitted to spare normal brain tissues from unnecessary radiation doses and avoid potential adverse neurocognitive effects. Patients undergo CNS imaging at planned intervals or if symptoms suggest progression. SRS is then used to treat new lesions.

This strategy has not yet been tested in a randomized trial for patients with brain metastases from melanoma. There are limited data that have included melanoma patients in the prospective evaluation of this treatment paradigm. For example, one prospective study assessed SRS as a single treatment modality in 41 patients with no more than 4 brain metastases [56]. Seven (16%) of the patients had melanoma primary tumors. Twenty-three of the enrolled patients (56%) experienced intracranial progression. Nine received salvage treatment with additional SRS and one with surgery and WBRT for persistent tumor. Eleven patients were treated with salvage WBRT due to an excessive number of new CNS lesions and two patients received non-radiotherapy palliative therapy. Intracranial recurrences were common in the absence of upfront WBRT; less than half of recurring patients (9/23) were eligible for salvage SRS therapy due to excessive number of new lesions, limited life expectancy or decreased performance status.

Data from a large, multi-institutional, retrospective study of 569 patients (16% with melanoma) support the feasibility of salvage SRS in replacement of upfront WBRT [57]. Of 268 patients treated initially with SRS alone, 98 received salvage therapy for CNS recurrence. Sixty-three (64%) of those needing salvage therapy received WBRT as part of the salvage regimen (which included SRS and/or surgery) and forty-seven (48%) received WBRT as the sole salvage therapy.

One retrospective study examined 45 patients (20 with melanoma, 44%) receiving SRS as salvage therapy [58]. Excellent local control at treated sites was achieved (92.4% at 52 weeks). Patients who received upfront WBRT were significantly less likely to require salvage therapy (p=0.008), although no survival benefit was reported.

A CNS metastasis management strategy in which SRS is used as sole initial therapy warrants continued evaluation, particularly for patients diagnosed with melanoma. The existing studies of this approach suggest that intracranial recurrence rates remain high with the omission of WBRT. Although salvage therapy with SRS may be planned initially, a large fraction of patients will require WBRT in the salvage setting to treat macroscopic recurrences, when WBRT is likely to be *least* effective

2.4.3. Neurocognitive effects of WBRT

A major argument against the use of adjuvant WBRT relates to its impact on NCF and higher executive neurologic functions, including learning, memory, calculation, and task planning. A variety of standardized neuropsychological tests measure global NCF, such as the MMSE. NCF impairment has a direct impact on overall QOL, affecting patients' ability to carry out activities of daily living, medical treatment compliance, and higher order planning and function [59].

One widely cited retrospective study examined patients treated at a single center for brain metastasis by either WBRT alone (n=370) or surgical metastectomy combined with WBRT (n=118) [60]. Radiation-associated dementia was reported at a rate of 1.9 (n=7) and 5.1% (n=5), respectively. Cases were defined as those patients treated for brain metastases with WBRT without evident CNS recurrence who subsequently developed "…a progressive dementing

illness." Neither baseline neurocognitive data information for the identified cases nor information regarding the source populations was provided. Among the 12 cases identified, a
variety of radiation dose and fractionation schemes were employed. The authors suggested
that the incidence of radiation-related leukoencephalopathy might have been underestimated
due to lack of sensitive tools for identifying neurocognitive dysfunction. Baseline neurocognitive dysfunction in patients with primary or secondary brain malignancy, however, is
present in as many as 90% of patients prior to treatment [61] due to the general debility of
patients with metastatic cancer, the neurocognitive effects of systemic chemotherapy and
supportive therapies, and the age of the patients. Thus, the results of this relatively old study
do not provide a clear picture of neurocognitive dysfunction associated with radiotherapeutic
treatment of brain metastases.

Fairly good evidence shows that radiation therapy of the brain leads to neurocognitive
dysfunction, which in some cases can be severe. A variety of patient-related factors play a role
in the development of risk for developing radiation-associated neurocognitive dysfunction.
These include patient age (children or those more than 50 years of age), other therapies received
(chemotherapy and/or anti-convulsants), and length of survival post radiation therapy (as seen
in survivors diagnosed with more favorable and indolent diseases, e.g., low-grade glioma)
[62-68]. Factors related to radiation therapy delivery include total dose received, dose per
fraction, and amount of cerebral volume irradiated [68-71].

More rigorous prospective assessments suggest that the neurocognitive impact of WBRT may
be modest. Data from the study of primary brain tumor patients, in which extracranial disease
and its treatment are not factors, may be relevant. For example, one study examined the dose-
dependency of radiotherapy-associated neurocognitive dysfunction in patients treated for
primary brain tumors [71]. Neuropsychological testing was undertaken up to 12 months after
completion of radiotherapy. No dysfunction was observed in patients receiving up to 30 Gy,
a typical dose used for adjuvant WBRT. Fraction size was not reported.

Another setting to examine the effects of WBRT is in diseases for which PCI is of proven benefit,
such as SCLC. In two large studies evaluating the role of PCI for good responders with SCLC,
there was no difference in NCF between those randomized to receive WBRT or not (24 Gy in
12 fractions-36 Gy in 18 fractions) [47, 48]. In the study by Gregor et al., both groups of patients
demonstrated baseline neurocognitive impairment versus normal controls, likely reflecting
effects of prior treatment. Among those without baseline impairment, impairment in cognitive
test performance was evident at 6 months and 1 year, but no obvious differences were seen
when comparing PCI-treated and –untreated patients. The authors did not, however, describe
rigorous statistical assessment of the longitudinal neurocognitive testing data [48].

Another prospective, non-randomized study showed no difference in cognitive function after
30-40 Gy of radiation therapy with 2-34 months of follow-up [72]. Again, a high degree of pre-
existing neurocognitive deficit was already present. This may have been attributable to
chemotherapy given prior to radiation therapy.

A non-randomized, prospective study of PCI was undertaken in NSCLC patients [73]. Seventy-
five patients received induction radiochemotherapy for locally advanced NSCLC. Forty-seven

received PCI (30 Gy over 3 weeks), while twenty-eight others did not. PCI reduced the overall rate of brain relapse from 54% to 13% at 3-4 years. In fifteen long-term survivors (10 PCI, 5 without PCI), no significant differences were noted in a battery of neuropsychological tests undertaken at a median of 47 (PCI) and 70 (no PCI) months.

A study recently presented short term follow-up of longitudinal NCF in patients having received PCI (small cell lung cancer; n=13), therapeutic cranial irradiation (TCI; brain meta-stases; n=16) or non-cranial irradiation (control: breast cancer; n=15) [74]. NCF was assessed prior to and during radiation treatment and 6-8 weeks after its completion. At 6-8 weeks after treatment, only verbal memory scores were lower in patients receiving cranial irradiation versus controls. Visual memory and attention were not affected. Pre-treatment verbal memory performance score was the major predictor of post-treatment outcome in univariate analysis, with a lesser contribution attributable to cranial irradiation. The data from this admittedly small study suggest that WBRT can have a negative impact on verbal memory, although other factors contributing to the baseline status seem dominant.

Aoyama and co-workers conducted a randomized trial of SRS with or without WBRT, discussed in detail above [75]. Baseline and follow-up MMSE scores were available for 110 and 92 of the 132 patients enrolled in the trial, respectively. Baseline MMSE scores were predicted by patient age, performance status, tumoral edema and total tumor volume, but not by the initial number of tumors.

Deterioration in MMSE occurred in equal proportions of each group (14/36 SRS + WBRT versus 12/46 SRS alone, p=0.21). Average time-to-deterioration was longer in the combined therapy group (13.6 months versus 6.8 months SRS alone, p=0.05). In the 14 members of the combined therapy group, the adjudged cause of deterioration was brain tumor progression in 3, toxic effects of radiotherapy in 5 and indeterminate in 6; in the group treated only with SRS, MMSE deterioration was due to brain tumor progression in 11 and indeterminate in 1 (combined vs. SRS, p<0.0001). The temporal trends in NCF between the two arms suggest that SRS-related cognitive decline may be associated with tumor recurrence, which may or may not be rever-sible with salvage therapy. Later dysfunction with WBRT is more variable in cause. Some may be attributable to CNS tumor recurrence, but other cases being attributable to late effects of radiation on normal brain tissue. Such treatment-associated damage would not be amenable to corrective therapy with further tumor-specific therapy.

The study of Chang and co-workers, discussed earlier, prospectively addressed NCF in the setting of adjuvant WBRT [50]. This study is notable in that the score on a specific neurocog-nitive test, HVLT, was the primary endpoint. Patients receiving adjuvant WBRT experienced greater rates of decline in their HVLT performance than those treated with SRS alone, despite decreased intracranial progression in the WBRT-treated patients.

The HVLT tests basic verbal learning capacity and is proposed as a screening test for mild dementia [76, 77]. The HVLT may have somewhat greater sensitivity for mild dementia than the MMSE, as well some logistical advantages [78]. In isolation, however, results from the HVLT must be judged cautiously, as it does not assess other more complex neurocognitive functions [79]. In studies of patients with brain metastases, the test is part of a battery of administered tests intended to develop a general overview of neurocognitive function [80, 81].

In the Chang study, a battery of neurocognitive function tests was administered, along with HVLT. Differences in performance on these other tests were not different between the two groups. The authors cautioned that the wide confidence intervals in the results of non-HVLT tests did not exclude a difference between the two test groups, but they also did not demonstrate a specific difference between the groups.

Studies of the effects of brain radiotherapy presented here vary in quality. They do not however give a clear picture suggesting severe adverse consequences of brain radiotherapy. Adverse effects are certainly identified in several studies, although their clinical significance is not certain and its cause is not clearly attributable to CNS radiotherapy. Intuitively, radiation therapy in and of itself is not beneficial for the nervous system. In the setting of brain metastasis treatment, however, the adverse effects of radiation therapy must be balanced against those of CNS tumor recurrence.

2.4.4. Neurocognitive effects of brain tumor progression

While little melanoma-specific data are available, the primary brain tumor literature reveals that there are significant negative cognitive effects from tumor progression. This literature is particularly useful, as cognitive deterioration in primary brain tumor patients is due entirely to incracranial disease and CNS treatment effects, as opposed to extracranial disease progression. Deterioration in MMSE was a strong predictor of impending intracranial tumor progression in a study of 1,244 glioma patients [82]. A change in MMSE score was seen even *prior* to radiographic progression. Decreased MMSE score also strongly correlated with performance status deterioration.

Another study in 445 brain metastasis patients (25 with melanoma) compared the drop in MMSE score before and after treatment with WBRT [83, 84]. The study was designed to assess the effect of the radiation fractionation schedules on survival, for which no effect was found. Tumor control was the primary factor in determining MMSE scores at 3 months. A 6.2 point drop (out of 30 possible) was seen in those with radiographic evidence of progression, compared to a 0.5 point drop in those with controlled tumors. In multivariate analysis, control of brain metastases was the only factor affecting MMSE score.

Another prospective brain metastasis study assessed a novel radiosensitizing agent combined with WBRT [85]. A detailed neurocognitive battery assessed NCF before and after therapy. Patients in the control arm, receiving WBRT alone, were subdivided into "good responders" (at least a 45% reduction in tumor size) and "poor responders" (less than a 45% reduction). Good responders had better NCF preservation rate, as well as a modest survival advantage (median survival 300 days versus 240 days; p=0.03).

These studies indicate that CNS tumor progression has adverse effects on neurocognitive status and QOL (reflected by performance status deterioration). While not melanoma-specific, there is no reason to believe that CNS progression of melanoma tumors would be any less adverse. These adverse effects of tumor progression must be balanced against those of adjuvant WBRT.

2.4.5. WBRT in advanced CNS melanoma

In some patients, disease in the CNS cannot reasonably be controlled using local treatment of brain metastases with surgery or SRS. At some point, lesion number becomes excessive, or lesions are present in locations that are not amenable to local treatment. Alternatively, a patient's extracranial disease may be so extensive that it is likely to be life-limiting, and the goal of CNS disease treatment is primarily symptom palliation. WBRT is often used in this circumstance, with the twin goals of improving survival and providing symptoms palliation.

No randomized, prospective studies are available to quantitate the benefit of WBRT, especially when compared to supportive care alone. A number of large retrospective case series have examined the questions specifically of survival, although these suffer from heterogeneous patient populations. In the study of Sampson and co-workers, 205 melanoma patients with brain metastases received systemic palliative chemotherapy, with median OS of 39 days, versus 120 days among the 180 patients treated only with whole brain radiotherapy (p=0.0006) [8]. Receipt of radiotherapy treatment was statistically significant in the multivariate analysis of another large retrospective study, with radiotherapy demonstrating median OS of 3.6 months, versus 1.3 months for those treated with corticosteroids alone (HR=0.38; p<0.001). In the study of Raizer and co-workers, 83 patients received no specific therapy for brain metastases, vesus 100 receiving WBRT alone [13]. Median OS was 2.0 and 4.0 months, respectively. The statistical significance of this difference was not reported.

The study of Fife and co-workers examined patients treated at a single center in Australia in the 1952-2000 date range [12]. For the 1985-2000 cohort, 210 patients received supportive care, versus 236 receiving radiotherapy alone. Median OS was 2.1 and 3.4 months in these two groups; in multi-variate Cox regression analysis, radiotherapy was associated with a decreased hazard ratio for death (HR-0.851; p=0.111). This may not have achieved statistical significance due to the heterogeneity of the patients in these two groups. In addition to treatment modality, other significant factors associated with survival were the presence of concurrent metastases at diagnosis, older age, and a longer time from initial melanoma diagnosis.

An older retrospective study identified 60 melanoma patients with cerebral melanoma metastases that were enrolled in two Radiation Therapy Oncology Group (RTOG) studies [86]. The study sought to determine the effects of WBRT on performance status, neurologic function, and neurologic symptoms. In the analysis, this study demonstrated that WBRT provided improvement of neurologic symptoms (including headache, motor loss, convulsion) in 76% of patients. Median survival in this uncontrolled report was 10-14 weeks, although the baseline clinical characteristics of the study population were quite variable.

Another retrospective study identified 87 patients who had received WBRT, of whom 46 (53%) had 3 or more metastases [87]. The majority of patients were already receiving dexamethasone before initiating radiation, and therefore it was difficult to isolate the effects of WBRT, since CNS signs and symptoms can be alleviated by corticosteroid treatment. The fraction of patients discontinuing corticosteroids due to symptom improvement served as a surrogate marker for palliative effects of WBRT. Upon completion of WBRT, 52% of all patients and 48% of symptomatic patients discontinued steroids. The same study demonstrated a small measurable response in tumor size following WBRT. Out of 87 patients, 65 had measurable disease at baseline; only 28 had at least one follow-up MRI scan to assess response. This may reflect a bias favoring follow-up scans being undertaken in those with responding disease. In these 28 patients at a median follow-up of 7 weeks, 75 tumors showed a median reduction in tumor size of 17%. The median OS of all patients evaluated in this study was 19 weeks. The median OS for patients who had undergone surgical resection prior to WBRT (22 patients) was 45 weeks, versus 16 weeks for those who did not undergo surgical resection (p<0.0001). Absence of extracranial disease (in 14 patients) was associated with higher median OS of 54 weeks, compared to 17 weeks in patients who had extracranial disease (p<0.0001).

Two prospective studies have combined WBRT with either temozolomide or fotemustine in melanoma patients with brain metastases [88, 89]. With temozolomide in a phase 2 study of 31 patients, only 3 (10%) demonstrated a response in the CNS, with median PFS in the CNS and OS of 2 and 6 months, respectively. In the phase 3 study of the combination with fotemustine, objective response rate (ORR) was 10% with median time-to-CNS-progression of 56 days and median OS of 105 days. These studies provide estimates of the clinical effect of WBRT, even though the relative contributions of WBRT and chemotherapy drug cannot be quantitated.

The use of WBRT in a patient with advanced CNS melanoma probably yields a modest survival benefit over supportive care alone. Symptom palliation is also probably a benefit of this therapy. There are many holes in the WBRT data set, many of which will never be answered definitively as melanoma treatment evolves. WBRT as a monotherapy has several signifcicant disadvantages, including its modest benefit at best, inability to undertake re-treatment, and lack of effect on extracranial disease. These limitations will likely be overcome only with the design of systemic therapy regimens, to be administered concurrently with, or in lieu of, WBRT.

2.5. Systemic therapy

Until the recent approvals in 2011 of ipilimumab [90, 91] and vemurafenib [92], no therapy tested in a randomized trial demonstrated an improvement in overall survival for metastatic melanoma patients. Dacarbazine had been the standard first-line systemic treatment since it was approved in the United States in 1975. Metastatic melanoma patients with intracranial or meningeal metastases were generally excluded from clinical trial participation for three reasons: 1) brain metastases were thought to portend a poor prognosis; 2) systemic therapies that were tested were not very effective in intracranial disease; and 3) it was presumed that most agents would not cross the blood-brain barrier. In this section, we will cover efforts to use chemotherapy, molecularly-targeted therapy, and immunotherapy for the management of melanoma brain metastases (Table 6) [88, 89, 93-99].

2.5.1. Chemotherapy

Several chemotherapeutic regimens failed to demonstrate benefit in melanoma brain meta-stasis, including regimens containing platinum-based compounds, dacarbazine, etoposide, and others [87, 100-109]. This may be largely due to the low efficacy of many of the tested agents in melanoma generally. It is probably unreasonable to expect agents with limited activity against extracranial disease to have activity in the CNS, with the added barrier of CNS penetration. Three chemotherapy agents with defined CNS activity in non-melanoma neo-plastic settings, namely temozolomide, thalidomide, and fotemustine have been investigated in some detail in melanoma [110, 111].

Temozolomide is metabolized to the same active metabolite as dacarbazine. It is orally bioavailable and penetrates the blood-brain barrier at clinically significant concentrations [111]. The drug is approved for the treatment of primary brain tumors, confirming its clinically significant penetration of the CNS. Since temozolomide is as effective as dacarbazine in treatment of metastatic melanoma and yields similar patient survival [112], several clinical trials evaluated its efficacy in melanoma patients with brain metastases.

A multicenter, open label, single-arm phase 2 study aimed to determine the efficacy and safety (both as primary endpoints) of temozolomide in metastatic melanoma patients who had developed brain metastasis [93]. The study enrolled 151 patients, comprising of 117 chemo-therapy-naïve and 34 previously treated. The clinical condition of the enrollees did not require immediate surgery or radiation therapy, justifying chemotherapy as the sole therapy.

For chemotherapy-naïve patients, eight patients (7%) achieved response, including one complete (CR) and seven partial responses (PR); 34 patients (29%) achieved stable disease (SD) in brain lesions for at least 4 weeks. Median OS was 3.5 months. In previously treated patients, 1 patient (3%) achieved PR, 6 (18%) had SD, and the median OS was 2.2 months. Notably, 25% of the chemotherapy-naïve and 21% of previously treated patients had extensive intracranial disease, defined as more than 4 radiologically evident brain lesions. The authors concluded that further evaluation was warranted, particularly in combination with other treatment modalities, but activity as a single agent in this setting was limited.

The combination of temozolomide and WBRT has been evaluated. A prospective phase 2 trial evaluated the combination in patients with CNS melanoma [88]. In 31 evaluable patients, temozolomide and WBRT combination yielded an overall ORR of 9.7%, comprising of one CR in the CNS lasting 4.5 months and two PR in the CNS lasting 2 months and 7 months. Although the combination of temozolomide and WBRT could be safely administered, its efficacy was limited.

Thalidomide, an anti-angiogenic agent crossing the blood-brain barrier, has been tested in combination with temozolomide to treat melanoma patients with brain metastases. In a phase 2 study, the combination of temozolomide and thalidomide was tested in chemotherapy-naïve patients [96]. The primary endpoint was ORR in the brain assessed every 8 weeks. Of the 26 patients treated, 16 patients were symptomatic and 25 had extracranial metastases. Treatment-associated toxicity, especially hemorrhage and thromboembolism was a problem: eleven patients discontinued treatment before completing one cycle of treatment due to intracranial hemorrhage (n=7), pulmonary embolism (n=2), deep vein thrombosis (n=1), and grade 3 rash (n=1). Of 15 evaluable patients, 3 (12% of the intent-to-treat population) achieved CR or PR, while 7 patients had minor response or SD in the brain. Of the 10 patients who derived benefit, however, 5 patients progressed at extracranial sites. Overall OS was 5 months in all 26 patients, while it was 6 months in the 15 evaluable patients. Given the limited efficacy and the toxicity associated with the temozolomide/thalidomide combination, its use in melanoma is not warranted, outside the setting of a clinical trial.

Temozolomide has also been evaluated in the adjuvant setting. A multicenter phase 3 study compared temozolomide to dacarbazine in the time to develop CNS metastasis [94]. The study randomized 150 patients to receive either oral temozolomide or intravenous dacarbazine in combination with cisplatin and interleukin-2. Compared to dacarbazine, temozolomide reduced the 1-year CNS failure from 31.1% to 20.6%, but was not statistically significant (p=0.22). The median OS was not different between the two arms. Even though temozolomide penetrates the CNS, it did not delay incidence of CNS failure. Thus it appears that temozolomide may not be very effective in the adjuvant setting.

Fotemustine is a chloroethyl-nitrosurea approved in Europe for the treatment of metastatic melanoma. Fotemustine demonstrates high CNS penetration; its efficacy in melanoma patients with intracranial disease has been evaluated in three major studies. A French multicenter phase 2 study evaluated 153 metastatic melanoma patients for response to single-agent fotemustine [97]. Previously treated patients were allowed in the study. Since fotemustine crosses the blood brain barrier, patients with intracranial metastases were enrolled.

Out of the 153 evaluable patients, 36 (23.5%) had cerebral metastasis as the dominant disease site. In patients with cerebral metastases, the drug yielded an ORR of 25% in the CNS, similar to the 24.2% ORR observed in extracranial disease. The median OS of all patients was 85 weeks, but survival of the brain metastases patients was not reported. This study suggests that fotemustine has activity in melanoma, including CNS metastases. The magnitude of the benefit is similar in the CNS and at extracranial sites.

To confirm the observed activity, a phase 3 trial randomized 229 patients with metastatic melanoma to receive either fotemustine or dacarbazine [113]. Dacarbazine is a useful and interesting comparator in this study, as prior studies had failed to demonstrate any significant activity in the CNS [100, 102, 104]. This study enrolled patients with and without pre-existing brain metastases. Forty-three patients with brain metastases enrolled, of whom 22 received fotemustine, while 21 patients received dacarbazine.

Among all patients, fotemustine yielded an ORR of 15% versus dacarbazine's 7% (p=0.043). The authors reported a trend to improved survival among fotemustine-treated patients, with median OS of 7.3 months versus 5.6 months in the dacarbazine arm (p=0.067). In the brain metastases sub-group, fotemustine yielded a 6% ORR, while dacarbazine produced no responses. While myelosuppression was the most common adverse event observed in both arms, fotemustine-induced myelosuppression was more frequent and severe. In the fotemustine arm, 71% (vs. 14% with dacarbazine) of patients experienced neutropenia, and 51% (vs. 5% with dacarbazine) of patients experienced grade 3- 4 neutropenia. Similarly, thrombocytopenia was observed in 94% of patients receiving fotemustine (vs. 57% with dacarbazine) and grade 3- 4 occurred in 43% of patients (vs. 6% with dacarbazine).

The responses of patients who had brain metastases in this study were not as impressive as previously reported in the phase 2 study discussed above, although this might be expected in a more rigorous phase 3 study setting. Although not quite statistically significant, fotemustine delayed the median time-to-develop first brain metastasis among those without pre-existing brain lesions to 22.7 months, versus 7.2 months for patients treated with dacarbazine (p=0.059), suggesting that fotemustine might have activity as an adjuvant treatment after surgical management of CNS metastases. This has not been tested, as of 2012.

A multicenter phase 3 trial randomized 76 patients to receive fotemustine alone or in combination with WBRT in brain metastasis patients and sought to determine the cerebral response and time-to-cerebral-progression [89]. The primary endpoints of this study was to compare the CNS ORR (CR+PR), CNS control rate (CR+PR+SD), and the time to CNS progression. Compared to fotemustine alone, the combination did not significantly improve the ORR or the control rate. The addition of WBRT, however, delayed CNS progression; it was 49 days (range 11–539 days) in the fotemustine-only arm and 56 days (range 19–348 days) in patients treated with fotemustine and WBRT (Wilcoxon test, p=0.028). The combination did not, however, significantly improve the clinical CNS control rate (after 7 weeks) or OS. In regards to safety, myelosuppression was similar in both arms, but alopecia was much higher in the combination arm (40% compared to 2.6% in the fotemustine-only arm).

2.5.2. Targeted agents

Approximately 40 to 50% of all melanomas harbor a mutation in *BRAF* [114]. Notably, 95% of *BRAF* mutations are at the valine in the amino acid position 600, and over 90% of these are substitutions to aspartic acid (depicted as V600E). *In vitro*, the V600E mutation causes a 500-fold increase in the activity of B-Raf kinase; its expression is sufficient to cause tumor formation by normal melanocytes injected into nude mice [114].

Vemurafenib, a small molecule inhibitor of the V600E-mutant, was approved in the United States in 2011 for the treatment of metastatic melanoma in patients harboring the V600E mutation [92]. Clinical trials leading up to its approval excluded patients who had active intracranial disease. Thus, the efficacy of vemurafenib is not well studied in patients with pre-existing intracranial disease.

A single-arm, open-label, pilot study was conducted in metastatic melanoma patients with the V600E mutation and unresectable brain metastases, who failed previous treatments of temozolomide and/or WBRT. Four patients, with extensive disease (3 to 10+ brain metastases), were enrolled. At the time of the abstract presentation, the staging reports for two of the four patients were available. The first patient had a confirmed PR in both intracranial and extracranial lesions, while the second patient had minor responses in intracranial and extracranial metastases. Although very limited data, vemurafenib exhibits preliminary evidence of activity in melanoma patients with brain metastases who failed prior therapy [115]. Additional studies are in progress to demonstrate efficacy of vemurafenib in melanoma patients with intracranial disease. For example, NCT01378975 is an open-label single-arm phase 2 study enrolling metastatic melanoma patients with BRAF V600 and measurable brain metastases (symptomatic or asymptomatic). Patients are enrolled regardless of prior systemic treatment history for brain metastases (except for previous treatment with BRAF or MEK inhibitors). The high response rate of patients harboring V600E mutations in melanoma (~50% vs. ~5% for dacarbazine) suggests that vemurafenib, and potentially other BRAF-targeted therapies, might be useful in post-surgical/SRS adjuvant therapy as an alternative to WBRT. This hypothesis should be tested, especially if CNS activity is confirmed.

Dabrafenib is another potent and selective BRAF V600E inhibitor that inhibits growth of B-Raf mutant melanoma and mutant B-Raf colorectal xenografts in mice [116]. In a phase 1 study, 184 patients with metatastic melanoma, untreated brain metastases, or other solid tumors received dabrafenib [117]. Only three patients with wildtype B-Raf were evaluated, with no evidence of benefit; such patients were subsequently excluded. The study included 156 metastatic melanoma patients, of whom 10 had pre-existing brain metastases. For patients with intracranial disease due to melanoma, 9 out of the 10 patients had reductions in the size of their brain lesions as well as their extracranial disease, with 4 of them achieving complete resolution of the CNS lesions.

A phase 2 study specifically assessing the response to dabrafenib in melanoma patients with intracranial disease harboring a V600E or V600K mutation was recently published [98]. The study enrolled 172 patients, of whom 89 patients had not received previous local treatment for brain metastases (cohort A) and 83 patients who progressed following previous local treatment (cohort B). In cohort A, the overall intracranial response rate (OIRR), which is the primary endpoint of this study, was 39.2% (29/74) in patients with the V600E mutation and 6.7% (1/15) in patients with the V600K mutation. In cohort B, the OIRR was 30.8% (20/65) in patients with the V600E mutation and 22.2% (4/18) in patients harboring the V600K mutation. These data suggest clinical activity in melanoma brain metastases patients harboring the V600E mutation and some activity in V600K patients, whether or not they received prior therapy for their brain metastases.

Given the limited activity of agents available up to this time, such as temozolomide, findings of CNS activity may not require formal confirmation in a phase 3 randomized trial. It is difficult to imagine what the comparator agent of such a trial would be. However, a study of the combination of either WBRT or SRS with concurrent B-Raf inhibitors (vemurafenib or dabrafenib) or with B-Raf inhibitors following radiotherapy would be important in the development of optimal therapy for patients with CNS metastases of melanoma.

2.5.3. Immunotherapy of melanoma in the central nervous system

Following the success, and subsequent FDA approval, of ipilimumab in the management of metastatic melanoma [90, 91], several anecdotal case reports highlighted the activity of ipilimumab in melanoma patients with brain metastases [118, 119]. For example, a retrospective analysis assessing the activity of ipilimumab in melanoma patients with brain metastasis who were enrolled in a phase 2 trial [120] identified 12 patients, of whom 2 achieved PR and

3 had SD in brain metastases. The median OS of all 12 patients was 14 months (range was 2.7 to 56.4 months).

Another retrospective study evaluated the outcome of 77 patients who underwent radiosurgery between 2002 and 2010 for melanoma brain metastases, of whom 27 (35%) received ipilimumab [121]. Ipilimumab–treated patients displayed a median OS of 21.3 months, versus 4.9 months for those not treated with ipilimumab. Even when adjusted for performance status, ipilimumab treatment was associated with a higher survival probability (HR 0.48, p=0.03). The median survival of ipilimumab-treated patients with poor prognosis (11/27 patients), who had Diagnosis-Specific Graded Prognostic Assessment (DS-GPA; discussed in more detail below) score of 0-2 was 15.7 months, while those with better prognosis (16/27 patients), DS-GPA score of 3-4 had a median survival of 25.2 months. The survival of patients who received ipilimumab was similar whether they received ipilimumab before or after developing brain metastases.

To determine the efficacy of ipilimumab prospectively, Margolin and colleagues designed a phase 2 study to assess the activity of ipilimumab in melanoma patients with brain metastasis [99]. The study segregated patients into two cohorts; cohort A included 51 patients who were neurologically asymptomatic, while cohort B included 21 patients with symptoms requiring corticosteroids, which continued during the course of the study, if necessary. The overall ORR in cohort A was 18% (9/51) and 5% (1/21) in cohort B. When assessing response in brain lesions alone, the ORR in cohort A was 24% (12/51) and 10% (2/21) in cohort B. The ORR of extracranial disease was similar in each group to the intracranial response: ORR was 27% (14/51) and 5% (1/21) in cohorts A and B, respectively. The median OS was 7 months for cohort A and 3.7 months in cohort B. Since the study did not specifically address the cause of deaths for patients enrolled in the study, it is not clear whether the variation in OS between the two cohorts was due to progression of intracranial or extracranial disease, or additional complications associated with symptomatic intracranial disease.

A number of observations can be made from the results of this study: a) the response of brain lesions was similar to responses in extracranial metastases; and b) patients with asymptomatic intracranial disease, not on corticosteroid treatment, tended to respond better. The authors of the study present two hypotheses that may explain the difference in response between the two cohorts: i) as suggested by survival data, patients with symptomatic intracranial disease requiring corticosteroids have inherently poorer prognosis; or ii) corticosteroids may potentially interfere with the effector lymphocyte activation induced by ipilimumab. The authors did contend that corticosteroid use with ipilimumab did not entirely abrogate its efficacy.

A single-arm phase 2 study conducted in seven Italian centers assessed the combination of ipilimumab and fotemustine in patients with metastatic melanoma, including patients with asymptomatic brain metastases [95]. The open-label, single-arm phase 2 study enrolled 86 metastatic melanoma patients, of whom 20 had brain metastases at baseline. The overall study population disease control rate (defined as immune-related CR, PR, or SD) was 46.5% (40/86 patients). Similarly, ten of the brain metastasis patients (50%) achieved disease control. This study provides preliminary evidence that the combination of ipilimumab and fotemustine is active in patients with metastatic melanoma, including those with intracranial disease. To confirm the activity of the combination, a randomized phase 3 trial is planned and will compare the activity of the combination versus fotemustine alone in patients with advanced melanoma and brain metastases (NIBIT-M2; CA184-192).

Study	Treatment	Evaluable Patients	Primary Endpoint	Response	Median Survival	Comments
Agarwala et al., 2004 [93]	TMZ	151 total 117 treatment naive 35 pts prior CTx	ORR in brain and toxicity	No prior CTx: ORR 7% SD 29% Prior CTx: PR 3% SD 18%	Treatment Naive: 3.5m Prior CTx: 2.2m	
Margolin et al., 2002 [88]	TMZ and WBRT	31 pts	ORR	CNS ORR 10% (1 CR and 2 PR)	PFS 2m OS 6m	
Hwu et al., 2005 [96]	TMZ + Thalidomide	26 pts 16 symptomatic 25 extensive extracranial mets	ORR in CNS	15 evaluable pts 3 CR or PR (12% by intent-to-treat)	OS 5m OS 6m (for evaluable pts)	15 pts completed ≥ 1 cycle. 11 discontinued before completing 1 cycle: 7 for intracranial hemorrhage, 2 for pulmonary embolism, 1 deep vein thrombosis, and 1 for Grade 3 rash
Chiarion-Sileni et al., 2011 [94]	CTI (TMZ + Cisplatin + IL2) vs. CDI (DTIC + Cisplatin + IL2 Phase 3	150 pts 118 evaluable (57 in CTI and 61 in CDI)	Time to CNS mets	CNS failure: CTI - 24/57 pts CDI 34/61 pts $P = 0.22$ 1y CNS failure rate CTI - 21% CDI - 31%	PFS CTI – 4.1m CDI – 3.9m $P=0.90$ OS CTI – 8.4m CDI – 8.7m 1y OS CTI – 31% CDI – 42%	
Jacquillat et al., 1990 [97]	Fotemustine	153 evaluable pts; 36 (23.5%) had CNS disease	ORR	ORR 25% CNS	NR for CNS pts.	The overall ORR in all pts was 24%
Mornex et al., 2003 [89]	Arm A: Fotemustine vs. Arm B: Fotemustine + WBRT Phase 3	76 pts Arm A: 39 pts Arm B: 37 pts	CNS ORR on day 50 CNS Control Rate (CR+PR +SD) on day 50	ORR 7.4% (arm A) 10.0% (arm B) $P = 0.73$ Control Rate 30% (arm A) 47% (arm B)	OS 86 days (arm A) 105 days (arm B). $P = 0.561$	

Study	Treatment	Evaluable Patients	Primary Endpoint	Response	Median Survival	Comments
			Time to objective CNS progression	$P = 0.19$ Time to CNS progression 49 days (arm A) 56 days (arm B) $P = 0.028$		
Long et al., 2012 [98]	Dabrafenib	172 pts Cohort A: no prior CNS therapy, 89 pts Cohort B: Prior CNS therapy, 83 pts	OIRR	Cohort A V600E 39% V600K 6.7% Cohort B V600E 31% V600K 22%	At 6 months, Cohort A: 27% Cohort B: 41%	Study limited to V600E and V600K BRAF mutated melanoma
Margolin et al., 2012 [99]	Ipilimumab	72 pts 51 Cohort A (no CNS symptoms) 21 Cohort B (CNS symptoms requiring corticosteroids) Phase 2	DCR (CR, PR, SD) at 12 wks	DCR Cohort A 18% Cohort B 5% DCR in CNS Cohort A – 24% Cohort B – 10%	OS Cohort A 7m Cohort B 3.7m	
Di Giacoma et al., 2012 [95]	Fotemustine + Ipilimumab	86 pts total 20 CNS disease at baseline	Immune-related DCR (CR, PR, SD) at 24 weeks	DCR Overall 46.5% CNS 50%	CNS PFS 4.5m CNS OS 13.4m At 1-yr, 54% of CNS pts alive	Out of the 10 brain responses 5 PR or SD 5 CR

CNS: Central Nervous System; CR: Complete response; CTx: Chemotherapy; DC: Disease control; DCR: Disease control rate; DTIC: Dacarbazine; NR: Not reported; OIRR: Overall intracranial response rate; ORR: Objective response rate; OS: Overall survival; PFS: Progression-free survival; PR: Partial response; SD: Stable disease; TMZ: Temozolomide; WBRT: Whole-brain radiation therapy

Table 6. Prospective trials of systemic therapy treatments for melanoma brain metastases

3. Risk stratification

Several systems estimate risk of recurrence and death in patients with brain metastases, including some with melanoma-specific data (Table 7). Recursive Partitioning Analysis (RPA) is one such system [122-124]. This combines age, performance status, and extracranial disease status to assign a class from I to III that estimates survival. Its original intention was to stratify patients for enrollment in clinical trials. Its clinically available factors are useful to consider in a discussion of brain metastasis patients.

RPA's initial description included 1200 patients, 200 of whom were affected by melanoma. Histology and tissue of origin were significant prognostic factors, with melanoma being unfavorable. The validity of RPA has since been confirmed in the melanoma subgroup [10, 19, 35, 42, 43].

While originally intended for stratification of patients in radiation therapy trials, RPA class also stratifies risk in patients undergoing surgical metastectomy [125, 126]. In 2004, the RTOG study enrolled 333 patients between 1996 and 2001, of whom 167 were assigned to WBRT and SRS and 164 received WBRT alone [15]. Median survival was longer in patients with a single brain metastasis for patients receiving WBRT+SRS combination compared to patients who only received WBRT (6.5 months *vs.* 4.9 months, p=0.0393). This study shed light on a limitation of RPA: it does not take into account the number of brain metastases present.

The Diagnosis-Specific Graded Prognostic Assessment (DS-GPA) was developed by retrospective analysis of 4,259 patients newly diagnosed with brain metastases [127]. In addition to the factors in RPA, it includes number of brain metastases and the underlying disease giving rise to brain metastases. In the melanoma subset, the analysis identified two significant prognostic factors: performance status (represented by KPS) and number of radiologically evident brain metastases. For KPS, a score of 90-100 is 2 points, 70-80 is 1 point, and less than 70 is 0 points. A single brain metastasis is 2 points, 2 to 3 metastasis is 1 point, and more than 3 metastases is 0 points. The DS-GPA score, calculated by adding the point values from a patient's KPS score and number of metastases, ranges from 0 (worst prognosis) to 4 (best prognosis). Median OS for melanoma patients ranges from 3.4 months (GS-GPA score of 0 to 1.0) to 13.2 months (GS-GPA score of 3.5 to 4.0).

Several other systems have been developed for use in specific sub-populations. The Basic Score for Brain Metastases (BS-BM) was developed by analyzing results from 110 SRS-treated patients [128]. The system generates a score based on KPS, control of primary tumor site, and extracranial disease status. Only 19 patients (17%) of the initial group of patients had melanoma. The system has not yet been studied in melanoma patients specifically and focuses on SRS treatment. Its applicability to other treatment modalities remains to be established.

The Score Index for Radiosurgery (SIR) was developed from the study of 65 SRS-treated patients with brain metastases from a variety of primary tumor types [129]. SIR derives a score from patient age, performance status, systemic disease status, maximum CNS lesion volume, and number of CNS lesions. In the population initially studied, SIR was more accurate in predicting survival than RPA. A retrospective study confirmed its utility in melanoma patients [38].

The Malignant Melanoma-Gamma Knife Radiosurgery score (MM-GKR) also assesses outcomes in metastatic melanoma patients treated with SRS [23]. Scoring is based on performance status, age, and CNS lesion location. The authors claim greater prognostic accuracy than with either RPA or SIR, particularly in identifying patients with an especially poor prognosis.

The Prognostic Index (PI) score estimates prognosis in patients treated with palliative WBRT [43]. Factors used in this system include number of extracranial metastatic sites, RPA class,

CNS disease progression prior to WBRT, and the presence of meningeal disease. This system is focused on those with extensive disease, not amenable to local therapy with SRS or surgery.

Median survival times predicted by studies of brain metastasis patients generally are similar to those reported for melanoma patients with CNS involvement. With minor differences, the systems described utilize similar and easily available data to arrive at their risk estimations. RPA has probably been examined in the widest array of clinical trial settings. It also does not seem to be specific to a given treatment modality. Its components are fairly simple to derive from clinical parameters. It will therefore be used for further discussion.

System	Prognostic Factors	Prognostic Classification				Median OS (all tumor types)	Median OS (melanoma)		Comments	References
RPA	KPS, age, extra-cranial disease status, control of primary disease site	Class I: KPS≥70, age<65 y., controlled primary disease site, no extra-cranial disease Class II: Not Class I or III Class III: KPS<70				Class I: 7.1 m Class II: 4.2 m Class III: 2.3 m	Class I: 6.5-10.5 m Class II: 3.5-5.9 m Class III: 1.8-2.5 m		Validated for radiation therapy and surgery.	Gaspar et al., 1997 [122] Gaspar et al., 2000 [123] Buchsbaum et al., 2002 [10] Lutterbach et al., 2002 [124] Harrison et al., 2003 [42] Morris et al., 2004 [43] Radbill et al., 2004 [35] Brown et al., 2002 [19]
PI	Number of ECM, RPA class (see above), PD on imaging prior to WBRT, presence of LM	Index= Number of ECM sites + (2 x RPA class) + (2 if PD on pre-WBRT imaging) + (4 if LM present)				NR	Score 2-4 5-6 7-8 9-10 11+	138 d 80 d 42 d 18 d 15 d	To determine outcome following palliative WBRT.	Morris et al., 2004 [43]
SIR	Age, KPS, extra-cranial disease status, volume of largest CNS lesion, number of CNS lesions	Factor Age KPS Systemic disease status Largest Lesion Volume (cm³)	0 ≥60 ≤50 PD °/>13	1 51-59 60-70 PR/SD 5-13	2 ≤50 ≥70 CR or NED <5	Score 0-3 4-7 8-10	Score 2.9 m 7 m 31 m	≤6 °/>6	4 m 7 m	Point values for individual factors are added to derive score. Intended for assessment of outcome after SRS.	Weltman et al., 2000 [129] Selek et al., 2004 [38]

System	Prognostic Factors	Prognostic Classification				Median OS (all tumor types)	Median OS (melanoma)	Comments	References
		# of CNS lesions	≥3	2	2				
MM-GKR	Age, KPS, Adverse CNS lesion locations (brainstem, posterior fossa, nuclei, cerebellum)	Factor	0	1	1.5 2	NR	Score	Intended for assessment of outcome after SRS.	Gaudy-Marqueste et al., 2006 [23]
		KPS	<80	-	- ≤80		0 → 7.1 m		
		Age	≤60	"/>60	- -		1-2 → 5 m		
		Adverse Location	No	-	Yes -		≥2.5 → 2.2 m		
BS-BM	KPS, control of primary tumor, presence of ECM	Factor	0	1		Score	NR	Not validated in melanoma, although study included 19 melanoma patients out of 110 total (17%). Score of 3 had OS not reaching median with 30 m of follow-up. Intended for assessment of outcome after SRS.	Lorenzoni et al., 2004 [128]
		KPS	50-70	"/>70		0 1.9 m			
		Primary tumor control	No	Yes		1 3.3 m			
						2 13.1 m			
		ECM	Yes	No		3 ND			
DS-GPA	RPA factors (KPS, age, extra-cranial disease status, control of primary disease site) and number of brain mets	Factor	0	1	2	0.0-1.0 3.4m	0.0-1.0 3.4m	In melanoma, only 2 significant prognostic factors: KPS (p<0.0001) and number of brain mets (p<0.0001)	Sperduto et al., 2010 [127]
		KPS	<70	70-80	90-100	1.5-2.5 6.4m	1.5-2.5 4.7m		
		# of brain mets	>3	2-3	1	3.0 11.6m 3.0	8.8m		
						3.5-4.0 14.8m 3.5-4.0	13.2m		

CNS: Central Nervous System; CR: Complete response; DS-GPA: Diagnosis-Specific Graded Prognostic Assessment; ECM: Extracranial metastases; KPS: Karnofsky performance status; LM: Leptomeningeal metastasis; MM-GKR: Malignant Melanoma-Gamma Knife Radiosurgery score; ND: Not defined; NED: No evidence of disease; NR: Not reported; OS: Overall survival; PD: Progressive disease; PI: Prognostic Index; PR: Partial Response; QOL: Quality of life; RPA: Recursive Partitioning Analysis; SD: Stable disease; SIR: Score Index for Radiosurgery

Table 7. Risk Stratification of Patients with Brain Metastases from Melanoma

An important caveat in discussing outcomes estimates derived using these risk stratification systems is that they all were first developed prior to 2011. Prior to that time, reliably effective and proven treatments for advanced melanoma were not available for general clinical use. Development of drugs with proven activity, such as ipilimumab and vemurafenib discussed above, are changing the outlook for melanoma patients. This includes patients with brain metastases. With these drugs, and more being developed with potentially even greater activity, the risk estimates of these systems will certainly change for the better. This is especially likely to be the case in patients with very high risk/poor prognosis disease. Treatment recommendations for the brain metastasis problem in melanoma will therefore likely be very fluid over the next several years, as new treatment paradigms for melanoma evolve.

4. Therapy of CNS disease

4.1. Unfavorable/poor risk

By definition, RPA class III patients have a KPS less than 70%. Often, they have multi-focal brain metastases, active extracranial disease, or both. Historically, their life expectancy was very limited. The PI prognostic system, intended to assess prognosis in this group as described above, uses days rather than months as the unit of time for its estimates [43].

Conventionally, surgery or SRS would only be used judiciously with palliative intent and well-defined goals. WBRT may be undertaken for symptom palliation and a very modest survival benefit [8, 12, 86, 130-132]. The anticipated duration of survival played an important part in designing any treatment approach, as even therapy of several weeks duration could consume a significant proportion of a patient's remaining lifespan. The burden of coming to repeated treatments (as might be the case with palliative WBRT, frequently administered as 10 treatments over 2 weeks) may lead to a significant QOL decrement in patients with poor performance status. By definition, RPA class III patients have such a poor performance status.

Prior to the approval in the United States of ipilimumab and vemurafenib in 2011, systemic therapy played a minimal role in this group. Exceptions included steroid therapy for tumor-associated edema and anti-convulsants for seizures. The low performance status and CNS disease in these patients excluded them from virtually all clinical trials. Activity of systemic agents with CNS penetration, such as temozolmide and fotemustine, was limited, with an onset of action too slow to benefit most patients with melanoma who were in this category.

As of 2011, BRAF mutational status serves as an important factor in making treatment decisions. This may be especially important in patients with RPA class III melanoma with CNS involvement. The BRAF inhibitors vemurafenib and dabrafenib, discussed above, have rapid onset of action, high response rates, preliminary evidence of CNS activity, oral administration and manageable toxicity profiles. As of November 2012, vemurafenib is approved in the United States and Europe, and debrafanib's approval is pending. For patients possessing an appropriate BRAF mutation, treatment with one of these agents would be reasonable to consider, even with RPA class III. Of course, the patient must be aware that information about this drug in the brain metastasis population is presently very limited. Data regarding combinations with radiotherapy is also very limited at this time. While a clinical trial would be the preferred setting to treat these patients, use of BRAF inhibition therapy would be reasonable to offer to BRAF-mutant melanoma patients with brain metastases and RPA class III.

For patients in whom a targetable BRAF mutation is not present, fewer options are available. Ipilimumab, discussed above, has a relatively slow onset of action, taking 3-4 months in phase 3 trials to confer a survival benefit versus controls [90, 91], with an overall low response rate.

For someone with a poor performance status unlikely to live that long, ipilimumab is unlikely to provide benefit, despite preliminary evidence of CNS activity. For these patients, further developments in melanoma therapy are awaited. Pallitative WBRT likely remains the standard therapy for these patients.

One peculiar circumstance remains: some patients present with RPA class III advanced disease, including brain metastases and poor performance status, but their BRAF mutational status is unknown. Given their overall condition and location of disease, obtaining a tumor specimen to determine BRAF mutation status may not be possible. A wait of 1-2 weeks for results of mutational testing may consume a significant portion of their remaining lifespan. In such patients, standard care would be supportive, potentially with the addition of WBRT. Given a frequency of BRAF mutations targeted by presently available drugs of about 50% and the lack of other proven options, a therapeutic trial of BRAF inhibition is unlikely to cause significant harm, and might lead to dramatic benefit if the patient possesses an appropriate mutation. Again, before embarking on such a treatment course, the patient must be aware of the limitations of our current dataset.

4.2. Favorable/good risk

Patients of RPA class I have a relatively good prognosis and warrant an aggressive treatment approach. Such patients are young, have a good performance status, and no active extracranial disease. However, among patients with metastatic melanoma, true RPA class I patients are infrequently encountered, especially those completely lacking detectable extracranial disease.

The major treatment decision for these patients relates to local therapy of existing brain lesions (Figure 1). The goal would be to treat all evident CNS disease by some form of definitive therapy (surgery or SRS). Traditionally, surgery was favored in cases involving one surgically accessible lesion, and benefit was reported in surgeries targeting up to 3 lesions [14, 133]. Surgery is also especially useful in specific situations where SRS is less favorable, such as large lesion size (> 3cm) or symptomatology (for example, bleeding). Surgery also yields a specimen to confirm the diagnosis and analyze for targetable alterations in the tumor, such as BRAF mutations status. In patients lacking any other evident disease, these data can be very important and only obtainable from a surgically resected CNS specimen. Otherwise, SRS is emerging as the preferred local therapy, both for its simpler administration and possibly for better local control [44]. SRS may also be able to provide definitive treatment at sites inaccessible to surgery. Surgery and SRS are not mutually exclusive: both may be necessary to provide definitive treatment of all lesions in multi-focal metastatic CNS disease.

SRS has been a remarkable addition to our armamentarium for treatment of brain metastases. Previously, surgery was the only approach to definitive treatment. If more than 3 lesions were present, or they were located in surgically inaccessible locations, surgery could not be used with the intention of long-term control. SRS allows treatment of multiple lesions, in sites inaccessible to surgery. It also offers the possibility of re-treatment. At some point, presumably, the number of lesions exceeds the ability of SRS to control the disease. The exact number is not defined, but some have advocated SRS to control up to five CNS lesions [37]. Beyond this, it may be unreasonable to expect a local treatment modality like SRS to control what is clinically widespread involvement in an organ system, even if limited to the CNS. Surgery and SRS may be able to control specific lesions that are symptomatic in such patients, but the overall treatment approach relies primarily on therapeutic WBRT and systemic therapy, discussed below under "Intermediate Risk."

In patients with RPA class I disease from melanoma, risk of failure in the CNS is high if treatment focuses solely on radiologically evident disease. This likely reflects the underlying biology, in which specific neurotropic sub-clones of melanoma develop that colonize the CNS, leading to brain metastases. Limiting treatment to surgery and/or SRS of only radiologically evident lesions ignores this biological reality. This observation is confirmed in the multiple randomized trials of adjuvant WBRT enrolling patients with multiple tumor types, including melanoma. Adjuvant WBRT decreases intracranial recurrence rates when combined with definitive local therapy. This effect is evident at both definitively treated macroscopic sites (treating residual contamination) and at distant sites within the CNS. At distant sites, adjuvant WBRT must accomplish this by either treating pre-existing radiologically undetectable micrometastatic disease or making the CNS less receptive to colonization from extracranial sites. The former is the more plausible biological explanation.

Approaches to address the problem of distant CNS recurrence have been discussed in detail earlier. Basically, these come down to either administering adjuvant WBRT up-front, or using an expectant management strategy, with regular imaging and re-treatment (primarily with SRS), at the time of CNS progression. Arguments against adjuvant WBRT include concern regarding its cognitive toxicity, its lack of clear survival benefit and inability to undertake re-treatment. As described earlier, cognitive effects of adjuvant WBRT, while not absent, are not unreasonable in the setting of CNS metastases, especially when balanced against the cognitive effects of tumor progression and those of re-treatment (as, for example, by SRS). Adjuvant WBRT is unlikely to be associated, in general, with an overall survival benefit overall due to extracranial disease as a competing cause of death. In the setting of RPA class I patients, who lack active extracranial disease, adjuvant WBRT may very well have a survival benefit [54, 134].

As noted above, the use of a salvage strategy, relying on SRS in the event of tumor progression, is associated with high rates of intracranial failure. The cognitive effects of such a strategy have not been assessed in detail, but the data regarding cognitive effects of allowing tumor progression have been reviewed and are clearly unfavorable. Whether the effects are better or worse than those due to adjuvant use of WBRT can only be answered by a randomized comparison of the two strategies.

We concede that the decision regarding use of adjuvant WBRT is not simple and clear-cut. To determine whether to recommend its use, the benefit of decreased intracranial progression rates must be balanced against its adverse effects. Overall, we believe that the published evidence generally supports the use of adjuvant WBRT in melanoma patients.

Systemic adjuvant therapy might be an alternative to adjuvant WBRT. Traditional cytotoxic therapy agents with known CNS activity, such as fotemustine or temozolomide, have not been shown clearly to impact the subsequent development of CNS disease in melanoma patients [113, 135]. In the setting of melanoma patients with CNS disease, their primary purpose was to treat extracranial disease, an important prognostic factor once CNS disease was controlled. By definition, true RPA class I patients have no active extracranial disease.

Newly developed agents, such as vemurafenib and ipilimumab, may have a role defined in the future for adjuvant therapy in patients with RPA class I CNS disease from melanoma. They may be able to affect both CNS recurrence rates and progression of extracranial disease. However, data supporting such use is not available at present. Their use as adjuvant therapies in this population is not warranted, outside the setting of a clinical trial.

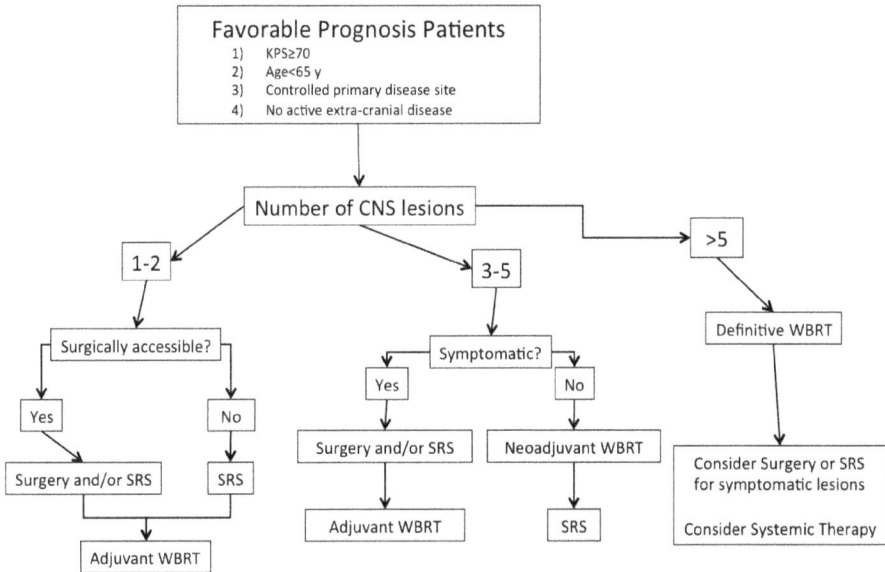

Figure 1. Treatment of melanoma patients with brain metastases with favorable risk profile, equivalent to RPA class I. In patients with more than one brain lesion who are to receive local therapy, it may be necessary to use both surgery and radiosurgery to treat all lesions. By definition, RPA class I patients have no active extracranial disease. Thus, systemic therapy is not indicated except in an experimental trial. CNS: central nervous system; KPS: Karnofsky performance status; RPA: Recursive Partitioning Analysis; SRS: stereotactic radiosurgery; WBRT: whole brain radiotherapy.

4.3. Intermediate risk

Treatment decisions in intermediate risk patients (equivalent to RPA class II) are probably most difficult of all (Figure 2). This relates to their variable clinical presentation. They have better performance status than those with unfavorable RPA class III. They are also of advanced age (according to RPA, anyone older than 65 years), have active extracranial disease, or both, conveying a negative prognosis relative to RPA class I. A logical way to divide this population is into those with CNS disease amenable to local definitive therapy and those with CNS disease too extensive for complete, definitive local therapy of all lesions.

Considerations regarding the use of adjuvant WBRT and the desirability for treatment in the context of a clinical trial are essentially the same as for favorable prognosis patients. The key differentiating question is whether local therapy of CNS lesions with surgery or SRS should be attempted at all. Several clinical situations argue against their use. Lesions may be inaccessible for surgery or too large for SRS or they may simply be too numerous. If definitive treatment of all CNS disease sites is possible, then it should be attempted. If CNS disease is not amenable to local therapy of all lesions, then treatment must rely on therapeutic WBRT and systemic therapy, with surgery or SRS reserved for large or symptomatic lesions.

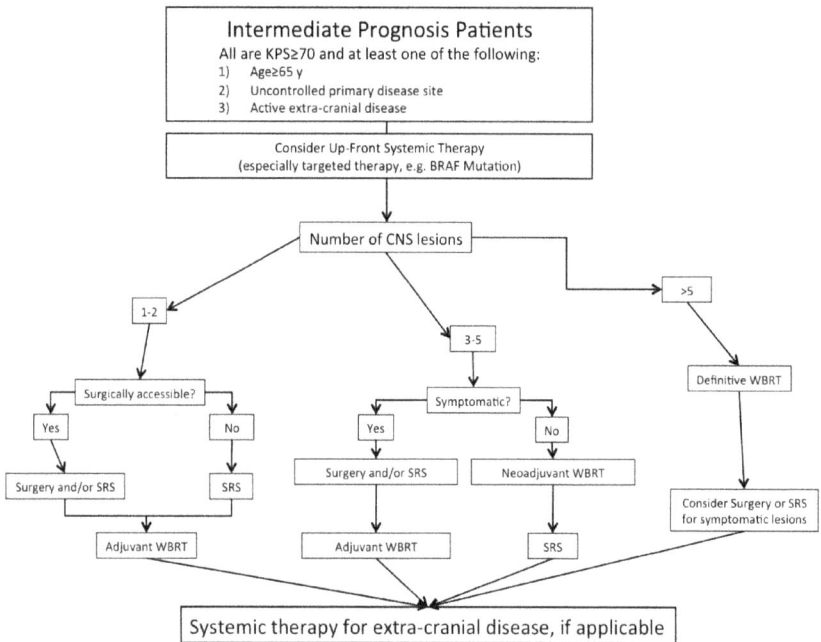

Figure 2. Treatment of melanoma patients with brain metastases with intermediate prognosis, equivalent to RPA class II. In patients with more than one brain lesion who are to receive local therapy, it may be necessary to use both surgery and radiosurgery to treat all lesions. Patients with active extracranial disease should be considered for systemic therapy. While in the past, few active systemic agents were available, newer therapies might have relevance early in the treatment of intermediate prognosis patients. For example, BRAF inhibition with vemurafenib has rapid onset of control, high response rates, and even preliminary evidence of CNS activity. Thus, early use of systemic therapy might be able to impact both CNS disease and extracranial disease. Extracranial disease activity is a consistent adverse prognostic factor in intermediate patients, once CNS disease is controlled. CNS: central nervous system; KPS: Karnofsky performance status; RPA: Recursive Partitioning Analysis; SRS: stereotactic radiosurgery; WBRT: whole brain radiotherapy.

In RPA class II patients with CNS melanoma, active extracranial disease status is a key prognostic factor. Disease outside the CNS represents a competing cause of death. Before the approval in 2011-2012 of agents with proven anti-melanoma activity (such as vemurafenib and ipilimumab), systemic therapy of the CNS was limited to temozolomide or fotemustine (in

Europe). Although these drugs treated extracranial disease as well, they were not highly active in either the CNS or extracranial compartments, and did not demonstrate clear or dramatic survival benefits.

Systemic therapy of melanoma in RPA class II patients is appearing brighter than it has in the past. Clinical trials are opening which permit these patients to enroll, and highly active agents, with CNS activity moreover, such as vemurafenib are available non-experimentally for patients with BRAF mutations. For patients lacking BRAF mutations, treatment with ipilimumab is a reasonable consideration, due to its survival benefit in a phase 3 trial, which included patients with pre-existing, treated brain metastases [90]. Most of these patients will live long enough to derive benefit from ipilimumab. As new agents are developed, their use in RPA class II melanoma patients is justified, even without demonstrable CNS activity, due to the active extracranial disease present in most of this population as a competing cause of death.

5. Directions for the future

Brain metastasis is part of the natural history of metastatic melanoma. It is a common problem and has a major adverse impact on treatment outcomes and QOL. The bulk of melanoma-specific research consists of retrospective analyses and single-center studies. Prospectively validated, comprehensive treatment paradigms do not yet exist. The preceding discussion suggests some important research questions for the future.

Optimal use of SRS technology remains undefined. One question relates to the treatment of multiple lesions. The only major randomized trial of SRS in brain metastasis therapy demonstrated a survival benefit in the presence of only a single brain metastasis [15]. No prospective data support a survival benefit from SRS when more than one lesion is present; retrospective data from several sources indicate that multiple CNS lesions are associated with worse survival [22, 26, 35].

At some point, the absolute number of CNS lesions poses a barrier to effective SRS therapy. Some argue that the presence of multiple lesions (up to about 5) should not preclude therapy, based on results indicating that the number of CNS melanoma lesions did not predict subsequent survival [39, 136]. Whether some threshold number of lesions exists is an unanswered question appropriate for investigation.

SRS itself is a generic term for a rapidly evolving technology. The relevance of even recently published results to current treatment technologies may be questioned. What is unlikely to change is the local nature of SRS therapy: SRS treats the radiated region, but not that which is unradiated. As discussed extensively, concurrent micrometastatic disease is not addressed by SRS, as it is also not by surgery. The use of adjuvant therapy after local treatment with surgery or SRS lacks melanoma-specific prospective data. Five randomized trials, described above, indicate that adjuvant WBRT can decrease intracranial recurrence rates, both at sites treated with surgery/SRS and at untreated sites. The adverse neurocognitive effects of WBRT and the efficacy of this modality in the metastatic melanoma population are valid questions. As noted above, such a study is in progress (NCT01503827) [55].

An alternative to the use of adjuvant WBRT is a planned radiosurgical salvage strategy. This presumably minimizes exposure of the CNS to WBRT and its adverse effects. Little data is available regarding this treatment approach. A randomized clinical trial would be most helpful, in which patients are randomized to receive immediate adjuvant WBRT after SRS therapy or undergo planned SRS salvage treatments, with WBRT only when SRS is not possible. This study would provide data to balance the neurocognitive consequences of immediate WBRT with those due to an increased rate of later macroscopic CNS progression. Further, some estimate of the neurocognitive cost of SRS re-treatment would be obtained.

SRS itself is used for adjuvant purposes after surgical metastectomy to treat residual disease at the resection site. The efficacy of this has not been defined. Additionally, such therapy does not treat occult disease at other sites within the CNS. A randomized trial comparing the efficacy of adjuvant SRS to either no adjuvant therapy or to adjuvant WBRT would be appropriate.

Finally, and perhaps most significantly, systemic therapy of melanoma is evolving rapidly, and those advances will have a major impact on treatment of CNS disease. Even now, convincing preliminary evidence of CNS activity of these several new agents has been presented. Previously, melanoma patients with CNS disease were excluded from clinical trials in the belief that the blood-brain barrier posed too great a hurdle to clinical efficacy. This no longer appears to be a valid assumption. As new agents emerge, their activity in the CNS should either be addressed in CNS-specific trials, or patients with CNS melanoma should be considered similar to any other melanoma patient, so long as their CNS disease is minimally or asymptomatic.

Much of this review has focused on the controversy of adjuvant therapy in the CNS. Adjuvant WBRT is not an optimal solution to this problem. It does not prevent CNS re-seeding from extracranial sites and cannot be used repeatedly. Adverse cognitive effects of WBRT are clearly demonstrable, even if their clinical impact is arguable. Critically, adjuvant WBRT also does not address the problem of extracranial disease, a major prognostic factor. Optimal adjuvant therapy to address these limitations is likely to be systemic. The development of highly active agents with CNS penetration opens the possibility of their use in melanoma patients after definitive treatment of brain metastases.

Several prior studies can provide necessary baseline data regarding rates of CNS progression for sample size calculations [113, 135]. Neurocognitive effects must be a secondary endpoint in any study, as it cannot be assumed that systemic agents are devoid of adverse neurocognitive effects. For example, case reports of melanoma patients treated with fotemustine reported toxic leukoencephalopathy with progressive dementia in several patients, [137, 138].

6. Conclusions

Brain metastasis is a frequent and serious problem for melanoma patients. New technologies, such as SRS and agents, such as vemurafenib and ipilimumab, are expanding our ability to treat this condition. Melanoma-specific studies guiding optimal employment of new technologies are limited. Most information regarding CNS treatment in melanoma is extrapolated from other conditions or is based on retrospective analyses from individual centers. Data from well-designed, prospective trials is lacking in many regards. This deficiency has been noted at least eight years previously by others [139]. At present, many of the same questions posed by those workers remain unanswered. Fortunately, melanoma treatment itself has not remained static, with new agents generating new questions regarding optimal treatment of the condition.

Well-designed, rigorous trials will allow our patients to receive the best and most cost-effective treatments available. Melanoma patients with brain metastases can look forward to a brighter future. We must, however, demand rigorous investigations to allow the best use possible of the arsenal being placed at our disposal to treat this challenging problem.

Abbreviations

BS-BM: Basic Score for Brain Metastases; CNS: Central Nervous System; CR: Complete Response; CT: Computed Tomography; DS-GPA: Diagnosis-Specific Graded Prognostic Assessment; Gy: Grey, unit of radiation dose; HVLT: Hopkin's Verbal Learning Test; KPS: Karnofsky Performance Status; MM-GKR: Malignant Melanoma-Gamma Knife Radiosurgery; MMSE: Mini-Mental Status Examination; MRI: Magnetic Resonance Imaging; NCF: Neurocognitive Function; NSCLC: Non Small Cell Lung Cancer; OIRR: Overall Intracranial Response Rate; ORR: Objective Response Rate; OS: Overall Survival; QOL: Quality-of-Life; PCI: Prophylactic Cranial Irradiation; PFS: Progression-Free Survival; PI: Prognostic Index; PR: Partial Response; RPA: Recursive Partitioning Analysis; RTOG: Radiation Therapy Oncology Group; SCLC: Small Cell Lung Cancer; SD: Stable Disease; SIR: Score Index for Radiosurgery; SRS: Stereotactic Radiosurgery; TCI: Therapeutic Cranial Irradiation; WBRT: Whole Brain Radiation Therapy

Author details

Sherif S. Morgan*[1], Joanne M. Jeter[1], Evan M. Hersh[1], Sun K. Yi[2] and Lee D. Cranmer*[1*]

*Address all correspondence to: lcranmer@azcc.arizona.edu

1 Section of Hematology and Oncology, Melanoma/Sarcoma Program, University of Arizona Cancer Center, University of Arizona, USA

2 Department of Radiation Oncology, College of Medicine, University of Arizona, USA

*Both of these authors contributed equally.

Conflict of Interest: The authors would like to disclose the following conflicts of interest: Sherif Morgan: None to disclose.
Evan Hersh: GlaxoSmithKline, Bristol-Meyers Squibb, Pfizer, Genentech/Roche, Celgene.

Joanne Jeter: None to disclose.
Sun K Yi: None to disclose.
Lee Cranmer: Bristol-Meyers Squibb, Merck, Genentech/Roche, Celgene, Prometheus Laboratories.

References

[1] Siegel, R., D. Naishadham, and A. Jemal, *Cancer statistics, 2012.* CA Cancer J Clin, 2012. 62(1): p. 10-29.

[2] Little, E.G. and M.J. Eide, *Update on the current state of melanoma incidence.* Dermatol Clin, 2012. 30(3): p. 355-61.

[3] Fidler, I.J., et al., *The biology of melanoma brain metastasis.* Cancer and Metastasis Rev, 1999. 18(3): p. 387-400.

[4] Madajewicz, S., et al., *Malignant melanoma brain metastases. Review of Roswell Park Memorial Institute experience.* Cancer, 1984. 53(11): p. 2550-2.

[5] Noordijk, E.M., et al., *The choice of treatment of single brain metastasis should be based on extracranial tumor activity and age.* Int J Radiat Oncol Biol Phys, 1994. 29(4): p. 711-7.

[6] Mintz, A.H., et al., *A randomized trial to assess the efficacy of surgery in addition to radiotherapy in patients with a single cerebral metastasis.* Cancer, 1996. 78(7): p. 1470-6.

[7] Patchell, R.A., et al., *A randomized trial of surgery in the treatment of single metastases to the brain.* N Engl J Med, 1990. 322(8): p. 494-500.

[8] Sampson, J.H., et al., *Demographics, prognosis, and therapy in 702 patients with brain metastases from malignant melanoma.* J Neurosurg, 1998. 88(1): p. 11-20.

[9] Wronski, M. and E. Arbit, *Surgical treatment of brain metastases from melanoma: a retrospective study of 91 patients.* J Neurosurg, 2000. 93(1): p. 9-18.

[10] Buchsbaum, J.C., et al., *Survival by radiation therapy oncology group recursive partitioning analysis class and treatment modality in patients with brain metastases from malignant melanoma: a retrospective study.* Cancer, 2002. 94(8): p. 2265-72.

[11] Zacest, A.C., et al., *Surgical management of cerebral metastases from melanoma: outcome in 147 patients treated at a single institution over two decades.* J Neurosurg, 2002. 96(3): p. 552-8.

[12] Fife, K.M., et al., *Determinants of outcome in melanoma patients with cerebral metastases.* J Clin Oncol, 2004. 22(7): p. 1293-300.

[13] Raizer, J.J., et al., *Brain and leptomeningeal metastases from cutaneous melanoma: survival outcomes based on clinical features.* Neuro Oncol, 2008. 10(2): p. 199-207.

[14] Bindal, R.K., et al., *Surgical treatment of multiple brain metastases.* J Neurosurg, 1993. 79(2): p. 210-216.

[15] Andrews, D.W., et al., *Whole brain radiation therapy with or without stereotactic radiosurgery boost for patients with one to three brain metastases: Phase III results of the RTOG 9508 randomised trial.* Lancet, 2004. 363(9422): p. 1665-72.

[16] Kondziolka, D., et al., *Stereotactic radiosurgery plus whole brain radiotherapy versus radiotherapy alone for patients with multiple brain metastases.* Int J Radiat Oncol Biol Phys, 1999. 45(2): p. 427-34.

[17] Manon, R., et al., *Phase II trial of radiosurgery for one to three newly diagnosed brain metastases from renal cell carcinoma, melanoma, and sarcoma: an Eastern Cooperative Oncology Group study (E 6397).* J Clin Oncol, 2005. 23(34): p. 8870-6.

[18] Friehs, G.M., et al., *Outcomes in patients treated with gamma knife radiosurgery for brain metastases from malignant melanoma.* Neurosurg Focus, 1998. 4(6): p. e1.

[19] Brown, P.D., et al., *Stereotactic radiosurgery for patients with "radioresistant" brain metastases.* Neurosurgery, 2002. 51(3): p. 656-65; discussion 665-7.

[20] 20.Chang, E.L., et al., *Outcome variation among "radioresistant" brain metastases treated with stereotactic radiosurgery.* Neurosurgery, 2005. 56(5): p. 936-945.

[21] Chen, J.C.T., et al., *Stereotactic radiosurgery in the treatment of metastatic disease to the brain.* Stereotact Funct Neurosurg, 1999. 73(1-4): p. 60-3.

[22] Christopoulou, A., et al., *Integration of gamma knife surgery in the management of cerebral metastases from melanoma.* Melanoma Res, 2006. 16(1): p. 51-7.

[23] Gaudy-Marqueste, C., et al., *Gamma knife radiosurgery in the management of melanoma patients with brain metastases: a series of 106 patients without whole-brain radiotherapy.* Int J Radiat Oncol Biol Phys, 2006. 65(3): p. 809-16.

[24] Gieger, M., et al., *Response of intracranial melanoma metastases to stereotactic radiosurgery.* Radiat Oncol Investig, 1997. 5(2): p. 72-80.

[25] Gonzalez-Martinez, J., et al., *Gamma knife radiosurgery for intracranial metastatic melanoma: a 6-year experience.* J Neurosurg, 2002. 97(5 Suppl): p. 494-8.

[26] Grob, J.J., et al., *Radiosurgery without whole brain radiotherapy in melanoma brain metastases. Club de Cancerologie Cutanee.* Eur J Cancer, 1998. 34(8): p. 1187-92.

[27] Hara, W., et al., *Cyberknife for brain metastases of malignant melanoma and renal cell carcinoma.* Neurosurgery, 2009. 64(2)(SUPPLEMENT): p. A26-A32.

[28] Herfarth, K.K., et al., *Linac-based radiosurgery of cerebral melanoma metastases.* Strahlenther Onkol, 2003. 179(6): p. 366-371.

[29] Koc, M., et al., *Gamma knife radiosurgery for intracranial metastatic melanoma: an analysis of survival and prognostic factors.* J Neurooncol, 2005. 71(3): p. 307-313.

[30] Lavine, S.D., et al., *Gamma knife radiosurgery for metastatic melanoma: an analysis of survival, outcome, and complications.* Neurosurgery, 1999. 44(1): p. 59-64.

[31] Liew, D.N., et al., *Outcome predictors of Gamma Knife surgery for melanoma brain metastases. Clinical article.* J Neurosurg, 2011. 114(3): p. 769-79.

[32] Mingione, V., et al., *Gamma surgery for melanoma metastases in the brain.* J Neurosurg, 2002. 96(3): p. 544-51.

[33] Mori, Y., et al., *Stereotactic radiosurgery for cerebral metastatic melanoma: factors affecting local disease control and survival.* Int J Radiat Oncol Biol Phys, 1998. 42(3): p. 581-589.

[34] Powell, J.W., et al., *Gamma knife surgery in the management of radioresistant brain metastases in high-risk patients with melanoma, renal cell carcinoma, and sarcoma.* J Neurosurg (Special Supplements), 2008. 109(6): p. 122-128.

[35] Radbill, A.E., et al., *Initial treatment of melanoma brain metastases using gamma knife radiosurgery: an evaluation of efficacy and toxicity.* Cancer, 2004. 101(4): p. 825-33.

[36] Redmond, A.J., et al., *Gamma knife surgery for the treatment of melanoma metastases: the effect of intratumoral hemorrhage on survival.* J Neurosurg (Special Supplements), 2008. 109(6): p. 99-105.

[37] Samlowski, W.E., et al., *Multimodality treatment of melanoma brain metastases incorporating stereotactic radiosurgery (SRS).* Cancer, 2007. 109(9): p. 1855-1862.

[38] Selek, U., et al., *Stereotactic radiosurgical treatment in 103 patients for 153 cerebral melanoma metastases.* Int J Radiat Oncol Biol Phys, 2004. 59(4): p. 1097-106.

[39] Seung, S.K., et al., *Gamma knife radiosurgery for malignant melanoma brain metastases.* Cancer J Sci Am, 1998. 4(2): p. 103-9.

[40] Somaza, S., et al., *Stereotactic radiosurgery for cerebral metastatic melanoma.* J Neurosurg, 1993. 79(5): p. 661-6.

[41] Yu, C., et al., *Metastatic melanoma to the brain: prognostic factors after gamma knife radiosurgery.* Int J Radiat Oncol Biol Phys, 2002. 52(5): p. 1277-87.

[42] Harrison, B.E., et al., *Selection of patients with melanoma brain metastases for aggressive treatment.* Am J Clin Oncol, 2003. 26(4): p. 354-7.

[43] Morris, S.L., et al., *A prognostic index that predicts outcome following palliative whole brain radiotherapy for patients with metastatic malignant melanoma.* Br J Cancer, 2004. 91(5): p. 829-33.

[44] Muacevic, A., et al., *Microsurgery plus whole brain irradiation versus gamma knife surgery alone for treatment of single metastases to the brain: a randomized controlled multicentre Phase III trial.* J Neurooncol, 2008. 87(3): p. 299-307.

[45] O'Neill, B.P., et al., *A comparison of surgical resection and stereotactic radiosurgery in the treatment of solitary brain metastases.* Int J Radiat Oncol Biol Phys, 2003. 55(5): p. 1169-1176.

[46] Bindal, A.K., et al., *Surgery versus radiosurgery in the treatment of brain metastasis.* J Neurosurg, 1996. 84(5): p. 748-754.

[47] Arriagada, R., et al., *Prophylactic cranial irradiation for patients with small-cell lung cancer in complete remission.* J Natl Cancer Inst, 1995. 87(3): p. 183-90.

[48] Gregor, A., et al., *Prophylactic cranial irradiation is indicated following complete response to induction therapy in small cell lung cancer: results of a multicentre randomised trial. United Kingdom Coordinating Committee for Cancer Research (UKCCCR) and the European Organization for Research and Treatment of Cancer (EORTC).* Eur J Cancer, 1997. 33(11): p. 1752-8.

[49] Aoyama, H., et al., *Stereotactic radiosurgery plus whole-brain radiation therapy vs. stereotactic radiosurgery alone for treatment of brain metastases: a randomized controlled trial.* JAMA, 2006. 295(21): p. 2483-91.

[50] Chang, E.L., et al., *Neurocognition in patients with brain metastases treated with radiosurgery or radiosurgery plus whole-brain irradiation: a randomised controlled trial.* Lancet Oncol, 2009. 10(11): p. 1037-44.

[51] Kocher, M., et al., *Adjuvant whole-brain radiotherapy versus observation after radiosurgery or surgical resection of one to three cerebral metastases: results of the EORTC 22952-26001 study.* J Clin Oncol, 2011. 29(2): p. 134-41.

[52] Patchell, R.A., et al., *Postoperative radiotherapy in the treatment of single metastases to the brain: a randomized trial.* JAMA, 1998. 280(17): p. 1485-9.

[53] Hagen, N.A., et al., *The role of radiation therapy following resection of single brain metastasis from melanoma.* Neurology, 1990. 40(1): p. 158-60.

[54] Skibber, J., et al., *Cranial irradiation after surgical excision of brain metastases in melanoma patients.* Ann Surg Oncol, 1996. 3(2): p. 118-123.

[55] Fogarty, G., et al., *Whole brain radiotherapy after local treatment of brain metastases in melanoma patients--a randomised phase III trial.* BMC Cancer, 2011. 11: p. 142.

[56] Chitapanarux, I., et al., *Prospective study of stereotactic radiosurgery without whole brain radiotherapy in patients with four or less brain metastases: incidence of intracranial progression and salvage radiotherapy.* J Neurooncol, 2003. 61(2): p. 143-149.

[57] Sneed, P.K., et al., *A multi-institutional review of radiosurgery alone vs. radiosurgery with whole brain radiotherapy as the initial management of brain metastases.* Int J Radiat Oncol Biol Phys, 2002. 53(3): p. 519-526.

[58] Chen, J.C., et al., *Radiosurgical salvage therapy for patients presenting with recurrence of metastatic disease to the brain.* Neurosurgery, 2000. 46(4): p. 860-6; Discussion 866-7.

[59] Spreen, O. and E. Strauss, *A compendium of neuropsychological tests: administration, norms, and commentary.* 1998, New York: Oxford University Press.

[60] DeAngelis, L.M., J.Y. Delattre, and J.B. Posner, *Radiation-induced dementia in patients cured of brain metastases.* Neurology, 1989. 39(6): p. 789-96.

[61] Tucha, O., et al., *Cognitive deficits before treatment among patients with brain tumors.* Neurosurgery, 2000. 47(2): p. 324-33; discussion 333-4.

[62] Duffner, P.K., *Long-term effects of radiation therapy on cognitive and endocrine function in children with leukemia and brain tumors.* Neurologist, 2004. 10(6): p. 293-310.

[63] Vigliani, M.-C., et al., *A prospective study of cognitive functions following conventional radiotherapy for supratentorial gliomas in young adults: 4-year results.* Int J Radiat Oncol Biol Phys, 1996. 35(3): p. 527-533.

[64] Kieffer-Renaux, V., et al., *Patterns of neuropsychological deficits in children with medulloblastoma according to craniospatial irradiation doses.* Dev Med Child Neurol, 2000. 42(11): p. 741-745.

[65] Postma, T.J., et al., *Radiotherapy-induced cerebral abnormalities in patients with low-grade glioma.* Neurology, 2002. 59(1): p. 121-123.

[66] Brown, P.D., et al., *Effects of radiotherapy on cognitive function in patients with low-grade glioma measured by the Folstein Mini-Mental State Examination.* J Clin Oncol, 2003. 21(13): p. 2519-2524.

[67] van Breemen, M.S., E.B. Wilms, and C.J. Vecht, *Epilepsy in patients with brain tumours: epidemiology, mechanisms, and management.* Lancet Neurol, 2007. 6(5): p. 421-430.

[68] Klein, M., et al., *Effect of radiotherapy and other treatment-related factors on mid-term to long-term cognitive sequelae in low-grade gliomas: a comparative study.* Lancet, 2002. 360(9343): p. 1361-1368.

[69] Surma-aho, O., et al., *Adverse long-term effects of brain radiotherapy in adult low-grade glioma patients.* Neurology, 2001. 56(10): p. 1285-1290.

[70] Imperato, J.P., N.A. Paleologos, and N.A. Vick, *Effects of treatment on long-term survivors with malignant astrocytomas.* Ann Neurol, 1990. 28(6): p. 818-822.

[71] Moretti, R., et al., *Neuropsychological evaluation of late-onset post-radiotherapy encephalopathy: a comparison with vascular dementia.* J Neurol Sci, 2005. 229-230: p. 195-200.

[72] Penitzka, S., et al., *Assessment of cognitive function after preventive and therapeutic whole brain irradiation using neuropsychological testing.* Strahlenther Onkol, 2002. 178(5): p. 252-8.

[73] Stuschke, M., et al., *Prophylactic cranial irradiation in locally advanced non-small-cell lung cancer after multimodality treatment: long-term follow-up and investigations of late neuropsychologic effects.* J Clin Oncol, 1999. 17(9): p. 2700-9.

[74] Welzel, G., et al., *Memory function before and after whole brain radiotherapy in patients with and without brain metastases.* Int J Radiat Oncol Biol Phys, 2008. 72(5): p. 1311-1318.

[75] Aoyama, H., et al., *Neurocognitive function of patients with brain metastasis who received either whole brain radiotherapy plus stereotactic radiosurgery or radiosurgery alone.* Int J Radiat Oncol Biol Phys, 2007. 68(5): p. 1388-1395.

[76] Frank, R.M. and G.J. Byrne, *The clinical utility of the Hopkins Verbal Learning Test as a screening test for mild dementia.* Int J Geriatr Psychiatry, 2000. 15(4): p. 317-324.

[77] Kuslansky, G., et al., *Detecting dementia with the Hopkins Verbal Learning Test and the Mini-Mental State Examination.* Arch Clin Neuropsychol, 2004. 19(1): p. 89-104.

[78] Hogervorst E, C.M., Lapuerta P, Rue J, Swales K, Budge M., *The Hopkins Verbal Learning Test and screening for dementia.* Dement Geriatr Cogn Disord, 2002. 13(1): p. 13-20.

[79] Lacritz, L.H. and C.M. Cullum, *The Hopkins Verbal Learning Test and CVLT: a preliminary comparison.* Arch Clin Neuropsychol, 1998. 13(7): p. 623-628.

[80] Regine, W.F., et al., *Feasibility of neurocognitive outcome evaluations in patients with brain metastases in a multi-institutional cooperative group setting: results of Radiation Therapy Oncology Group Trial BR-0018.* Int J Radiat Oncol Biol Phys, 2004. 58(5): p. 1346-1352.

[81] Herman, M.A., et al., *Neurocognitive and functional assessment of patients with brain metastases: a pilot study.* Am J Clin Oncol, 2003. 26(3): p. 273-279.

[82] Brown, P.D., et al., *Detrimental effects of tumor progression on cognitive function of patients with high-grade glioma.* J Clin Oncol, 2006. 24(34): p. 5427-33.

[83] Regine, W.F., et al., *Neurocognitive outcome in brain metastases patients treated with accelerated-fractionation vs. accelerated-hyperfractionated radiotherapy: an analysis from Radiation Therapy Oncology Group Study 91-04.* Int J Radiat Oncol Biol Phys, 2001. 51(3): p. 711-7.

[84] Murray, K.J., et al., *A randomized Phase III study of accelerated hyperfractionation vs. standard in patients with unresected brain metastases: a report of the Radiation Therapy Oncology Group (RTOG) 9104.* Int J Radiat Oncol Biol Phys, 1997. 39(3): p. 571-574.

[85] Li, J., et al., *Regression after whole-brain radiation therapy for brain metastases correlates with survival and improved neurocognitive function.* J Clin Oncol, 2007. 25(10): p. 1260-6.

[86] Carella, R.J., et al., *Value of radiation therapy in the management of patients with cerebral metastases from malignant melanoma: Radiation Therapy Oncology Group Brain Metastases Study I and II.* Cancer, 1980. 45(4): p. 679-83.

[87] Franciosi, V., et al., *Front-line chemotherapy with cisplatin and etoposide for patients with brain metastases from breast carcinoma, nonsmall cell lung carcinoma, or malignant melanoma: a prospective study.* Cancer, 1999. 85(7): p. 1599-605.

[88] Margolin, K., et al., *Temozolomide and whole brain irradiation in melanoma metastatic to the brain: a phase II trial of the Cytokine Working Group.* J Cancer Res Clin Oncol, 2002. 128(4): p. 214-8.

[89] Mornex, F., et al., *A prospective randomized multicentre phase III trial of fotemustine plus whole brain irradiation versus fotemustine alone in cerebral metastases of malignant melanoma.* Melanoma Res, 2003. 13(1): p. 97-103.

[90] Hodi, F.S., et al., *Improved survival with ipilimumab in patients with metastatic melanoma.* N Engl J Med, 2010. 363(8): p. 711-23.

[91] Robert, C., et al., *Ipilimumab plus dacarbazine for previously untreated metastatic melanoma.* N Engl J Med, 2011. 364(26): p. 2517-26.

[92] Chapman, P.B., et al., *Improved survival with vemurafenib in melanoma with BRAF V600E mutation.* N Engl J Med, 2011. 364(26): p. 2507-16.

[93] Agarwala, S.S., et al., *Temozolomide for the treatment of brain metastases associated with metastatic melanoma: a phase II study.* J Clin Oncol, 2004. 22(11): p. 2101-7.

[94] Chiarion-Sileni, V., et al., *Central nervous system failure in melanoma patients: results of a randomised, multicentre phase 3 study of temozolomide- and dacarbazine- based regimens.* Br J Cancer, 2011. 104(12): p. 1816-21.

[95] Di Giacomo, A.M., et al., *Ipilimumab and fotemustine in patients with advanced melanoma (NIBIT-M1): an open-label, single-arm phase 2 trial.* Lancet Oncol, 2012.

[96] Hwu, W.J., et al., *Temozolomide plus thalidomide in patients with brain metastases from melanoma: a phase II study.* Cancer, 2005. 103(12): p. 2590-7.

[97] Jacquillat, C., et al., *Final report of the French multicenter phase II study of the nitrosourea fotemustine in 153 evaluable patients with disseminated malignant melanoma including patients with cerebral metastases.* Cancer, 1990. 66(9): p. 1873-8.

[98] Long, G.V., et al., *Dabrafenib in patients with Val600Glu or Val600Lys BRAF-mutant melanoma metastatic to the brain (BREAK-MB): a multicentre, open-label, phase 2 trial.* Lancet Oncol, 2012. 13(11): p. 1087-95.

[99] Margolin, K., et al., *Ipilimumab in patients with melanoma and brain metastases: an open-label, phase 2 trial.* Lancet Oncol, 2012. 13(5): p. 459-65.

[100] Beretta, G., et al., *Comparative evaluation of three combination regimens for advanced malignant melanoma: results of an international cooperative study.* Cancer Treat Rep, 1976. 60(1): p. 33-40.

[101] Christodoulou, C., et al., *Temozolomide (TMZ) combined with cisplatin (CDDP) in patients with brain metastases from solid tumors: a Hellenic Cooperative Oncology Group (HeCOG) Phase II study.* J Neurooncol, 2005. 71(1): p. 61-5.

[102] Costanza, M.E., et al., *Results with methyl-CCNU and DTIC in metastatic melanoma.* Cancer, 1977. 40(3): p. 1010-5.

[103] Daponte, A., et al., *Temozolomide and cisplatin in avdanced malignant melanoma.* Anticancer Res, 2005. 25(2B): p. 1441-7.

[104] Fletcher, W.S., et al., *Evaluation of cisplatin and DTIC in inoperable stage III and IV melanoma. A Southwest Oncology Group study.* Am J Clin Oncol, 1993. 16(4): p. 359-62.

[105] Kolaric, K., et al., *Phase II clinical trial of cis dichlorodiammine platinum (Cis DDP) in metastatic brain tumors.* J Cancer Res Clin Oncol, 1982. 104(3): p. 287-93.

[106] Krown, S.E., et al., *Phase II study of temozolomide and thalidomide in patients with metastatic melanoma in the brain: high rate of thromboembolic events (CALGB 500102).* Cancer, 2006. 107(8): p. 1883-90.

[107] Larkin, J.M., et al., *A phase I/II study of lomustine and temozolomide in patients with cerebral metastases from malignant melanoma.* Br J Cancer, 2007. 96(1): p. 44-8.

[108] Madajewicz, S., et al., *Phase II study--intra-arterial BCNU therapy for metastatic brain tumors.* Cancer, 1981. 47(4): p. 653-7.

[109] Reiriz, A.B., et al., *Phase II study of thalidomide in patients with metastatic malignant melanoma.* Melanoma Res, 2004. 14(6): p. 527-31.

[110] Carlino, M.S., G.B. Fogarty, and G.V. Long, *Treatment of melanoma brain metastases: a new paradigm.* Cancer J, 2012. 18(2): p. 208-12.

[111] Agarwala, S.S. and J.M. Kirkwood, *Temozolomide, a novel alkylating agent with activity in the central nervous system, may improve the treatment of advanced metastatic melanoma.* Oncologist, 2000. 5(2): p. 144-51.

[112] Middleton, M.R., et al., *Randomized phase III study of temozolomide versus dacarbazine in the treatment of patients with advanced metastatic malignant melanoma.* J Clin Oncol, 2000. 18(1): p. 158-66.

[113] Avril, M.F., et al., *Fotemustine compared with dacarbazine in patients with disseminated malignant melanoma: a Phase III study.* J Clin Oncol, 2004. 22(6): p. 1118-25.

[114] Dhomen, N. and R. Marais, *BRAF signaling and targeted therapies in melanoma.* Hematol Oncol Clin North Am, 2009. 23(3): p. 529-45, ix.

[115] Dummer, R., et al., *An open-label pilot study of vemurafenib in previously treated metastatic melanoma patients with brain metastases.* ASCO Meeting Abstracts, 2011. 29(15_suppl): p. 8548.

[116] Laquerre, S., et al., *A selective Raf kinase inhibitor induces cell death and tumor regression of human cancer cell lines encoding B-RafV600E mutation.* Molecular Cancer Therapeutics, 2009. 8(12 Suppl; abstract B88).

[117] Falchook, G.S., et al., *Dabrafenib in patients with melanoma, untreated brain metastases, and other solid tumours: a phase 1 dose-escalation trial.* Lancet, 2012. 379(9829): p. 1893-901.

[118] Schartz, N.E., et al., *Complete regression of a previously untreated melanoma brain metastasis with ipilimumab.* Melanoma Res, 2010. 20(3): p. 247-50.

[119] Hodi, F.S., et al., *CTLA-4 blockade with ipilimumab induces significant clinical benefit in a female with melanoma metastases to the CNS.* Nat Clin Pract Oncol, 2008. 5(9): p. 557-61.

[120] Weber, J.S., et al., *Safety and clinical activity of ipilimumab in melanoma patients with brain metastases: retrospective analysis of data from a phase 2 trial.* Melanoma Res, 2011. 21(6): p. 530-4.

[121] Knisely, J.P., et al., *Radiosurgery for melanoma brain metastases in the ipilimumab era and the possibility of longer survival.* J Neurosurg, 2012. 117(2): p. 227-33.

[122] Gaspar, L., et al., *Recursive partitioning analysis (RPA) of prognostic factors in three Radiation Therapy Oncology Group (RTOG) brain metastases trials.* Int J Radiat Oncol Biol Phys, 1997. 37(4): p. 745-51.

[123] Gaspar, L.E., et al., *Validation of the RTOG recursive partitioning analysis (RPA) classification for brain metastases.* Int J Radiat Oncol Biol Phys, 2000. 47(4): p. 1001-6.

[124] Lutterbach, J., et al., *Patients with brain metastases: hope for recursive partitioning analysis (RPA) Class 3.* Radiother Oncol, 2002. 63(3): p. 339-45.

[125] Agboola, O., et al., *Prognostic factors derived from recursive partition analysis (RPA) of Radiation Therapy Oncology Group (RTOG) brain metastases trials applied to surgically resected and irradiated brain metastatic cases.* Int J Radiat Oncol Biol Phys, 1998. 42(1): p. 155-9.

[126] Tendulkar, R.D., et al., *RPA classification has prognostic significance for surgically resected single brain metastasis.* Int J Radiat Oncol Biol Phys, 2006. 66(3): p. 810-7.

[127] Sperduto, P.W., et al., *Diagnosis-specific prognostic factors, indexes, and treatment outcomes for patients with newly diagnosed brain metastases: a multi-institutional analysis of 4,259 patients.* Int J Radiat Oncol Biol Phys, 2010. 77(3): p. 655-61.

[128] Lorenzoni, J., et al., *Radiosurgery for treatment of brain metastases: estimation of patient eligibility using three stratification systems.* Int J Radiat Oncol Biol Phys, 2004. 60(1): p. 218-224.

[129] Weltman, E., et al., *Radiosurgery for brain metastases: a score index for predicting prognosis.* Int J Radiat Oncol Biol Phys, 2000. 46(5): p. 1155-61.

[130] Broadbent, A.M., et al., *Survival following whole brain radiation treatment for cerebral metastases: an audit of 474 patients.* Radiother Oncol, 2004. 71(3): p. 259-65.

[131] Stone, A., et al., *A comparison of survival rates for treatment of melanoma metastatic to the brain.* Cancer Invest, 2004. 22(4): p. 492-7.

[132] Ellerhorst, J., et al., *Whole brain irradiation for patients with metastatic melanoma: a review of 87 cases.* Int J Radiat Oncol Biol Phys, 2001. 49(1): p. 93-7.

[133] Barker II, F.G., *Surgical and radiosurgical management of brain metastases.* Surg Clin North Am, 2005. 85(2): p. 329-45.

[134] Regine, W.F., et al., *Risk of symptomatic brain tumor recurrence and neurologic deficit after radiosurgery alone in patients with newly diagnosed brain metastases: results and implications.* Int J Radiat Oncol Biol Phys, 2002. 52(2): p. 333-8.

[135] Chiarion-Sileni, V., et al., *Temozolomide (TMZ) as prophylaxis for melanoma brain metastases (BrM): Results from a Phase III, multicenter study.* J Clin Oncol (Meeting Abstracts), 2008. 26(15_suppl): p. 20014.

[136] Samlowski, W.E., *Multimodality treatment of patients with metastatic melanoma with brain metastases,* in *American Society of Clinical Oncology Educational Book: 43rd Annual Meeting,* R. Govindan, Editor. 2007, American Society of Clinical Oncology: Alexandria, VA. p. 519-522.

[137] Gruss, C., et al., *Severe neurological disabilities after complete remission of advanced malignant melanoma following fotemustine therapy in combination with total brain irradiation.* Melanoma Res, 2002. 12(4): p. 403-4.

[138] Khalil, Z., et al., *Neurological toxicity during metastatic melanoma treatment with fotemustine.* Melanoma Res, 2005. 15(6): p. 563-4.

[139] Douglas, J. and V. Sondak, *RE: A comparison of survival rates for treatment of melanoma metastatic to the brain,* in *Cancer Invest.* 2004. p. 643-644.

Chapter 2

Management of In-Transit Malignant Melanoma

Paul J. Speicher, Douglas S. Tyler and Paul J. Mosca

Additional information is available at the end of the chapter

1. Introduction

In-transit melanoma is a unique pattern of recurrence that occurs in up to ten percent of patients with melanoma. In-transit disease denotes multifocal tumor deposits occurring between the site of the primary lesion and its regional draining lymph node basin [1, 2]. It is an independent adverse prognostic factor and is frequently associated with distant metastasis. This pattern of recurrence represents a challenging management problem, but provides unique treatment modalities as well. In addition, studying in-transit melanoma has the potential to shed additional light on melanoma biology. The goal of this chapter is to discuss the presentation, underlying disease biology, and various current treatment strategies for this unique pattern of recurrence in melanoma.

2. Background

2.1. Nomenclature and staging

The nomenclature used for in-transit melanoma can be confusing, in part because a number of different terms have traditionally been used in the literature to describe what is most likely the same oncologic process. Historically, terms such as locoregional recurrence, satellitosis, and in-transit disease have all been used with varying definitions and intentions. Historically, satellitosis has been defined as locoregional recurrence, not lying within the regional nodal basin, that is located within either 5cm of the initial lesion or 2cm of the excision scar, whereas the term in-transit disease has been defined as such a recurrence occurring at greater distances from the initial lesion or scar, respectively. In either case, such lesions likely represent tumor deposits growing along routes of lymphatic drainage. More recently, it has become apparent that for locoregional recurrence, distance from the primary lesion to the site of recurrence does not carry significant prognostic value [3-6]. Accordingly, the most recent AJCC staging system for melanoma does not differentiate between in-transit lesions and satellitosis in the assignment of stage, both being designated as N2 or N3 disease, depending on regional node status [7]. Thus, in an effort to address the ambiguity arising from nomenclature, many authors have advocated for eliminating the term satellitosis, instead referring to all regional non-nodal metastatic disease as in-transit disease.

Stage	T	N	M
IIIA	Any depth, *Without* ulceration	1-3 nodes (not clinically detectable)	No distant disease
IIIB	Any depth, *With* ulceration	1-3 nodes (not clinically detectable)	No distant disease
	Any depth, *Without* ulceration	1-3 nodes (clinically detectable), *OR* in-transit lesions	No distant disease
IIIC	Any depth, *With* ulceration	1-3 nodes (clinically detectable), *OR* in-transit lesions, *OR* any combination of positive nodes and in-transit disease, *OR* greater than 4 positive nodes	No distant disease

Table 1. Breakdown of AJCC staging for stage III melanoma [7].

An additional and equally important point of clarification is the distinction between actual local recurrence and in-transit disease. True local recurrence is defined as a primary tumor that recurs as a result of incomplete primary excision, and is confined to or contiguous with an excision scar and bearing an in situ component [8]. As this carries a much better prognosis, it must be distinguished from potentially similar appearing in-transit disease found in close proximity to a prior excisional scar.

2.2. Presentation

By definition, in-transit melanoma represents advanced stage disease, and such recurrences are typically discovered months after the initial management of a primary lesion. In most series, this disease-free interval to recurrence as in-transit disease ranges from 12-16 months [9, 10]. The clinical presentation can be quite variable, but usually involves anywhere from one to upwards of one-hundred small cutaneous or subcutaneous nodules. The lesions themselves can differ significantly in size, ranging from sub-millimeter diameter to well over one centimeter. They may take the form of superficial cutaneous (also called epidermotropic) or deeper subcutaneous tumors. For extremity-based disease, the lesions may be clustered near the primary lesion, or may involve the entire extremity extending between the primary tumor and its lymphatic drainage basin. For non-extremity disease, the distribution can be even more variable, with widespread tumor burden on the head, neck or trunk, depending on the location of the primary melanoma.

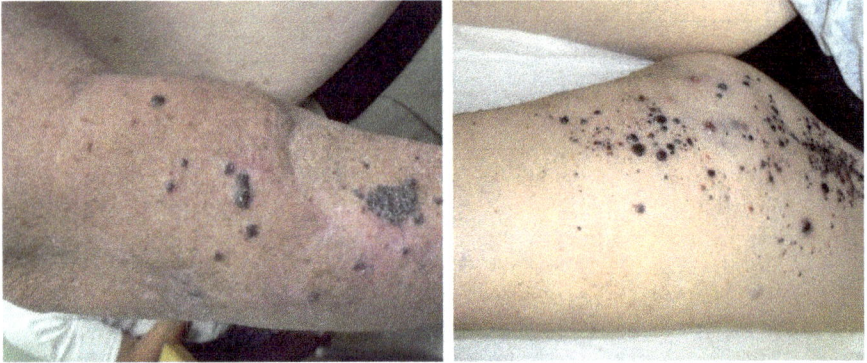

Figure 1. Examples of in-transit melanoma of the arm (left) and leg (right). Note the distribution and extent of disease, making these presentations very poor candidates for surgical excision. On the left, there is evidence of in-transit metastases both within the area of previous skin flap, as well as extending more proximally along its course of lymphatic drainage. On the right, there is extensive disease extending up to the inguinal crease.

2.3. Incidence

In-transit melanoma is a relatively uncommon phenomenon, with fewer than 10% of melanomas recurring as in-transit disease [1, 11]. This accounts for approximately 12-22% of all recurrences, although this number is difficult to determine with accuracy due to ambiguity regarding terminology used to describe local recurrence versus regional in-transit disease [12-14]. Stage of disease appears to be the most important factor that predicts the development of in-transit metastasis. The presence of associated nodal disease significantly increases risk of in-transit recurrence, with one study reporting incidence as high as 31% when three or more positive nodes were present [12]. Location itself also appears to be a factor, with a higher incidence of in-transit disease in the lower extremities compared to the upper extremities [15]. Of note, some earlier authors observed that surgical lymph node dissection may lead to increased risk of recurrence as in-transit disease, an area of some debate. This is postulated to be a result of lymphatic trapping, whereby dissection of the draining lymph node basin removes the potential outflow of lymphatic tumor deposits, possibly leading to increased likelihood of in-transit disease. In larger, more recent studies, however, neither sentinel lymph node biopsy nor lymphadenectomy were found to have any effect on the incidence of in-transit metastases [16-19].

2.4. Outcomes

The presence of in-transit metastases indicates either N2 or N3 status under the current AJCC TNM system, and is classified as stage IIIB or C disease, respectively. In-transit melanoma carries a poor prognosis, with 5-year survival rates ranging from 25% to 30% in most reports [12, 20, 21]. Additionally, the presence or absence of regional lymph node disease is of significant prognostic value; the combination of nodal metastasis and in-transit melanoma comprise stage IIIC disease, which is associated with a poorer outcome than stage IIIB (40% vs. 59% five-year survival, respectively) [7]. There is a high incidence of occult distant metastasis in the presence of in-transit melanoma, but this is not universally the case. Studies examining the outcomes of major amputation for the treatment of this pattern of recurrence have identified a number of patients who experience a complete and durable response and have demonstrated five-year survival rates ranging from 21-32% [22-26]. This indicates that a significant minority of patients with in-transit metastases have disease that is truly limited to the extremity at the time of detection. Nonetheless, it is essential that distant metastases be ruled out when staging patients with in-transit melanoma, since treatment options and prognosis may differ substantially when measurable distant disease is present.

3. Biology of in-transit disease

The underlying biology of in-transit melanoma is believed to be related to lymphatic dissemination of small tumor emboli along the lymphatic drainage from the primary tumor. It is generally accepted that these migrating tumor cells become trapped in the dermal and subdermal lymphatics, typically, though not always, somewhere between the primary lesion and the draining regional lymph nodes. These cells are thought to remain static along this route, eventually progressing to a clinically detectable lesion. Consistent with this theory, in-transit melanoma is often described as an ongoing process, with increasing disease burden over time. Although the lymphatic route is the most likely biological explanation, some authors have suggested other mechanisms. One alternate explanation describes in-transit disease as a manifestation of systemic disease resulting from hematogenous spread, similar to distant metastases [27, 28]. Proponents of this argue that in the lymphatic theory, wider margins of primary excision would be expected to include more static occult cells, with subsequent improved clinical outcomes, yet this has not been shown to be the case. It is difficult to reconcile this theory, however, with the significant differences in survival observed in stage III versus stage IV melanoma.

4. Therapy for in-transit disease

Treatment of locoregionally recurrent melanoma depends on a number of important factors, including tumor size, multiplicity, and anatomic location. Although in-transit melanoma is often followed by metastatic disease, it is important that the surgeon choose an appropriate therapy based on clinical presentation, history, technical experience, and patient preference.

4.1. Local management

Distinguishing in-transit disease from true local recurrence is of great importance, as the management and prognosis differ substantially. Local recurrence, or tumor confined to or contiguous with an excision scar and bearing an in situ component, should be managed similarly to the primary lesion with wide local excision. For in-transit disease, however, it is generally accepted that the wide local excision margin guidelines applicable to primary melanomas need not be applied. In-transit metastases are generally very clearly demarcated histologically from surrounding tissue, and complete macroscopic excision with negative surgical margins is usually all that is required.

In addition to wide local excision, there has been significant interest in other forms of local therapy for melanoma lesions, including laser ablation, external beam radiation, and intralesional injections. Irrespective of modality, these should all be thought of as equivalents to local surgical excision regarding indications and prognosis.

Laser therapy was first described in 1973, and has gained favor in the local treatment of in-transit disease that is not amenable to surgical excision, such as when the disease is too extensive [29]. It is most useful in patients with a large number of small in-transit lesions, but its advantages and utility decrease as lesions increase in size [30]. For tumors smaller than approximately 3mm, the entire lesion can be ablated using a carbon dioxide laser, though larger lesions must be circumscribed using the laser and subsequently excised with forceps.

Intralesional injections have also been used in the treatment of in-transit melanoma with some success. The most commonly used therapies include bacillus Calmette-Guérin (BCG), dinitrochlorobenzene (DNCB), and interferon-alpha (INF-α), and IL-2. Small studies have demonstrated complete response rates of 31-63% (overall response 45-91%), although long-term survival, when reported, remained unfortunately low [31-33]. This suggests that if surgical excision is not a viable option, intralesional injection is a reasonable alternative. More recently, electrochemotherapy (ECT) has gained popularity as local alternative to radiotherapy and laser ablation. This technique relies on using high intensity electric pulses to allow intracellular delivery of cytotoxic drugs, such as cisplatin and bleomycin, via intralesional injection [34]. Complete response rates have been reported as 53-89% (overall response 84-99%), with minimal systemic toxicity [35-37]. Unfortunately, regardless of which method is employed, local management of in-transit melanoma remains suboptimal in many situations.

4.2. Radiation therapy

Early in-vitro and clinical studies suggested that melanoma tumors exhibited significant intrinsic resistance to ionizing radiation, and as such, radiotherapy has not traditionally been considered to have a major role in the treatment of in-transit melanoma [38, 39]. More recent studies, however, have suggested radiotherapy may be of value in certain subsets of individuals, particularly those with one or few metastatic lesions that are not amenable to surgical excision [40]. As a primary treatment, radiotherapy is largely reserved for palliation of patients with incurable symptomatic lesions, particularly in cases that are not amenable to surgical excision. Generally speaking, when unresectable in-transit melanoma is amenable to regional chemotherapy, this should be considered prior to employing radiotherapy.

While some studies have demonstrated potential benefit of adjuvant radiation therapy in patients with nodal melanoma metastases, there are very little data regarding the use of adjuvant radiation therapy in the setting of in-transit disease [41, 42]. Treatment depends on area and location of involvement. While not routine practice, adjuvant radiotherapy should be considered in patients with head and neck disease, and in those with positive margins that are not amenable to re-excision [43-45].

4.3. Regional therapy

Given the high rate of local treatment failure and frequently increased burden of in-transit disease, regionally focused modalities offer potential strategies to obtain more durable treatment responses. Regional chemotherapy is a promising therapeutic option for suitable patients with extremity in-transit melanoma and is currently the focus of exciting research. This modality involves vascular isolation of the affected area, after which chemotherapy is then delivered at doses 10-20 times higher than doses that can be achieved and tolerated systemically, with dosing based on affected limb volume. As regional therapy requires complete vascular isolation of the affected body area, obvious anatomic limitations are involved. The inflow and outflow vessels to the area of interest must be selectively cannulated, and the treatment region must then be isolated from the systemic circulation, usually by means of a tourniquet.

There remains significant debate as to whether regional chemotherapy produces an overall survival benefit over other therapeutic modalities, but studies have demonstrated a survival benefit in patients who exhibited a clinical response [46-48]. Originally described in the 1950s, two primary forms of regional chemotherapy have evolved: hyperthermic isolated limb perfusion (HILP) and isolated limb infusion (ILI).

	HILP	ILI
Drug delivery	Cardiopulmonary bypass	Manual pump with three-way stopcock
Circuit pressure	High; with significant risk for systemic leak	Low; significantly reduced risk of systemic leak
Vessel access	Open surgical exposure; large diameter cannulas	Percutaneous access under fluoroscopic guidance, smaller diameter cannulas
Limb pH	Physiologic	Acidotic
Limb oxygenation	Active membrane oxygenation	No external oxygenation; profound hypoxia
Temperature	39-40°C	37.8-38.5°C
Duration of treatment	60 minutes	30 minutes
Technical demand	Technically complex, difficult re-operation	Technically simpler, re-do operation without difficulty

Table 2. Comparison of technique and parameters between hyperthermic isolated limb perfusion (HILP) and isolated limb infusion (ILI).

4.4. Regional chemotherapy agents

Melphalan is typically the drug of choice for regional chemotherapy. It is an alkylating agent derived from phenylalanine, an amino acid preferentially taken up by melanocytes due to its key role in melanin synthesis. Theoretically, melphalan should produce selective toxicity in melanocytes and melanin-containing melanoma cells. As a systemic agent, however, melphalan is ineffective despite its theoretical benefits, as its allowable dose is significantly less than its effective dose. For regional therapy, in contrast, this much higher effective dose is achieved without systemic toxicity.

Other agents have been employed either alone or in combination with melphalan in the treatment of in-transit melanoma. An essential quality of any agent considered for regional therapy is the constraint that it must not require metabolic transformation to take on a biologically active form. Cisplatin is another alkylating agent that held significant promise in preclinical studies of regional chemotherapy. Early clinical reports were favorable regarding response rates, but were plagued by concerns over toxicity [49-51]. Subsequent studies confirmed significant limb-threatening toxicity with the use of cisplatin, and as such most authors recommend against its routine use in regional therapy [52, 53]. Similarly, TNFα has exhibited some potential, particularly when combined with interferon-gamma, but widespread use of TNFα-based regimens have been tempered by significant concerns regarding toxicity [54]. The 2006 ACOSOG Z0020 trial comparing melphalan with melphalan plus TNFα was terminated early after interim analysis demonstrated a significant increase in toxicity with the addition of TNFα and yet a similar clinical response rate compared to melphalan alone [55]. Temozolomide is a newer alkylating agent that could have potential application in regional chemotherapy, as it also does not require hepatic conversion to become active. Early results in animal models reported superior tumor growth delay compared to regional melphalan, and a phase 1 clinical trial is currently underway, enrolling patients at Duke University Medical Center [56].

4.5. Isolated limb perfusion

Isolated limb perfusion (ILP) was first described in Creech and colleagues in 1958, basing their technique on advances in cardiopulmonary bypass developed for cardiac surgery in the 1950s [57]. They utilized an extracorporeal oxygenator as part of the isolated limb circuit to deliver high dose chemotherapy while maintaining normal oxygen tension and pH of the treated limb. Ten years later, Stehlin and coworkers added the effects of hyperthermia to the treatment protocol, now called hyperthermic isolated limb perfusion (HILP), enhancing the cytotoxicity of the chemotherapy and increasing efficacy [58]. The technical aspects of HILP vary somewhat among surgeons and institutions, but the basic technique is similar.

The procedure is performed under general anesthesia, and the vasculature supplying the affected limb is exposed and cannulated. During this exposure, one typically performs a regional lymphadenectomy, which aids vascular exposure (particularly in the case of the iliac vessels) and is often indicated from an oncologic standpoint. The target limb is isolated from the systemic circulation using a proximal tourniquet. Perfusion is then initiated via the cannulated vessels, utilizing a membrane oxygenator and cardiopulmonary bypass apparatus to maintain limb oxygen tension and pH at physiologic levels. The perfusion treatment is generally continued for 60 to 90 minutes, depending on the protocol. External warming blankets and heated melphalan perfusate are used to achieve hyperthermia. During HILP, it is important to monitor for leakage of the perfusate into the systemic circulation, particularly when high dose TNF-alpha is employed, as systemic leakage can lead to significant morbidity or mortality. Traditionally this monitoring was performed using intravenous fluorescein and watching for staining proximal to the tourniquet. A more precise method involves the administration of radiolabeled tracer into the HILP circuit, followed by continuously monitored systemic radiation exposure using a gamma probe placed over the chest. After completion of chemotherapy perfusion, a 30-minute washout period with crystalloids follows to remove the active agents.

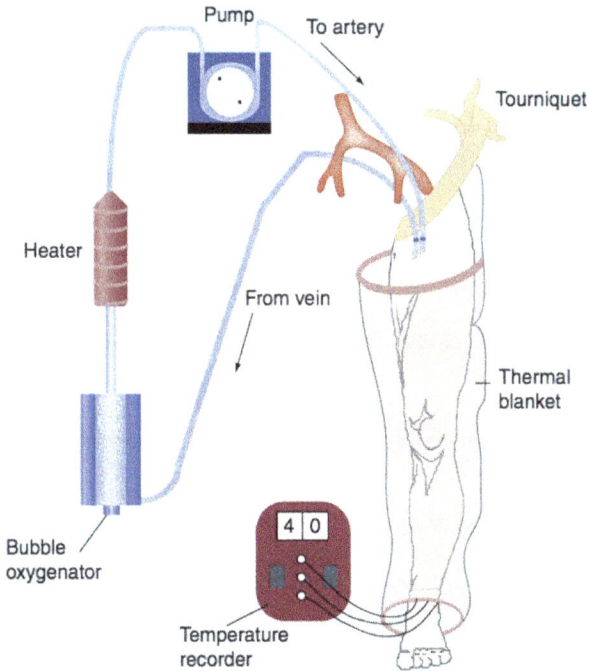

Expert Rev. Anticancer Ther. © Future Science Group (2009)

Figure 2. Hyperthermic isolated limb perfusion. Surgical exposure of the proximal vasculature is followed by cannulation and circulation of chemotherapy perfusate. Acid-base status and oxygenation is maintained throughout the procedure. Reproduced with permission.

Results of HILP vary widely, perhaps depending on the patient population and adjunctive agents employed. In single-center studies, overall response rates of 81-100% and complete response rates of 39-82% [46, 48, 59-62] have been reported. However, the previously mentioned multi-center ACOSOG Z0020 study demonstrated complete response rates of only 25%, significantly lower than what had been previously reported [55]. Overall, recurrence rates are 50-60% within one year, and overall 5-year survival rates remain in the 30-40% range [63]. As such, while HILP may be the best treatment option for suitable patients with in-transit extremity melanoma, there remains significant room for therapeutic improvement.

Study (year) [ref]	Patients (n)	CR (%)	PR (%)	OR (%)
Minor (1985) [60]	18	82	18	100
Storm (1985) [62]	26	50	31	81
Di Filippo (1989) [59]	69	39	43	82
Cornett (2006) [55]	58	25	39	64
Sanki (2007) [48]	120	69	15	84
Raymond (2011) [61]	62	55	26	81

Table 3. Response rates following HILP in patients with in-transit melanoma. Adapted with permission from Coleman et al., Expert Rev. Anticancer Ther. 2009;9(11):1599-1602. CR: Complete response; PR: Partial response; OR: Overall response.

4.6. Isolated limb infusion

Isolated limb infusion (ILI) was developed by Thompson and coworkers at the Sydney Melanoma Unit as a less invasive alternative to HILP. This technique employs percutaneous catheters inserted under fluoroscopic guidance as a means to cannulate the target limb vessels. An external tourniquet is used to isolate the limb, which is then wrapped in heating blankets. The key difference with ILI as compared to HILP is the lack of a perfusion pump and membrane oxygenator. The melphalan solution is instead manually circulated via the arterial catheter using a syringe and three-way stopcock. Consequently, during ILI the limb is not maintained at normal pH and oxygen tension, and becomes markedly hypoxic and acidotic during the course of the procedure. Some authors propose that the acidosis and hypoxia may serve to augment melphalan action [64]. In addition, while external and internal warming are performed in ILI, limb temperatures achieved with ILI are lower than those in HILP and generally do not exceed 38.5 degrees centigrade [65, 66].

From a technical standpoint, ILI is appreciably simpler and easier to perform and learn. The infusion treatment is continued for about 30 minutes, followed by a similar washout period with crystalloid. Lower doses of melphalan are typically used, often in combination with dactinomycin, and regional morbidity is reduced, particularly with respect to incidence of severe toxicity. In light of these factors, ILI is generally well tolerated, and is often offered to frail patients with multiple comorbidities who would not tolerate the longer and more invasive groin exposure required for HILP. Along similar lines, due to its simplicity and lower morbidity, ILI can be safely offered as a repeat procedure. Although theoretically attractive as a means of obtaining fractionated regional chemotherapy, elective repeat ILI has not been shown to improve survival compared to single ILI [67]. However, repeat ILI can be very valuable in the management of recurrent or progressive in-transit disease after primary regional therapy.

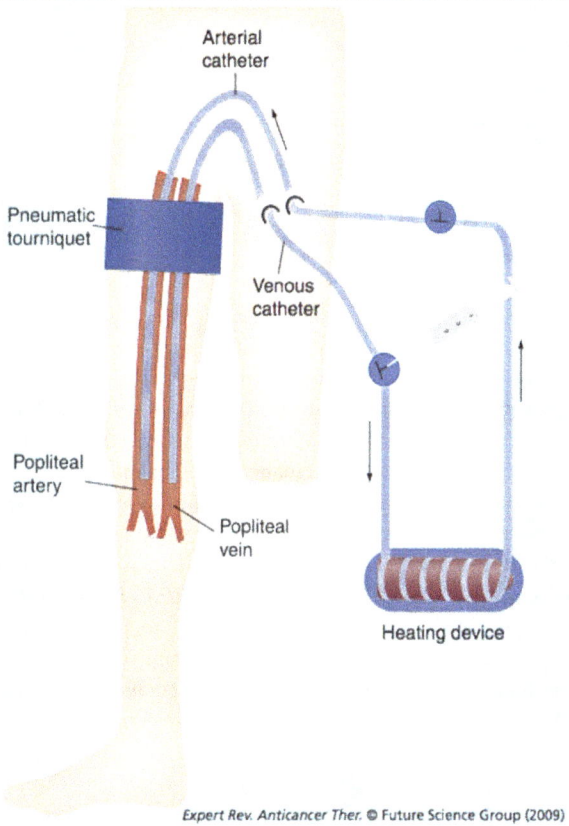

Expert Rev. Anticancer Ther. © Future Science Group (2009)

Figure 3. Isolated limb infusion. Catheters are placed percutaneously, and chemotherapy is circulated by hand without active oxygenation, leading to profound hypoxia and acidosis.

Outcomes after ILI are generally inferior to HILP, with complete response ranging from 23-44% and overall response ranging from 43-100% [47, 61, 65, 66, 68-70]. In one of the largest studies explicitly comparing patterns of recurrence, ILI was found to have both significantly higher probability of recurrence (85% vs. 65%) and shorter time to first recurrence (8 months vs. 23 months) as compared to HILP [71]. Notably, there was no statistically significant difference in overall survival between the two groups, although there was a trend in favor of HILP.

Study (year) [ref]	Patients (n)	CR (%)	PR (%)	OR (%)
Mian (2001) [70]	9	44	56	100
Lindner (2002) [66]	128	41	44	85
Brady (2006) [69]	22	23	27	50
Kroon (2008) [47]	185	38	46	84
Beasley (2009) [68]	128	31	33	64
Raymond (2011) [61]	126	30	13	43

Table 4. Response rates following ILI in patients with in-transit melanoma. Adapted with permission from Coleman et al., Expert Rev. Anticancer Ther. 2009;9(11):1599-1602. CR: Complete response; PR: Partial response; OR: Overall response.

4.7. Post-treatment complications

As a result of the high concentration of chemotherapies administered in regional therapy, some degree of tissue toxicity is often seen. Multiple grading systems have been developed to score regional toxicity after treatment, with one of the most prominent being that developed by Wieberdink and colleagues. In this system scores range from Grade I, or no evidence of significant reaction, to Grade V, representing reaction severe enough to warrant possible amputation [72]. Up to 85% of patients will exhibit Grade I or II level of toxicity, but as a result of careful drug dosing based on limb volume rather than total body weight, fortunately overall less than 1% of patients develop Grade V toxicity [73]. While the spectrum of toxicity is similar between patients undergoing ILI and HILP, the risk of significant toxicity is greater among those undergoing HILP. Furthermore, HILP carries a higher risk of limb loss from amputation as compared to ILI. Regardless of modality, most adverse reactions are transient, with almost all patients demonstrating some skin erythema and edema that peaks in the first month post-operatively. Rare but more serious complications include severe muscle toxicity and the development of compartment syndrome, necessitating fasciotomy.

4.8. Amputation

Amputation is almost never indicated in the standard treatment of in-transit melanoma. As mentioned previously, historical treatment of in-transit disease by means of limb amputation has led to long-term survival rates of 20-30 percent, which would suggest that a significant minority of patients with locoregional disease have recurrence that is in fact confined entirely to the affected extremity. Recent advancements in aggressive local management, regional therapy and systemic treatment have rendered extremity amputation obsolete except for the most intractable disease, particularly in light of comparable five-year survival rates among patients undergoing these therapies. Thus, amputation should generally only be offered with palliative intent or in patients who refuse or are not candidates for regional chemotherapy or other less morbid therapies [22, 26].

4.9. Systemic treatment

While a comprehensive discussion regarding systemic therapy for the treatment of melanoma is beyond the scope of this chapter, when appropriate this modality should be considered in the management of in-transit disease. Systemic therapy is typically applied in cases of in-transit disease in the presence of distant metastases – that is, stage IV disease [74]. Similarly, patients with non-extremity in-transit metastases – such as in-transit disease involving the head and neck, truncal or genitalia – present a difficult management problem and are often palliated best with systemic treatment options. Systemic therapy should also be considered for in-transit metastases in patients with recurrent or progressive disease who are not candidates for repeat local or regional therapy. Unfortunately, systemic therapy for the treatment of patients with advanced melanoma has historically been quite poor. A large meta-analysis of 42 trials of systemic treatments demonstrating a median progression free survival of 1.7 months with only 14.5% of patients being progression-free at 6 months [75]. Despite this poor track record, newer approaches to systemic treatment of regional disease may hold promise, including vascular regulating agents, signal targeting therapies and immune modulation therapy.

Current strategies have focused on attempting to increase tumor sensitivity to chemotherapeutics, improve local drug delivery, or target apoptotic pathways in an attempt to augment response to regional therapy. The BRAF enzyme inhibitor vemurafenib, as well as the immune modulating anti-CTLA-4 antibody ipilimumab, have recently shown promise in phase III trials, although neither is likely to provide durable disease-free survival [76, 77]. Another newer agent is bevacizumab, a monoclonal antibody to vascular endothelial growth factor (VEGF), which is believed to normalize immature and shunt-dominated tumor vasculature, leading to improved delivery of chemotherapeutics to tumor cells. A recent preclinical animal study demonstrated that systemic treatment with bevacizumab prior to regional therapy increased delivery of melphalan to the tumors of interest [78]. Another vascular targeting agent of recent interest is ADH-1, a pentapeptide that targets and disrupts N-cadherin adhesion complexes, which are predominantly expressed by melanocytes after malignant transition into melanoma [79, 80]. ADH-1 is believed to increase blood vessel permeability, increasing chemotherapy drug delivery [81]. A recent phase II clinical trial studying pre-treatment systemic ADH-1 administration prior to ILI with melphalan demonstrated a reassuring complete response rate of 38% and an overall response rate of 60%, although no significant progression free survival was appreciated [82]. The role of all of these agents as systemic adjuncts to regional chemotherapy remains to be seen, and is being defined in ongoing trials.

5. Conclusions

In-transit melanoma is a distinctive form of tumor recurrence, and is an indicator of late-stage disease. It is very distressing to patients, often requiring multiple treatments, procedures and hospitalizations. As such, management of this disease can be challenging and frustrating to clinicians as well. Similar to systemic melanoma, in-transit disease is notoriously resistant to chemotherapy, and treatment outcomes remain unsatisfactorily poor. Local therapies often tout impressive initial response rates, but are plagued by recurrence. Over the past half-century, advances have been made in regional approaches to chemotherapy, including isolated limb perfusion and isolated limb infusion. While some of these methods have demonstrated limited success, significant improvements in patient outcomes will require further advances in both regional and systemic treatment of melanoma.

Author details

Paul J. Speicher, Douglas S. Tyler and Paul J. Mosca

Division of Surgical Oncology, Department of Surgery, Duke University Medical Center, Durham, USA

References

[1]   Pawlik TM, Ross MI, Johnson MM, Schacherer CW, McClain DM, Mansfield PF, et al. Predictors and natural history of in-transit melanoma after sentinel lymphadenectomy. Annals of surgical oncology. 2005;12(8):587-96. Epub 2005/07/16.

[2]   Meier F, Will S, Ellwanger U, Schlagenhauff B, Schittek B, Rassner G, et al. Metastatic pathways and time courses in the orderly progression of cutaneous melanoma. The British journal of dermatology. 2002;147(1):62-70. Epub 2002/07/09.

[3]   Singletary SE, Tucker SL, Boddie AW, Jr. Multivariate analysis of prognostic factors in regional cutaneous metastases of extremity melanoma. Cancer. 1988;61(7):1437-40. Epub 1988/04/01.

[4]   Karakousis CP, Temple DF, Moore R, Ambrus JL. Prognostic parameters in recurrent malignant melanoma. Cancer. 1983;52(3):575-9. Epub 1983/08/01.

[5]   Roses DF, Karp NS, Oratz R, Dubin N, Harris MN, Speyer J, et al. Survival with regional and distant metastases from cutaneous malignant melanoma. Surgery, gynecology & obstetrics. 1991;172(4):262-8. Epub 1991/04/01.

[6]   Haffner AC, Garbe C, Burg G, Buttner P, Orfanos CE, Rassner G. The prognosis of primary and metastasising melanoma. An evaluation of the TNM classification in 2,495 patients. British journal of cancer. 1992;66(5):856-61. Epub 1992/11/01.

[7]   Balch CM, Gershenwald JE, Soong SJ, Thompson JF, Atkins MB, Byrd DR, et al. Final version of 2009 AJCC melanoma staging and classification. Journal of clinical oncolo-

gy : official journal of the American Society of Clinical Oncology. 2009;27(36): 6199-206. Epub 2009/11/18.

 [8] Brown CD, Zitelli JA. The prognosis and treatment of true local cutaneous recurrent malignant melanoma. Dermatologic surgery : official publication for American Society for Dermatologic Surgery [et al]. 1995;21(4):285-90. Epub 1995/04/01.

 [9] Lee YT. Loco-regional recurrent melanoma: I natural history. Cancer treatment reviews. 1980;7(2):59-72. Epub 1980/06/01.

[10] Wong JH, Cagle LA, Kopald KH, Swisher SG, Morton DL. Natural history and selective management of in transit melanoma. Journal of surgical oncology. 1990;44(3): 146-50. Epub 1990/07/01.

[11] Roses DF, Harris MN, Rigel D, Carrey Z, Friedman R, Kopf AW. Local and in-transit metastases following definitive excision for primary cutaneous malignant melanoma. Annals of surgery. 1983;198(1):65-9. Epub 1983/07/01.

[12] Cascinelli N, Bufalino R, Marolda R, Belli F, Nava M, Galluzzo D, et al. Regional non-nodal metastases of cutaneous melanoma. European journal of surgical oncology : the journal of the European Society of Surgical Oncology and the British Association of Surgical Oncology. 1986;12(2):175-80. Epub 1986/06/01.

[13] McCarthy WH, Shaw HM, Thompson JF, Milton GW. Time and frequency of recurrence of cutaneous stage I malignant melanoma with guidelines for follow-up study. Surgery, gynecology & obstetrics. 1988;166(6):497-502. Epub 1988/06/01.

[14] Soong SJ, Harrison RA, McCarthy WH, Urist MM, Balch CM. Factors affecting survival following local, regional, or distant recurrence from localized melanoma. Journal of surgical oncology. 1998;67(4):228-33. Epub 1998/05/14.

[15] Karakousis CP, Balch CM, Urist MM, Ross MM, Smith TJ, Bartolucci AA. Local recurrence in malignant melanoma: long-term results of the multiinstitutional randomized surgical trial. Annals of surgical oncology. 1996;3(5):446-52. Epub 1996/09/01.

[16] Kang JC, Wanek LA, Essner R, Faries MB, Foshag LJ, Morton DL. Sentinel lymphadenectomy does not increase the incidence of in-transit metastases in primary melanoma. Journal of clinical oncology : official journal of the American Society of Clinical Oncology. 2005;23(21):4764-70. Epub 2005/07/22.

[17] Morton DL, Thompson JF, Cochran AJ, Mozzillo N, Elashoff R, Essner R, et al. Sentinel-node biopsy or nodal observation in melanoma. The New England journal of medicine. 2006;355(13):1307-17. Epub 2006/09/29.

[18] Pawlik TM, Ross MI, Thompson JF, Eggermont AM, Gershenwald JE. The risk of in-transit melanoma metastasis depends on tumor biology and not the surgical approach to regional lymph nodes. Journal of clinical oncology : official journal of the American Society of Clinical Oncology. 2005;23(21):4588-90. Epub 2005/07/22.

[19] van Poll D, Thompson JF, Colman MH, McKinnon JG, Saw RP, Stretch JR, et al. A sentinel node biopsy does not increase the incidence of in-transit metastasis in pa-

tients with primary cutaneous melanoma. Annals of surgical oncology. 2005;12(8): 597-608. Epub 2005/07/16.

[20] Calabro A, Singletary SE, Balch CM. Patterns of relapse in 1001 consecutive patients with melanoma nodal metastases. Archives of surgery (Chicago, Ill : 1960). 1989;124(9):1051-5. Epub 1989/09/01.

[21] Zogakis TG, Bartlett DL, Libutti SK, Liewehr DJ, Steinberg SM, Fraker DL, et al. Factors affecting survival after complete response to isolated limb perfusion in patients with in-transit melanoma. Annals of surgical oncology. 2001;8(10):771-8. Epub 2002/01/05.

[22] Jaques DP, Coit DG, Brennan MF. Major amputation for advanced malignant melanoma. Surgery, gynecology & obstetrics. 1989;169(1):1-6. Epub 1989/07/01.

[23] Karakousis CP, Choe KJ, Holyoke ED. Biologic behavior and treatment of intransit metastasis of melanoma. Surgery, gynecology & obstetrics. 1980;150(1):29-32. Epub 1980/01/01.

[24] McPeak CJ, McNeer GP, Whiteley HW, Booher RJ. Amputation for Melanoma of the Extremity. Surgery. 1963;54:426-31. Epub 1963/09/01.

[25] Pack GT, Gerber DM, Scharnagel IM. End results in the treatment of malignant melanoma; a report of 1190 cases. Annals of surgery. 1952;136(6):905-11. Epub 1952/12/01.

[26] Turnbull A, Shah J, Fortner J. Recurrent melanoma of an extremity treated by major amputation. Archives of surgery (Chicago, Ill : 1960). 1973;106(4):496-8. Epub 1973/04/01.

[27] Griffiths RW, Briggs JC. Incidence of locally metastatic ('recurrent') cutaneous malignant melanoma following conventional wide margin excisional surgery for invasive clinical stage I tumours: importance of maximal primary tumour thickness. The British journal of surgery. 1986;73(5):349-53. Epub 1986/05/01.

[28] Heenan PJ, Ghaznawie M. The pathogenesis of local recurrence of melanoma at the primary excision site. British journal of plastic surgery. 1999;52(3):209-13. Epub 1999/09/04.

[29] Kaplan I, Ger R, Sharon U. The carbon dioxide laser in plastic surgery. British journal of plastic surgery. 1973;26(4):359-62. Epub 1973/10/01.

[30] Strobbe LJ, Nieweg OE, Kroon BB. Carbon dioxide laser for cutaneous melanoma metastases: indications and limitations. European journal of surgical oncology : the journal of the European Society of Surgical Oncology and the British Association of Surgical Oncology. 1997;23(5):435-8. Epub 1997/12/11.

[31] Green DS, Bodman-Smith MD, Dalgleish AG, Fischer MD. Phase I/II study of topical imiquimod and intralesional interleukin-2 in the treatment of accessible metastases in malignant melanoma. The British journal of dermatology. 2007;156(2):337-45. Epub 2007/01/17.

[32] Radny P, Caroli UM, Bauer J, Paul T, Schlegel C, Eigentler TK, et al. Phase II trial of intralesional therapy with interleukin-2 in soft-tissue melanoma metastases. British journal of cancer. 2003;89(9):1620-6. Epub 2003/10/30.

[33] von Wussow P, Block B, Hartmann F, Deicher H. Intralesional interferon-alpha therapy in advanced malignant melanoma. Cancer. 1988;61(6):1071-4. Epub 1988/03/15.

[34] Testori A, Faries MB, Thompson JF, Pennacchioli E, Deroose JP, van Geel AN, et al. Local and intralesional therapy of in-transit melanoma metastases. Journal of surgical oncology. 2011;104(4):391-6. Epub 2011/08/23.

[35] Glass LF, Pepine ML, Fenske NA, Jaroszeski M, Reintgen DS, Heller R. Bleomycin-mediated electrochemotherapy of metastatic melanoma. Archives of dermatology. 1996;132(11):1353-7. Epub 1996/11/01.

[36] Heller R, Jaroszeski MJ, Reintgen DS, Puleo CA, DeConti RC, Gilbert RA, et al. Treatment of cutaneous and subcutaneous tumors with electrochemotherapy using intralesional bleomycin. Cancer. 1998;83(1):148-57. Epub 1998/07/09.

[37] Mir LM, Glass LF, Sersa G, Teissie J, Domenge C, Miklavcic D, et al. Effective treatment of cutaneous and subcutaneous malignant tumours by electrochemotherapy. British journal of cancer. 1998;77(12):2336-42. Epub 1998/07/02.

[38] Adair FE. Treatment of melanoma: report of four hundred cases. Surgery, gynecology & obstetrics. 1936;62:406-8.

[39] Barranco SC, Romsdahl MM, Humphrey RM. The radiation response of human malignant melanoma cells grown in vitro. Cancer research. 1971;31(6):830-3. Epub 1971/06/01.

[40] Overgaard J, Gonzalez Gonzalez D, Hulshof MC, Arcangeli G, Dahl O, Mella O, et al. Hyperthermia as an adjuvant to radiation therapy of recurrent or metastatic malignant melanoma. A multicentre randomized trial by the European Society for Hyperthermic Oncology. International journal of hyperthermia : the official journal of European Society for Hyperthermic Oncology, North American Hyperthermia Group. 1996;12(1):3-20. Epub 1996/01/01.

[41] Burmeister BH, Henderson MA, Ainslie J, Fisher R, Di Iulio J, Smithers BM, et al. Adjuvant radiotherapy versus observation alone for patients at risk of lymph-node field relapse after therapeutic lymphadenectomy for melanoma: a randomised trial. The lancet oncology. 2012;13(6):589-97. Epub 2012/05/12.

[42] Corry J, Smith JG, Bishop M, Ainslie J. Nodal radiation therapy for metastatic melanoma. International journal of radiation oncology, biology, physics. 1999;44(5):1065-9. Epub 1999/07/27.

[43] Ballo MT, Bonnen MD, Garden AS, Myers JN, Gershenwald JE, Zagars GK, et al. Adjuvant irradiation for cervical lymph node metastases from melanoma. Cancer. 2003;97(7):1789-96. Epub 2003/03/26.

[44] O'Brien CJ, Petersen-Schaefer K, Stevens GN, Bass PC, Tew P, Gebski VJ, et al. Adjuvant radiotherapy following neck dissection and parotidectomy for metastatic malignant melanoma. Head & neck. 1997;19(7):589-94. Epub 1997/10/10.

[45] Stevens G, Thompson JF, Firth I, O'Brien CJ, McCarthy WH, Quinn MJ. Locally advanced melanoma: results of postoperative hypofractionated radiation therapy. Cancer. 2000;88(1):88-94. Epub 2000/01/05.

[46] Aloia TA, Grubbs E, Onaitis M, Mosca PJ, Cheng TY, Seigler H, et al. Predictors of outcome after hyperthermic isolated limb perfusion: role of tumor response. Archives of surgery (Chicago, Ill : 1960). 2005;140(11):1115-20. Epub 2005/11/23.

[47] Kroon HM, Moncrieff M, Kam PC, Thompson JF. Outcomes following isolated limb infusion for melanoma. A 14-year experience. Annals of surgical oncology. 2008;15(11):3003-13. Epub 2008/05/30.

[48] Sanki A, Kam PC, Thompson JF. Long-term results of hyperthermic, isolated limb perfusion for melanoma: a reflection of tumor biology. Annals of surgery. 2007;245(4):591-6. Epub 2007/04/07.

[49] Wile AG, Guilmette E, Friedberg H, Mason GR. A model of experimental isolation perfusion using cis-platinum. Journal of surgical oncology. 1982;21(1):37-41. Epub 1982/09/01.

[50] Aigner K, Hild P, Henneking K, Paul E, Hundeiker M. Regional perfusion with cisplatinum and dacarbazine. Recent results in cancer research Fortschritte der Krebsforschung Progres dans les recherches sur le cancer. 1983;86:239-45. Epub 1983/01/01.

[51] Roseman JM. Effective management of extremity cancers using cisplatin and etoposide in isolated limb perfusions. Journal of surgical oncology. 1987;35(3):170-2. Epub 1987/07/01.

[52] Santinami M, Belli F, Cascinelli N, Rovini D, Vaglini M. Seven years experience with hyperthermic perfusions in extracorporeal circulation for melanoma of the extremities. Journal of surgical oncology. 1989;42(3):201-8. Epub 1989/11/01.

[53] Thompson JF, Gianoutsos MP. Isolated limb perfusion for melanoma: effectiveness and toxicity of cisplatin compared with that of melphalan and other drugs. World journal of surgery. 1992;16(2):227-33. Epub 1992/03/01.

[54] Fraker DL, Alexander HR, Andrich M, Rosenberg SA. Treatment of patients with melanoma of the extremity using hyperthermic isolated limb perfusion with melphalan, tumor necrosis factor, and interferon gamma: results of a tumor necrosis factor dose-escalation study. Journal of clinical oncology : official journal of the American Society of Clinical Oncology. 1996;14(2):479-89. Epub 1996/02/01.

[55] Cornett WR, McCall LM, Petersen RP, Ross MI, Briele HA, Noyes RD, et al. Randomized multicenter trial of hyperthermic isolated limb perfusion with melphalan alone compared with melphalan plus tumor necrosis factor: American College of Surgeons

Oncology Group Trial Z0020. Journal of clinical oncology : official journal of the American Society of Clinical Oncology. 2006;24(25):4196-201. Epub 2006/09/01.

[56] Ueno T, Ko SH, Grubbs E, Yoshimoto Y, Augustine C, Abdel-Wahab Z, et al. Modulation of chemotherapy resistance in regional therapy: a novel therapeutic approach to advanced extremity melanoma using intra-arterial temozolomide in combination with systemic O6-benzylguanine. Molecular cancer therapeutics. 2006;5(3):732-8. Epub 2006/03/21.

[57] Creech O, Jr., Krementz ET, Ryan RF, Winblad JN. Chemotherapy of cancer: regional perfusion utilizing an extracorporeal circuit. Annals of surgery. 1958;148(4):616-32. Epub 1958/10/01.

[58] Stehlin JS, Jr. Hyperthermic perfusion with chemotherapy for cancers of the extremities. Surgery, gynecology & obstetrics. 1969;129(2):305-8. Epub 1969/08/01.

[59] Di Filippo F, Calabro A, Giannarelli D, Carlini S, Cavaliere F, Moscarelli F, et al. Prognostic variables in recurrent limb melanoma treated with hyperthermic antiblastic perfusion. Cancer. 1989;63(12):2551-61. Epub 1989/06/15.

[60] Minor DR, Allen RE, Alberts D, Peng YM, Tardelli G, Hutchinson J. A clinical and pharmacokinetic study of isolated limb perfusion with heat and melphalan for melanoma. Cancer. 1985;55(11):2638-44. Epub 1985/06/01.

[61] Raymond AK, Beasley GM, Broadwater G, Augustine CK, Padussis JC, Turley R, et al. Current trends in regional therapy for melanoma: lessons learned from 225 regional chemotherapy treatments between 1995 and 2010 at a single institution. Journal of the American College of Surgeons. 2011;213(2):306-16. Epub 2011/04/16.

[62] Storm FK, Morton DL. Value of therapeutic hyperthermic limb perfusion in advanced recurrent melanoma of the lower extremity. American journal of surgery. 1985;150(1):32-5. Epub 1985/07/01.

[63] Grunhagen DJ, Brunstein F, Graveland WJ, van Geel AN, de Wilt JH, Eggermont AM. One hundred consecutive isolated limb perfusions with TNF-alpha and melphalan in melanoma patients with multiple in-transit metastases. Annals of surgery. 2004;240(6):939-47; discussion 47-8. Epub 2004/12/01.

[64] Siemann DW, Chapman M, Beikirch A. Effects of oxygenation and pH on tumor cell response to alkylating chemotherapy. International journal of radiation oncology, biology, physics. 1991;20(2):287-9. Epub 1991/02/01.

[65] Beasley GM, Petersen RP, Yoo J, McMahon N, Aloia T, Petros W, et al. Isolated limb infusion for in-transit malignant melanoma of the extremity: a well-tolerated but less effective alternative to hyperthermic isolated limb perfusion. Annals of surgical oncology. 2008;15(8):2195-205. Epub 2008/06/06.

[66] Lindner P, Doubrovsky A, Kam PC, Thompson JF. Prognostic factors after isolated limb infusion with cytotoxic agents for melanoma. Annals of surgical oncology. 2002;9(2):127-36. Epub 2002/03/13.

[67] Lindner P, Thompson JF, De Wilt JH, Colman M, Kam PC. Double isolated limb infusion with cytotoxic agents for recurrent and metastatic limb melanoma. European journal of surgical oncology : the journal of the European Society of Surgical Oncology and the British Association of Surgical Oncology. 2004;30(4):433-9. Epub 2004/04/06.

[68] Beasley GM, Caudle A, Petersen RP, McMahon NS, Padussis J, Mosca PJ, et al. A multi-institutional experience of isolated limb infusion: defining response and toxicity in the US. Journal of the American College of Surgeons. 2009;208(5):706-15; discussion 15-7. Epub 2009/05/30.

[69] Brady MS, Brown K, Patel A, Fisher C, Marx W. A phase II trial of isolated limb infusion with melphalan and dactinomycin for regional melanoma and soft tissue sarcoma of the extremity. Annals of surgical oncology. 2006;13(8):1123-9. Epub 2006/06/23.

[70] Mian R, Henderson MA, Speakman D, Finkelde D, Ainslie J, McKenzie A. Isolated limb infusion for melanoma: a simple alternative to isolated limb perfusion. Can J Surg. 2001;44(3):189-92. Epub 2001/06/16.

[71] Sharma K, Beasley G, Turley R, Raymond AK, Broadwater G, Peterson B, et al. Patterns of Recurrence Following Complete Response to Regional Chemotherapy for In-Transit Melanoma. Annals of surgical oncology. 2012. Epub 2012/04/06.

[72] Wieberdink J, Benckhuysen C, Braat RP, van Slooten EA, Olthuis GA. Dosimetry in isolation perfusion of the limbs by assessment of perfused tissue volume and grading of toxic tissue reactions. European journal of cancer & clinical oncology. 1982;18(10):905-10. Epub 1982/10/01.

[73] Klaase JM, Kroon BB, van Geel BN, Eggermont AM, Franklin HR, Hart GA. Patient- and treatment-related factors associated with acute regional toxicity after isolated perfusion for melanoma of the extremities. American journal of surgery. 1994;167(6):618-20. Epub 1994/06/01.

[74] Li Y, McClay EF. Systemic chemotherapy for the treatment of metastatic melanoma. Seminars in oncology. 2002;29(5):413-26. Epub 2002/10/31.

[75] Korn EL, Liu PY, Lee SJ, Chapman JA, Niedzwiecki D, Suman VJ, et al. Meta-analysis of phase II cooperative group trials in metastatic stage IV melanoma to determine progression-free and overall survival benchmarks for future phase II trials. Journal of clinical oncology : official journal of the American Society of Clinical Oncology. 2008;26(4):527-34. Epub 2008/02/01.

[76] Hodi FS, O'Day SJ, McDermott DF, Weber RW, Sosman JA, Haanen JB, et al. Improved survival with ipilimumab in patients with metastatic melanoma. The New England journal of medicine. 2010;363(8):711-23. Epub 2010/06/08.

[77] Sosman JA, Kim KB, Schuchter L, Gonzalez R, Pavlick AC, Weber JS, et al. Survival in BRAF V600-mutant advanced melanoma treated with vemurafenib. The New England journal of medicine. 2012;366(8):707-14. Epub 2012/02/24.

[78] Turley RS, Fontanella AN, Padussis JC, Toshimitsu H, Tokuhisa Y, Cho EH, et al. Bevacizumab-induced alterations in vascular permeability and drug delivery: a novel approach to augment regional chemotherapy for in-transit melanoma. Clinical cancer research : an official journal of the American Association for Cancer Research. 2012;18(12):3328-39. Epub 2012/04/13.

[79] Qi J, Chen N, Wang J, Siu CH. Transendothelial migration of melanoma cells involves N-cadherin-mediated adhesion and activation of the beta-catenin signaling pathway. Molecular biology of the cell. 2005;16(9):4386-97. Epub 2005/07/01.

[80] Hsu MY, Meier FE, Nesbit M, Hsu JY, Van Belle P, Elder DE, et al. E-cadherin expression in melanoma cells restores keratinocyte-mediated growth control and down-regulates expression of invasion-related adhesion receptors. The American journal of pathology. 2000;156(5):1515-25. Epub 2000/05/04.

[81] Augustine CK, Yoshimoto Y, Gupta M, Zipfel PA, Selim MA, Febbo P, et al. Targeting N-cadherin enhances antitumor activity of cytotoxic therapies in melanoma treatment. Cancer research. 2008;68(10):3777-84. Epub 2008/05/17.

[82] Beasley GM, Riboh JC, Augustine CK, Zager JS, Hochwald SN, Grobmyer SR, et al. Prospective multicenter phase II trial of systemic ADH-1 in combination with melphalan via isolated limb infusion in patients with advanced extremity melanoma. Journal of clinical oncology : official journal of the American Society of Clinical Oncology. 2011;29(9):1210-5. Epub 2011/02/24.

Chapter 3

Surgical Treatment of Nevi and Melanoma in the Pediatric Age

Andrea Zangari, Federico Zangari,
Mercedes Romano, Elisabetta Cerigioni,
Maria Giovanna Grella, Anna Chiara Contini and
Martino Ascanio

Additional information is available at the end of the chapter

1. Introduction

Surgical care of children affected by melanocytic lesions is a complex area of pediatric surgery, where psychosocial aspects, involving parents and children of different ages, overlap with oncologic implications. In this challenging field results may be frustrating despite knowledge and experience.

Due to its rarity, the occurrence of malignant melanoma in children may be underestimated by involved professionals. Melanoma in children is rare, but it does exist and every effort should be done to assure proper treatment, which should be guaranteed in a pediatric tertiary care center by a multi-specialist approach.

The role of dermatologists is essential to achieve proper selection of indications to surgery, by clinical follow up and dermatoscopy techniques. On the other hand surgeon is expected to share a profound knowledge of indications and techniques of treatment. In fact, the awareness that simple excision of a nevus may represent the first and most important therapeutic intervention of a MM, before knowing the definitive diagnosis, is sometimes lacking even among pediatric care professionals and the occasional occurrence of a MM diagnosis may be confounding and cause of an incomplete care strategy.

Decisions about surgical treatment of congenital giant nevi in some cases may need psychological assessment because of complex relationships between patient's and parents' awareness and willingness.

Pediatric anesthesia offers a variety of techniques that can be personalized to suite patients from the newborn to the adolescent.

The intent of this chapter is to contribute to knowledge of this multifaceted field of pediatric surgery.

2. Nevomelanocytic lesions in the pediatric age

Current strategies for the treatment of nevomelanocytic lesions in children mostly derived from the more extensive experience in adults. Nevertheless, further knowledge and experience in this field have shown some peculiarities that require special considerations relevant to the pediatric age. In fact, due to the multifaceted field of congenital nevi, to the rarity of melanoma in children and to peculiar features of some nevic lesions in this age range, important implications related to treatment emerge.

2.1. Congenital nevi

Congenital nevi are present at birth and occur approximately in 1% of newborn infants. They result from a proliferation of benign melanocytes in the dermis, epidermis, or both. Occasionally, nevi that are histologically identical to congenital nevi may develop approximately during the first 2 years of life. These are referred to be considered tardive congenital nevi [1].

The etiology of congenital melanocytic nevi remains unclear. The melanocytes of the skin originate in the neuroectoderm, although the specific cell type from which they derive remains controversial [3, 4, 5].

One hypothesis is that pluripotential nerve sheath precursor cells migrate from the neural crest to the skin along paraspinal ganglia and peripheral nerve sheaths and differentiate into melanocytes upon reaching the skin [6]. There are many reports of familial aggregation of congenital nevi.

One study found that the MC1R (melanocortin-1-receptor) genotype, which corresponds to a red-haired genotype and a tendency to increased birthweight, was overrepresented in a cohort of congenital melanocytic nevi affected Northern European patients. How MC1R variants promote growth of congenital melanocytic nevi and the fetus itself is unknown as is the application of this finding to non-european and more darkly pigmented races [7].

Congenital nevi have been stratified into 3 groups according to size. Small nevi are less than 1.5 cm in greatest diameter, medium nevi are 1.5-19.9 cm in greatest diameter, and large or giant nevi are greater than 20 cm. Giant nevi are often surrounded by several smaller satellite nevi.

Large congenital nevi of the head or posterior midline may also be seen as a component of neurocutaneous disorder, with cranial and/or leptomeningeal melanosis. Neurocutaneous melanosis may result from an error in the morphogenesis of the neuroectoderm, which gives rise to the melanotic cells of both the skin and meninges. Clinically, patients may present with increased intracranial pressure due to hydrocephalus or a mass lesion. The prognosis of patients with symptomatic neurocutaneous melanosis is very poor, even in the absence of malignancy [8]. Significant association is between giant congenital nevi and neurofibromatosis, with development of neurofibromas [9]. The histology is characterized by the presence of melanocytes in the epidermis ordered in theques and/or malanocytes in the dermis as sheets, nests, cords and/or single cells [10].

The histology of large congenital nevus may be delivered into nevus cell, neuroid, epithelioid cell and/or spindle cell, dermal melanocytic and mixed [11].

In the *nevus cell type* histology may appear identical to acquired nevi, but in the congenital nevus melanocytes are more in the lower two-thirds of the reticular dermis or deeper and more associated with neurovascular structures in the reticular dermis. In the *neuroid type* of giant congenital nevi, the dermis imelanocyte cells appear to be arranged in palisaded around a cellular mass of homogeneous material (Varocay Body) and sheating of nerves by neuroid tissue (neuroid tubes). The neuroid type of giant congenital nevus may be associated with congenital anomalies of bone (club foot, spina bifida, atrophy). In the *Spindle cell and/or epithelioid cell type* of giant congenital nevus, the dermis is infiltrated in whole or in part by nests or sheets of epithelioid and/or spindle cells, but unlike acquired variety is involved deeper the reticular dermis, with neuroid elements. Sometime, in giant congenital nevi, architectural and cellular features may be so atypical making differentiation with melanoma very difficult. In the *dermal melanocytic type* of giant congenital nevi, appearance may be that of a giant blue nevus.

In large congenital nevi are occasionally present, within melanocytes, trace of other tissue like muscle, bone, placenta. Other tissues occasionally present intermixed with melanocytic elements are hemangiomas, increased numbers of mast cells, cartilage, calcificacion. Associated tumors include schwannoma, neuroid tumors, lipoma, rhabdomyosarcoma, neurofibroma, sebaceous nevus, blue nevus, hemangioma, lymphangioma and mastocytoma, nevi of Ota and Ito, Spitz nevus [12]. The etiology of congenital melanocytic nevi has not been elucidated. One possible cause is a mutation. An association between infantile hemangiomas and congenital melanocytic nevi has been suggested [13]. Future investigation may yield more definitive causative factors. A review of dermoscopy patterns in congenital nevi found that most nevi demonstrate a reticular, globular, or reticuloglobular pattern. The findings varied with age and the anatomic location of the nevus, with the globular pattern found more often in younger children and the reticular pattern found in patients aged 12 years or older [14]. The role of dermoscopy in congenital nevi is currently recruiting.

2.2. Association between congenital nevi and melanoma

The risk of melanoma development is proportional to to the size of congenital nevus., with a clear evidence of increased risk in patients with congenital nevi involving over 5% of the body surface. For giant congenital melanocytic nevi, the risk of developing melanoma has been reported to be as high as 5-7% [15]. Risk for the development of melanoma in smaller nevi has not been well quantified and the matter is still controversial (Fig.1). Also suggested is that melanoma developing within smaller congenital nevi usually occurs at puberty or later and develops more superficially in the skin, where it is easier to detect clinically. The lifetime risk of melanoma for patients with very large congenital nevi has benn estimated, approximately and considering variations in several countries and studies, at least 6%.

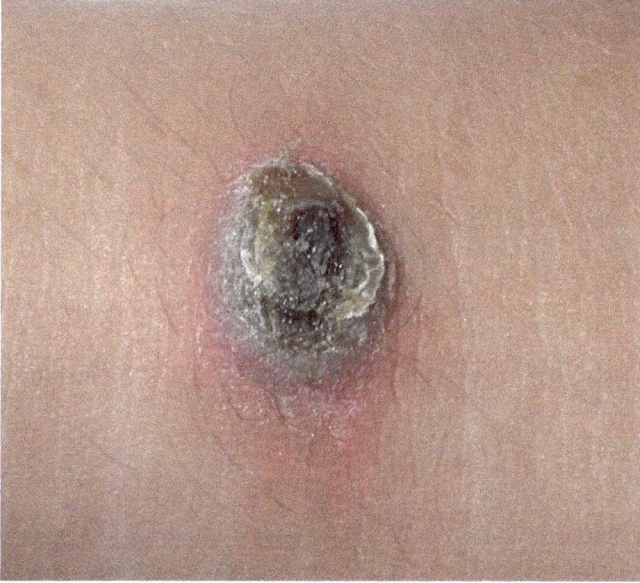

Figure 1. Malignant melanoma diagnosed in a small congenital lesion of the dorsal foot

2.3. Spitz nevus

It is also defined by other terms, including epithelioid cell and/or Spindle cell nevus, juvenile melanoma, benign juvenile melanoma. It occurs normally in children, but may appear in 15% of adolescents and adults. Spitz nevus is a unique, acquired, usually benign melanocytic tumor, so alarming in its clinical presentation and sometimes histologically confused with melanoma. It is possible that some lesions regress spontaneously. It can appear pink or tan, as a papule, often with teleangiectasies on the surface (Fig.2). A variety called Reed nevus, more frequent In adults, may also be confused with melanoma, but histologically is an acquired, predominantly spindle cells variety, darkly pigmented [16].

2.4. Common acquired melanocytic nevus

Acquired melanocytic nevus is a common disorder of melanocytes, occurring as a pigmented benign lesion, possibly localized in every part of the skin (palmoplantar areas included) and

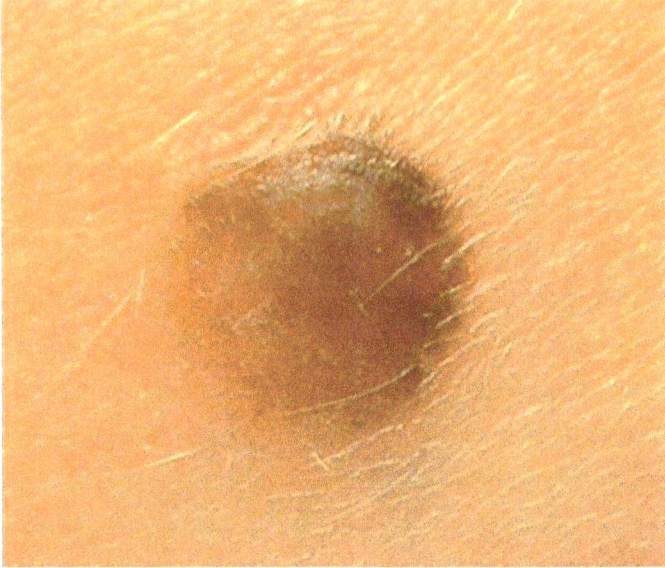

Figure 2. Spitz nevus

oral, ocular, genital mucosae. They first can appear after 6-12 months of life. Histology classifies acquired melanocytic nevi as a collection of melanocytic cells in the epidermis (Junctional), dermis (Intradermal), or both (Compound), disposed in isolated elements (epidermal variety, lentiginous pattern) or aggregated (junctional, intradermal and compound variety). There is evidence that number and size of common acquired nevi is associated with familiarity. Studies documented an increased number of nevi for pale skin, blond hair, blue or green eyes, tendency to sunburn. Typical acquired nevi usually have a round or oval, symmetric shape and relatively well-demarcated, smooth borders. The surface of nevi may be flat-topped, dome-shaped, papillomatous or peduncolated. More elevated acquired nevi tend to be more lightly pig-mented, and flatter acquired nevi tend to be more darkly pigmented. More elevated and less pigmented lesions tend to have a prominent intradermal melanocytic component, whereas flatter and darker lesions have a more prominent junctional melanocytic component and a less prominent dermal component. Changes in acquired melanocytic nevi can be physiologic in puberty, pregnancy, corticosteroid administration and sun exposure; also changes may occur slowly during the years as normal evolution of nevi. Though most of times changes are benign, in presence of alterations of symmetry, color, borders, extension or regression, especially in a short time (months), a periodic monitoring of all nevi on the skin and mucosa is necessary, preferably with dermoscopy. When melanoma occurs on a melanocytic acquired nevi, changes may be global or, most of times, partial, that is the reason why asymmetry is a predominant parameter to be evaluated [17].

2.5. Blue nevus

The blue nevus consists of an acquired or congenital blue, blue-gray or blue-black papule, plaque or nodule, histologically composed by dermal dendritic, fibroblast-like cells containing melanin. Most of times it is localized on dorsa of hands and feet, usually singular. Common blue nevi remain unchanged or possibly regress. Particular types of blue nevi are:

- Cellular blue nevus is a blue-gray nodule or plaque 1 to 3 cm diameter mostly located on the buttock or sacrum.

- Combined blue nevus-melanocytic nevus, sometimes confused with atypical nevi or melanoma.

Malignant blue nevus, may develop in contiguity with cellular blue nevus, nevus of Ota, or de novo [18].

2.6. Dysplastic melanocytic nevi

Dysplastic nevus is an acquired, usually atypical-appearing melanocytic tumor, characterized histologically by epidermic and/or dermal melanocytic dysplasia. Dysplasia refers to abnormal tissue development. When applied to melanocytic tumors, dysplasia is referred to a disordered melanocytic proliferation in association with discontinuous and variable cellular atypia (mild, moderate and severe). About this spectrum of atypia, from slight to marked may be said that intraepidermal melanocytes in dysplastic melanocytic nevi occupy an intermediate position between typical and malignant, basing on nuclear and cytoplasmic features. Not all atypical-appearing melanocytic lesions have an atypical histology. It is generally believed that a melanocytic nevus appearing asymmetric, irregular in borders and pigmentation and with a diameter equal or more than 6 mm is considered dysplastic, but these characteristics are referred to "Atypical acquired Nevus", also called "Clark Nevus". Although the diagnosis of dysplastic nevus is suspected because of the atypical appearing, histological confirmation is required to establish the presence or not of dysplasia. It is important to define if atypical nevus is dysplastic, because it is a potential histogenic precursor of melanoma and marker of increased melanoma risk.

2.7. Halo nevi

Halo nevus, also referred as "Sutton's nevus" or "leukoderma acquisitum centrifugum", is a nevus surrounded by a macule of leukoderma (hypopigmented or apigmented area). It occurs in up to 1% of general population, with a peak of incidence in the second decade. It is commonly composed of a central pigmented nevus and an acquired surrounding depigmented halo. From 25 to 50% of patients have more than one halo nevi. Nevus regression can be complete and is caused by a lymphocytic aggression against nevus melanocytes with involvement of sur-rounding epidermal melanocytes. Association with vitiligo needs clinical and anamnestic analysis as a history for melanoma.

2.8. Nevus of Ota and Ito

Ota first described this nevus and called it "nevus fuscocaeruleus ophtalmomaxillaris. Nevus of Ota is usually congenital but may appear in early childhood or in puberty. It is usually characterized by unilateral, flat, blue-black macules in the skin innervated by the first and second branches of the trigeminal nerve. Oral, nasal and pharingeal mucosae, conjunctivae and tympanic membranes may be involved. More rarely pigmentation may extend to cornea, optic nerve, fundus oculi, retrobulbar fat and periosteum. Enlargement and darkening may be observed over time. Histology shows stellate melanocytes widely scattered in the reticular dermis. Overlying melanocytes may be reduced in size and contain increased melanin. Nevus of Ota does not improve with time. 66 cases of melanoma development in nevus of Ota have been reported. Effective treatment is photothermolysis with Q-Switched LASER needing multiple sessions, with good results. Nevus of Ito is analogous to nevus of Ota and may coexist in the same patient. The difference between the two types of nevi is that nevus of Ito involves the distribution of the lateral supraclavicular and brachial nerves.

2.9. Melanoma

Melanoma is a malignant tumor resulting from the trasformation of melanocytes of the skin and less frequently of mucosae. During embryonic life, melanoblasts migrate from neural crest to the basal-cell layer of epidermis and a minus part to skin appendages and dermis. Melanoma can arise from melanocytes located in these sites.

Risk for the development of melanoma remains low in pre-pubertal age, with an annual incidence of 0.7 cases per million children aged 0-9 years. Reaching adolescence the incidence of melanoma increases, with a rate of 13.2 cases per million children aged 15-19 years [2]. Prevention and early recognition of melanoma is mainly applied to adults through periodic clinical and dermoscopic controls. Only in recent years data documented alarm about increasing incidence of melanoma in adolescents. This increase, combined with other data about congenital nevi, allow physicians in the last years to play a crucial role in the identification of children at risk for melanoma, with particular regard to detection of risk factors in children and adolescents, and education about sun and artificial ultraviolet exposure.

3. Types of primary melanoma of the skin

3.1. Lentigo maligna

Lentigo maligna is a precursor lesion that may progress into invasive melanoma. It appears as a macular, freckled-like lesion of irregular shape, occurring most often in *elderly patients* (age over 60 years) in sun exposed and sun-damaged, atrophic skin. Lentigo maligna normally grows slowly for long periods (years) with a prolonged radial growth phase, before evolution in Lentigo Maligna Melanoma. Hstopathology reveals atrophic epidermis and increased numbers of atypical basilar melanocytes that may extend down the hair follicles and skin appendages.

3.2. Lentigo maligna melanoma

It is a melanoma in situ slow growing progressing to invasive melanoma with nests of malignant melanocytes invading the dermis. Lentigo Maligna Melanoma represents 4 to 15 % of all melanoma.

3.3. Superficial spreading melanoma

SSM is the most frequent type of melanocytic malignancy representing 70% of all melanomas.

Most commonly it occurs on the upper back of men and on the legs of women, although it can develop at any site, mucosa included. The usual history is that of slow change (months to 1-5 years) of a preexisting melanocytic lesion or can arise "de novo".

SSM most frequently presents as a macule asymmetric, variegated pigmentation (from brown to black, with variable presence of blue-gray, gray-white or pink areas as sign of regression along the borders or inside the lesion. Borders may present intact initially in presence of a precursor melanocytic nevus, but mostly are irregular. Dermoscopy can reveal better all these alterations, and more other parameters typical of SSM (salt-peppering areas, star-bust aspect, pseudopodes at borders, blue-white veil and so on). Diagnosis of SSM may be done from a macroscopic view, but dermoscopy helps much for *confirmation diagnosis* and for *early diagnosis*, when it is difficult to find macroscopically some alterations typical of melanoma.

Histopathology reveals a "pagetoid" distribution of atypical large melanocytes thruoughout the epidermis. The large cells may occur singularly or in nests and have a monomorphous appearance. In the dermis areas of invasion of atypical melanocytes are present.

3.4. Nodular melanoma

The second most common subtype of melanoma is nodular melanoma with a frequency of 15 to 30 percent of all types. NM is remarkable for its rapid evolution and may arise from melanocytic nevi or normal skin (de novo), but in lack of an apparent radial growth phase. NM is more common to arise "de novo" than from a preexisting nevus.

NM appears typically as a blue-black, blue-red or amelanotic nodule or papule. In certain cases it may be difficult to diagnose especially when it appears as an amelanotic reddish lesion.

Histopathology may demonstrates a little tendency for intraepidermal growth, but it typically arises at dermal-epidermal junction and from its onset with extention to the dermis, composed of large epithelioid cells, spindle cells, small cells, or a mix of these different cells.

3.5. Acral lentiginous melanoma

ALM is more common in darker skin individuals (60 to 72 percent in blacks, 29 to 46 percent in asians). In white skin people it represents only 2 to 8 percent of melanomas. ALM occurs on palms and more often on soles, or beneath the nail plate.

The biologic behavior of ALM is traditionally considered more aggressive with a poorer prognosis and this may be due to late diagnosis and/or to the different biologic origin of it.

3.6. Melanoma of the mucosa

It involves oral, nasal, vulva, anorectal, conjunctival mucosae and it may occur with or without a radial growth phase.

3.7. Desmoplastic melanoma

It is a rare subtype of melanoma, locally aggressive and with high rates of local recurrence. It may arise in association with LM, ALM and mucosal melanoma or "de novo". DM may appear as a pigmented macule, papule, nodule or reddish. Histologically it is caracterized by fibrous tissue and atypical spindle-shaped melanocytes that show a propensity to infiltrate cutaneous nerves.

The incidence of malignant melanoma is rapidly increasing in the last decades. The surveillance, epidemiology and results program (SEER) has documented a 32,7% increased in mortality rates over the period 1973 to 1995. on the other hand, the overall survival rate has been improving for melanoma in the last decades. Currently, cutaneous melanoma accounts for approximatively 1% of all cancer deaths [19, 20, 21, 22].

More recent studies indicate that the rate of increase in all age groups was 2.8% per year from 1981 to 2001 and in children (age < 20 years) was 1.1% per year from 1975 to 2001.1 The diagnosis is often delayed in children since melanoma is rare (300 to 420 new cases per year), and benign lesions, especially Spitz nevus, may mimic melanoma. The prognosis is good when there is prompt identification and wide local excision of early disease, but poor for those with advanced disease at presentation [23]. Case-control studies in adults have identified multiple host and environmental factors associated with increased risk of malignant melanoma. Host factors include fair skin, white race, blond or red hair, light eye color, tendency to burn with UV radiation exposure, increased number of benign nevi, dysplastic nevi, family history of melanoma, and xeroderma pigmentosum.6,7 Environmental factors include sunburns, often as a child, and increased exposure to UV radiation. Proposed risk factors for paediatric melanoma include congenital, dysplastic, or increased number of nevi; inability to tan; blue eyes; facial freckling; family history of melanoma; disorders of DNA excision repair like xeroderma pigmentosum; acquired or congenital immunosuppression and a previous history of malignancy [24, 25, 26].

Analysis regarding children and young adults with melanoma between 1973 and 2001 show how older age, more recent year of diagnosis, female sex, white race, and increased environmental UV radiation were all associated with a significant increase in the risk of melanoma. In the first year of life, the incidence of melanoma is similar by race, but it diverges by age 5 to 9 years and is more than 40-fold higher in white individuals by age 20 to 24 years.

The increase in incidence of melanoma in children, especially in adolescents, is similar to that seen in young adults. This may reflect increased cumulative UV exposure during childhood or adolescence, greater awareness and more frequent diagnosis of melanoma (eg, versus atypical Spitz nevus), differences in genetic predisposition, and/or other environmental factors. The increased risk of melanoma in girls, particularly on the lower extremities, may be a result of increased UV exposure. In adults, sun-related behaviours differ between men and women. [22] The increased rates of melanoma in adolescent and young women may reflect sunbathing or the widespread (> 25%) practice of indoor tanning [28].

Prognosis for young children, adolescents, and young adults with melanoma appears to be similar. Also increased is the risk of death in male children, those with regional or distant metastasis, primary sites other than the extremities or torso, increasing thickness of the primary lesion, earlier year of diagnosis, and previous cancer.

Melanoma-specific survival in children has improved by approximately 4% per year during the last 3 decades. It is difficult to explain this dramatic improvement. Although earlier diagnosis could be associated with improved survival, there has been no decrease in lesion thickness over the last decade. Furthermore, survival has improved for all stages of paediatric melanoma. The most notable improvement has been in the "unstaged" group, likely due to more complete staging. There are important differences in young children (age < 10 years) with melanoma compared with adolescents and young adults that may reflect distinct tumor biology and/or host characteristics.

Published large series of paediatric melanoma report 5-year survival rates of 74% to 80%. This is significantly worse than the 91% 5-year overall survival seen in recent analysis, after the exclusion of cases of melanoma in situ [29, 30]. Accepted prognostic factors in adult melanoma include primary lesion thickness, ulceration, and non-extremity site; increased age; regional lymph node involvement; satellite or in-transit metastases; elevated serum lactate dehydrogenase level; visceral or brain metastases.[4,9 However, prognosis and prognostic factors in children are less defined. In a recent review of more than 300 cases, the outcome for paediatric patients (5-year survival of 74%) was slightly worse than that of young adults, but these survival estimates have limitations. In a large European registry study of children, male sex, unfavorable site (lesions on the trunk), and/or second primary or regional or distant metastasis. [10] Advanced stage has been associated with poor prognosis in other paediatric studies [27].

In summary, paediatric melanoma is an important and increasing problem. Factors conferring risk of adult melanoma, including older age, white race (blue eyes, blond or red hair, freckling tendency, liability to tan and tendence to sunburn), family history of melanoma, elevate number of acquired melanocytic nevi (double risk in 50 to 99 of acquired melanocytic nevi), dysplastic nevi, environmental exposure to UV radiation, congenital or acquired immunosuppression are also important in paediatric melanoma.

4. Indications for excision of nevi

Indication for excision are usually assessed by dermatologists, paediatric surgeons, paediatrician and physicians.

Nevi can be divided into congenital and acquired. In turn congenital nevi can be small, intermediate and large (>20cm). Melanoma risk in small congenital nevi is debated, although in some reports it seems to be of importance [32] Some studies demonstrated an increased risk of malignant melanoma in small lesions as well as in intermediate lesions, but this is still a matter of controversy. In the lack of consensus about systematic removal of small congenital nevi, careful dermatologic monitoring and prompt excision after clinical changing is recommended [33] In the Literature there is a large agreement on the excision of large congenital nevi. In fact they show an increased risk for development of malignant melanoma, varying from 1% to 31%. Nonetheless malignancy is reported to occur despite complete excision and may be not preventable [34, 35]

Indications for surgical excision [36] of acquired nevi are mainly related to lesions resembling malignant melanoma, such as atypical nevi, Spitz nevi, and lesions presenting clinical signs and symptoms as diameter of more than 5 mm or increasing diameter, irregular margins, border notching, irregular pigmentation, asymmetry, rapid onset or increase in diameter, ulceration, bleeding, pain and itching. These last signs seem to represent the presentation symptoms of malignant melanoma in 85% of cases [37] Although the risk of malignant melanoma is higher in familial atypical nevi rather than in nonfamilial, features of atypical nevi have been reported to be the most frequent indication to surgery [38]

Some special consideration is given to Spitz nevus for possible misdiagnosis with MM. Most dermatologists and physicians recommend biopsy. In an interview with dermatologists, most responding specialists (93%) recommended the biopsy of suspected Spitz nevi. Sixty-nine percent of physicians would completely excise a lesion that was histologically diagnosed as an incompletely removed Spitz nevus. Seventy percent of general dermatologists and 80% of pediatric dermatologists would recommend excision with a 1- to 2-mm margin of normal-appearing skin around a Spitz nevus [39]. The lack of consensus about the nature and the ideal management of Spitz nevus reflects the uncertainty in histopathologic distinction between Spitz nevus and melanoma, and such a concern influences management. By some authors 2 mm margins excisional biopsy of clinically appearing Spitz nevus, as of any nevic lesion, is recommended

In some cases nevi located in sites of clinically difficult monitoring or placed in sites of exposure to frequent trauma are an indication for excision [38, 40]

5. Treatment of acquired nevi

Acquired melanocytic nevi begin to appear after the first 6 months of life and increase in number during childhood and adolescence, typically reaching a peak count in the third decade and then slowly regressing with age. They are classified as junctional nevi if the nests of melanocytes are in the dermal – epidermal junction, intradermal nevi if the nests are in dermis and compound nevi if the nests are located in both sites.

They usually have a diameter of less than 6 - 8 mm, a homogeneous surface, pigmentation, round or oval shape, regular outline, and demarcated border, sometimes with pigmentary stippling or perifollicular hypopigmentation.

These are rarely complicated by evolution in malignant melanoma so conservative treatment, that is clinical periodic control, is usually enough.

However, when removal of a naevus is necessary we have to do some considerations especially in order to the characteristics of the nevus and its position.

5.1. Anesthesia

Indications and surgical techniques of the excision of a skin lesion are similar to the adult and so the actual difference with children is the anesthetic management.

Analgesics are commonly administered prior to surgical procedure in children. The concept of preemptive analgesia is still controversial and its effectiveness may depend on the type of surgery. Nowadays the most commonly used medications are acetaminophen alone or with codeine, but also non – steroidal anti – inflammatory medications (ibuprofen) are effective analgesics for perioperative pain, but less used for the impact on bleeding.

In association with analgesics and anesthetic medicament the use of sedative is very common and useful also in children as in the adult. Midazolam is very convenient in children because not only alleviates the anxiety of surgery, but also induces an anterograde amnesia, useful for treatments requiring multiple visits. Furthermore, it can be administrated in various vehicles via the nasal, rectal, sublingual that are less traumatic than intramuscular injection in children.

Fentanyl is 100 times more potent than morphine and has less influence on GI motility than morphine, so reducing the effect of emesis and oxygen desaturation becoming more tolerable in children.

General anaesthesia is used in the excisional surgery of large lesions and occasionally in non – cooperative children. It is a very safe procedure, but the rate of complication increases in case of surgery in the first year of life and when the anesthesiologist has no pediatric experience.

In recent years the use of topical anesthetics, especially EMLA cream (eutectic mixture of local anesthetics), knows an important development in office procedures in children, although the incorrect use of EMLA causes failure in reducing pain of dermatologic procedure. In particular for an effective absorption of the anesthetic into the skin an occlusive dressing is useful.

5.2. Surgery

Any skin lesion presenting features of malignant melanoma are biopsied. Although melanoma in children is rare, the most frequent indication for excision of an acquired nevus is early diagnostic evaluation because of melanoma concern.

Excisional biopsy is the treatment of choice. It may be elliptical, wedge or circular, but the first is the most commonly used.

5.2.1. Simple excision

Skin incisions should be planned along or parallel to the relaxed skin tension lines (RSTLs). This allows, on one hand, a better wound healing, an easier matching of edge of the wound and lower tension of the sutures and, on the other hand, to hide the wound in a skin fold.

The elliptical excisional biopsy, as the other type of excisional biopsy, must include a portion of healthy tissue of 0,2 cm wideness from the perimeter of the lesion and the subcutaneous tissue. The possible exuberant tissue, called "dog - ear" can be corrected by extending the ellipse or removing the excess skin with a L or Y incision.

The wedge excisional biopsy is usually utilized for the lesions located on or close to the free margin of some particular structures as eyelid, lip, nose and ear. In the eyelids it is possible to make an incision along the edge and remove only the skin, although some lesions require excision of full thickness eyelid. 1/4 of eyelid or 1/3 of the lower lip can be completely excised and the defect closed with a simple suture without elaborated reconstructions.

The circular excisional biopsy is used when a skin limited incision is needed as in the case of nose or in the anterior region of the auricle. The defect can be closed with a skin graft or a skin flap.

When repairing the loss of substance by combination of skin edges is impossible, other techniques are necessary:

Grafts, rarely used for the excision of acquired nevi

5.2.2. Flaps

A flap is a portion of one or more tissues transferred from a donor site to a receiver maintaining a neurovascular connection ("pedicle").

The use of flap has many advantages including that of allow the repair of the defect by means of tissue similar or equal to those of the receiving site. It is very important for specialized tissues as lip or eyelid.

The skin flap, composed by skin only or including subcutaneous tissue, is transferred from one part of the body to another with its neurovascular pedicle or attached by just a margin to preserve vascular support.

There are two types of skin flap: those which rotate around a pivot point (rotation, transposition and interpolation flaps) and advancement flaps (single pedicle, V – Y, Y – V and bi – pedunculated.

The rotation flap is a semicircular flap that rotates from its pivot point to the receiving site (Fig.3). If tension is too high, the incision can be extended by a reverse incision from pivot point along the base of the flap (backcut).

The transposition flap is composed by a rectangle or square of skin and subcutaneous tissue that rotate around a pivot point close to lesion.

The advancement flap is brought forward on the lesion without rotation.

This can have only one pedicle, so feeding is maintained by exploiting the elasticity of the skin.

The advancement V – Y flap more than a flap is a V incision whose sides are closed in such a way that the final suture gives a Y.

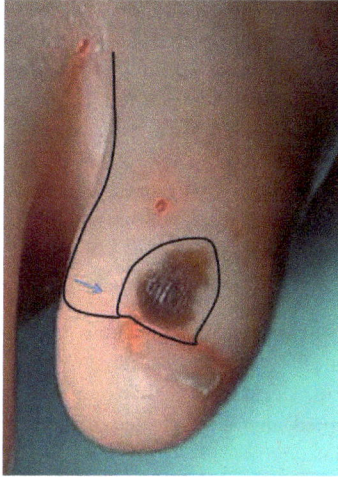

Figure 3. Rotational flap to excise a peliungueal nevus

6. Treatment of congenital nevi in the pediatric age

6.1. Indications and timing

Surgery of congenital nevi is predominantly indicated for preventive reasons, related to the risk of developing a malignant melanoma within the lesion during life. This indication has been discussed more extensively elsewhere in the chapter. Evaluation of all small and medium CNN for prophylactic excision should take place before the patient is aged 12 years. After this age, malignant potential rises sharply. Some authors advocate prophylactic excision of all CNN [35, 41, 42],

whereas others advocate clinical monitoring of small [38] or both small and medium nevi [43] The incidence of malignant melanoma appears higher in large congenital nevi, in the scalp, back, and buttocks and requires removal first. This increase in incidence is likely secondary to the total body surface area. The presence of an enlarging nodular mass indicates malignant change and requires immediate treatment. This mass may represent a rare neuroectodermal sarcoma.

The other important indication to treatment is the possible discomfort due to the presence of a visible difference or even disfigurement. Psychological implications of this condition can involve both parents and children, in a different manner for different ages. Parents feelings about their child's appearance are likely to influence the child's perception of his or her disfigurement, the developing body image and feelings of self-worth [44]. Parental strategies to deal with a physical difference vary considerably. Some discuss it openly, others may act as if it does not exist, parents may be over-protective or children may avoid issues related to their appearance for fear of upsetting their parents 45. Most children with a visible difference often experience appearance-related teasing and bullying during the course of their school career [46]. A link between appearance-related teasing, body dissatisfaction and general psychological disturbance has been discussed by Gilbert and Thompson [47]. The physical and psychological changes associated with adolescence increase the importance of physical appearance, and having a disfigurement during this period may present particular challenges. Image counts in the dating game, and joining an acceptable social grouping can be difficult if social confidence has been in some way weakened. Harter [48] reported that teenagers who believed their appearance determined their self-worth had lower self-esteem and greater depression than adolescents who believed their self-worth determined their feelings about their appearance.

Nonetheless, indications to surgical treatment should be carefully evaluated when the motivation of patient is doubtful. Treatment decisions made during childhood, adolescence and adulthood can be stressful. Deciding whether or not to undergo appearance-altering surgery may not be easily accepted, and those affected can question any motivation for putting themselves through the associated stress [49] Furthermore, expectations about outcomes may be unrealistic, and can generate disappointment when the aesthetic result becomes apparent. Given the multifaceted nature of surgical adjustment, the prevailing model of care needs to be expanded to offer psychosocial support and intervention as routine adjuncts or alternatives to surgical treatment. Interventions need to be carefully planned to take account of individual physical (e.g. growth) and social issues and the child with a visible difference or disfiguring lesion should receive continuing psychological support, preoperative assessment and follow up during the course of treatment.

Surgical excision with reconstruction, is the mainstay of treatment. If direct closure after complete excision is not possible, reconstruction may include excision with skin grafts, skin flaps, tissue expansion with subsequent flap rotation or full thickness skin grafting, autologous cultured human epithelium, artificial skin replacement, and free tissue transfer after tissue expansion [50, 51, 52] Chemical peels, dermabrasion, and laser treatments are adjunctive treatment choices, that have not been demonstrated to decrease the malignant potential, because of incomplete removal of cells in the treated area. If surgical excision is not feasible, management consists of examination and high-quality photographic documentation for life.

Serial excision of large congenital nevi by skin expansion should preferably start in early months of life, for their malignant potential and for their size, requiring many surgical stages. It is usually addressed at age 6 months, to decrease anesthetic and surgical risks [52, 53, 54]. Attempts to complete the treatment of particularly disfiguring lesions is preferably carried out before age 5, when possible, or at least in the pre-adolescent, to prevent important psychosocial implications linked to the different developmental stages of the child and to parental behavior [55]. The goals of treatment are to remove all or as much as feasible of the CNN and reconstruct the defect, preserving function and maintaining the aesthetic appearance. Each case requires tailoring of the operations to fit the anatomic defect and to respect anatomic units and relaxed skin tension lines when possible. Excision begins in the 6-9 month range, placing procedures 3-6 months apart.

6.2. Surgical techniques

Technical choices vary depending on nevus size and anatomical site and may be challenging in some cases of giant nevi.

General considerations, including anatomical and surgical principles, should be remembered.

Incisions are planned according to the orientation of the relaxed skin tension lines (RSTL) when possible, with attention to the most favorable and less visible site of the resulting scar, especially when the use of skin expanders is required.

A variable amount of subcutaneous tissue should be included in the excision, for its diagnostic value in the rare occasional finding of melanoma in the specimen. This amount is thinner in facial areas, to avoid nerve injuries, but enough to include hair follicles.

6.2.1. Small congenital nevi

Excision of small congenital nevi (diameter ≤1.5 cm) is usually performed with 2 mm margins of normally appearing skin, by simple excision. In special areas, as some parts of the nose, lip, eyelid or ear, serial excision or rotation, advancement or transposition flaps are often necessary.

6.2.2. Medium size congenital nevi

Excision of medium size nevi (diameter >1.5 <19 cm) can be achieved by serial excision or tissue expansion.

Serial excision

The efficacy of serial excision for the treatment of medium size congenital nevi has been reported by different authors [56] and it is the indication of choice when the procedure can be easily planned in 2 stages [57].

In children this indication can be extended to larger lesions, requiring more than 2 stages, when considering the possibility of avoiding morbidity related to tissue expansion, longer operating time of every stage, multiple expanding percutaneous injections and poor compliance by the patient. When surgical planning suggests too many operations to complete the removal of the lesion, tissue expansion should be seriously considered as an alternative.

Techniques of serial excision:

A symmetric, fusiform ellipse is drawn within the lesion, parallel to the RSTLs and the margins are undermined enough to obtain a tension free suture (Fig. 4)

In the subsequent period the surrounding skin is going to stretch and and adapt, releasing tension on the scar. After a minimum of 3 months a second excision is performed to complete nevus removal.

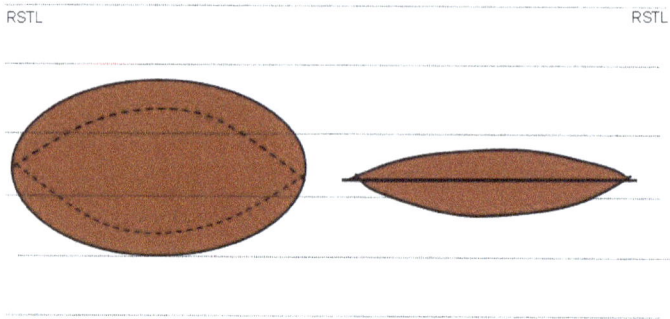

Figure 4. First stage of serial excision with the long axis of the lesion parallel tothe RSTL

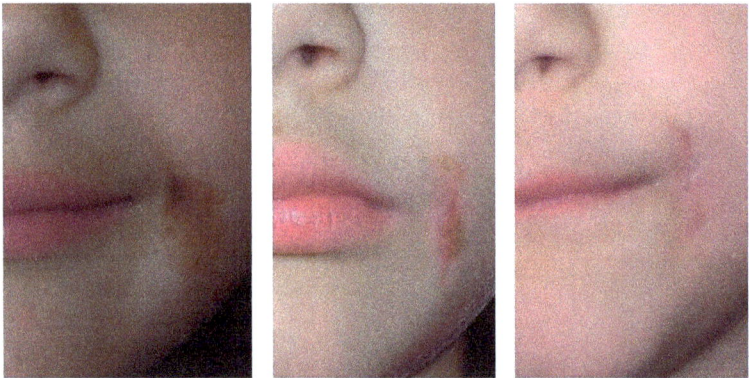

Figure 5. Serial excision of medium size congenital nevus, with final positioning of the scar in the nasogenien crease

When the resulting scar is desired to fall in a crease or for the treatment of particular anatomical sites, as nasal ala, oral commissure, lateral canthus, some modifications may be required. The fusiform excision may be planned to be eccentric and the skin undermined more on one side, to move the tissue in one direction rather than the opposite one. The direction of the prevalent movement can be towards a natural crease, the border of an aesthetic unit or an anatomical area not to be distorted, as nasal ala or oral commissure (Fig.5)

Flap surgery

In difficult anatomical sites and for wider intermediate sized lesions flap surgery is also indicated to obtain excision without tissue loss or distortion. An advancement flap may be used when its incision lines can be drawn along the borders of different aesthetic units. For example, in the case of a round nevus on the lateral aspect of nasal pyramid, incisions of an advancement flap could be outlined on the infraorbital and nasogenien folds to hide scars in

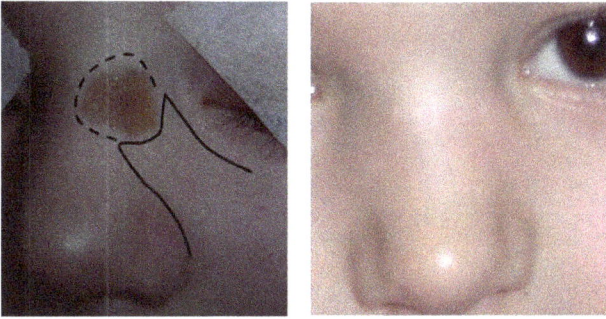

Figure 6. An advancement flap is drawn in the infraorbital area along infraorbital and nasogenien creases.

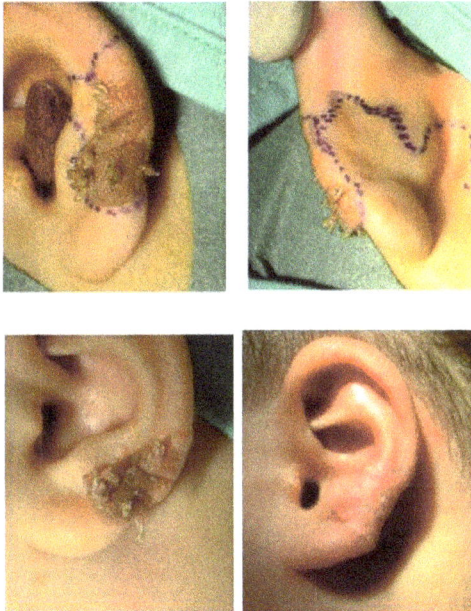

Figure 7. A bilobed flap is transposed from the retroauricular crease.

these creases (Fig.6). On the auricle, due to the adherence of local skin, a sufficient amount of tissue can be obtained from the retroauricular fold by a transposition flap (Fig.7).

6.2.3. Large or giant congenital nevi

Treatment of large or giant congenital melanocytic nevi (CGMN) (diameter>19 cm) always requires multiple surgical stages and complex strategies.

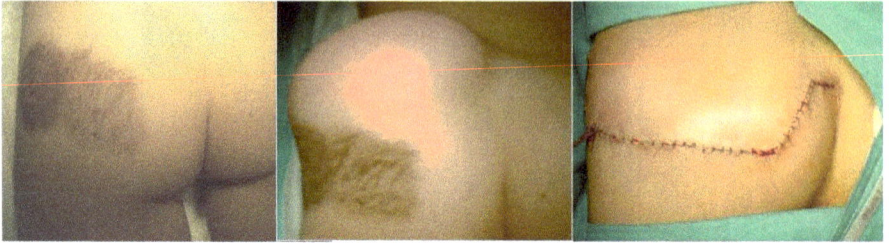

Figure 8. Skin expansion to excise a large congenital nevus of the gluteal region

6.2.4. Tissue expansion technique

Although multistaged direct excision, described elsewhere about medium size nevi, is sometimes feasible for the treatment of large lesions, skin expansion is the treatment of choice and will be discussed in more detail. In general terms, expansion of tissue is used to improve rotation, transposition or advancement of local or regional flaps, or to increase the harvest of full-thickness skin grafts. In adults, aside from their use in breast reconstruction, tissue expanders are used primarily for secondary burn and trauma reconstruction in the head and neck region. In the pediatric population, expanders have been used in a variety of reconstructive procedures. The most common indication in children is to reconstruct defects left by excision of giant congenital nevi (Fig.8).

Tissue expansion is contraindicated in infected skin. Although expansion is possible in radiated or scarred tissue, it is associated with a much higher complication rate and should be avoided whenever possible.

Surgical technique of skin expansion relies on the ability of skin and soft tissues to grow by generation of new tissue in response to tension. Tensive impulse is generated by implanting a subcutaneous device (expander) that is inflated over a period of weeks; new tissue is generated in response to the constant stretch caused by the progressive inflation. An increase in skin surface area after expansion is due to generation of new tissue rather than the stretching of existing skin, as supported by numerous studies. Fibroblast and epidermal hyperplasia induced by mechanical stress have been observed in culture. Histological response to expansion is similar in adult and pediatric skin. Within 1-3 weeks of expansion, the epidermis begins to thicken and the dermis thins while skin appendages do not change. The subcutaneous fat atrophy. Cellular proliferation reduces the resting tension of the skin over time, enabling further expansion to take place. Once the process is complete, the expanded skin eventually returns to its baseline thickness. The vessels of the skin and subcutaneous tissue also resume their pre-expanded size and number [58, 59].

Expanders are available in a variety of shapes and sizes, and there is no absolute ideal expander for a given site or condition. Expanders have different types of filling ports. These can be internal to the expander or remote and connected by a tube of various length, that is usually adjustable by the surgeon. Most experienced surgeons recommend using remote ports. These should be placed away from the expander. Internal ports have both a higher failure rate and a greater incidence of accidental expander rupture. In children, the use of internal ports is associated with a higher rate of exposure of the expander due to the pressure exerted on the skin by the port. As a rule, expansion proceeds best when the expander rests on a firm base like the ribs or skull. When placed within the abdominal wall, for example, expansion tends to be tess predictable. The incisions for expander placement and the remote port should be placed where they will not interfere with later advancement or compromise the blood supply to the expanded tissue. If possible the incisions for expander placement are placed in the proposed area to be excised. Incisions are never placed parallel to the edges of the expander. This creates a situation that increases implant exposure, additional scar tissue outside the lesion, possible stretching of the scar and a delay in inflation of expander. Incisions should be radial or almost perpendicular to the expander or in the form of a V or W

The broad base of the V or W should be directed toward the expander, thus facilitating implant insertion and inflation because the lines of tension are perpendicular to the wound. The open end of the V should be at least 2 to 3 cm from the pocket to accommodate expansion. In addition, a sigma (lazy S) incision can also be beneficial in instances where partial excision of some of the lesion might be helpful during the insertion phase. By this approach, partial excision can be done while an expander is placed. Once the wounds heal, the expander can then be inflated without worry because the end of the incision is almost radial to the expansion process [60]. The expander should be placed on top of the deep fascia (or subgaleal in the scalp), unless the plan is to incorporate muscle into the expanded flap. The pocket should always be larger than the base diameter of the expander. Blunt dissection in a single fascial plane is safest for preserving blood supply. Filling the expanders intraoperatively with sufficient saline to eliminate dead space can prevent postoperative bleeding and hematoma. An alternative to traditional prolonged expansion is immediate intraoperative expansion combined with broad undermining of the defect. In rapid expansion, the skin initially expands due to its elasticity and the displacement of interstitial fluid. Within minutes, the alignment of the collagen fibers changes due to the stretch. This process yields up to 20% more tissue for flap coverage. Intraoperative expansion is indicated for relatively small defects, such as in coverage of defects of the ear.

The rate of inflation is variable and largely based on surgeon preference. Patient comfort and signs of tissue perfusion, such as tension, color, and capillary refill, guide the filling rate. Filling is usually initiated 7-10 days postoperatively and performed once or twice a week, based on the above mentioned criteria and patient tolerance. The rate of expansion depends both on the body site as well as patient factors. Some skin is more amenable to expansion, and some patients can tolerate the discomfort better than others [61]. Tissue expansion should continue until the expanded area is larger than the defect, usually up to 2 months. As a general rule, the diameter of the expanded flap should be 2-3 times the diameter of the skin that is to be excised

Most surgeons overinflate tissue expanders beyond the manufacturer's recommended maximum capacity. Studies have demonstrated that significant overinflation is possible before weakening or rupturing.

The use of rotation and transposition flaps enables the transfer of tension from the tip of the flap more proximally to its base. A single or double back-cut can be performed prior to inset in order to gain extra length. The donor site should be closed in layers after the implant capsule is excised.

Scalp. Although tissue expansion does not increase the number of hair follicles, the size of the hair-bearing region can be doubled without a noticeable decrease in hair density. As such, tissue expansion may be used to reconstruct the scalp when removal of a medium or large nevus is needed. Expanders are most commonly placed in the occipital or posterior parietal regions. They are placed under the galea, superficial to the periosteum. It usually requires up to 12 weeks to complete the expansion in children. Radial scoring of the galea at the time of surgery can facilitate the process. Once the expansion is complete, flaps are advanced or transposed, based on named arteries of the scalp. It is important to orient flaps so that the correct direction of hair growth is maintained. Although galeal scoring or capuslotomy incisions can be useful, wide undermining is a safer method of recruiting tissue.

Forehead. The brow position is the most important structure to preserve during forehead expansion. When possible, two or more expanders are used with incisions hidden within the hairline.

Midforehead nevi are best treated using an expansion of bilateral normal forehead segments and medial advancement of the flaps, placing scars along the brow and at or posterior to the hairline. Hemiforehead nevi often require serial expansion of the uninvolved area of the forehead to reduce the need for a back-cut. Nevi of the supraorbital and temporal forehead can be treated with a transposition of the expanded normal skin medial to the nevus. When the temporal scalp is minimally involved with nevus, the parietal scalp can be expanded and advanced to create the new hairline. When the temporoparietal scalp is also involved with nevus, a combined advancement and transposition flap provides the proper hair direction for the temporal hairline and allows significantly greater movement of the expanded flap. Once the brow is significantly elevated on either the ipsilateral or contralateral side from the reconstruction, it can only be returned to the preoperative position with the interposition of additional, non–hair-bearing forehead skin. The largest expander possible beneath the uninvolved forehead skin should always be used, occasionally even carrying the expander under the lesion [62].

Face and Neck. The skin of the neck and face is relatively thin. Therefore, multiple expanders with smaller volumes are preferable to a single large expander. In general, however, a single larger expander is preferable to several smaller expanders. Careful planning is essential in determining where to place the expanders, and where incisions should be located in order to preserve aesthetic units, facial symmetry and matching skin color and to avoid distortion of the eyelids and oral commissure. The expander is usually placed above the platysma muscle to avoid risk of facial nerve injury and to keep the flap from being excessively bulky. The expanded flaps are positioned by advancement, rotation, or transposition. Incisions should be placed in skin creases such as the nasolabial fold or along the margins of aesthetic units. Expanding the hairless skin adjacent to the mastoid region can increase the available tissue for reconstructive procedures of the ear. The skin above the clavicle can be expanded to provide full-thickness skin grafts to the face.

Trunk. Unlike the head and neck, there are very few critical landmarks on the trunk that must be preserved. Aside from the breast and nipple-areola complex, distortion of the skin and soft tissues of the trunk is well-tolerated. For defects requiring excision, multiple expanders surrounding the defect are often employed. Expanders can also be used to expand the skin of the abdomen for use as a donor site of full-thickness skin grafts.

Extremities. Tissue expansion in the extremities has been reported to have a higher complication rate, in comparison to other regions and therefore, especially in children, should not be a first choice. Blood supply and drainage of the extremities is inferior to that of the trunk and head. This predisposes limbs, especially below the knee, to an increased rate of wound complications such as infection, dehiscence and prosthesis extrusion. Multiple expanders are usually required in the extremites.

Complications. Among all patients, the major complication rate is about 10% and includes implant exposure, deflation, and wound dehiscence. Minor complications also occur in about 10% of patients. These include filling port problems, seroma, hematoma, infection and delayed healing.

Patients under the age of 7 have the highest risk of complications. One explanation for this is that young children are more prone to expander rupture due to external pressure on the expanded skin. Expansion in the extremities caries twice the risk of complication compared to other regions. The use of tissue expansion in congenital nevi has a 5-7% complication rate. Tissue that has undergone serial expansion (two or more prior expansions) is at a higher risk for a major complication.

7. Surgery of primary melanoma

Pediatric melanoma is rare but increasing in incidence [63] limited options are possible for treatment. Early diagnosis and surgical management are the cornerstone of therapy and must adhere to the guidelines estabilished by the American Joint Committee on Cancer (AJCC) [64] Diagnosis of melanoma in children is more difficult than in adults, it relates to a number of variables, so many criteria used in adults are of limited value, for example the natural evolution of congenital and acquired nevi during childhood and adolescence [65] Historically, a wide excision with 5-cm margins with regional lymph node dissection was recommended for all melanomas. This indication, dating back 1907, was based on evaluations following a single necropsy, on a patient with advanced melanoma, assuming that in this way, all possible neoplastic foci would have been eliminated.

Furthermore, the indications suggested to extend the excision below the fascia, so as to also remove the superficial vascular and lymphatic structures.

This attitude has remained unchanged, until Breslow and Match described the treatment of melanoma with narrow margins [66]

Once decided to remove a suspicious lesion, it is recommended to perform a 1- to 2-mm circumferential margin. There are no prospective data to provide an evidence-based approach in this setting.

It has long been suggested that malignant cells may be shed into the bloodstream during any given surgical procedure for cancer. While there is no evidence to suggest that an incisional biopsy does cause local spread of melanoma, it is generally not advocated. [67]

There may be times that the incision is to big that the tissue are not able to cover the skin defect, in this case is possible to use a skin graft, or in order to avoid a graft, the surgical defect may be closed using a rotational or advancement flap

The orientation of the incision should follow the relaxed skin tension lines (RSTLs, also known as lines of Langer), however, at the level of the limbs incisions parallel to the major axis of the limb are used, not to alter the paths of lymphatic drainage.

In the setting of dysplastic changes or once the diagnosis of melanoma is established, in children, surgical excision should be performed with the same excision margins recommended for adults by the National Comprehensive Cancer Network (NCCN) in 2007, and depends on the Breslow depth of the primary lesion, Clark's level of tumor invasion may provide additional prognostic value for thin melanomas [68].

The basic oncologic criteria of surgery are: the resection margins and the depth of the skin excision.

When there is an in situ melanoma, excision should include 0,5 centimeter of normal skin surrounding the tumor and takes off the skin layers down to the fat; in removing an invasive melanoma that is 2 mm thick the margins are extended to 1 cm and the excision goes through all skin layers and down to the fascia; margins are 2 cm for lesions greater than 2 mm in thickness. [69]

The depth of excision can reach muscolaris fascia, whose removal has no oncological meaning, furthermore the preservation of the fascia allows a better aesthetic result.

An exception is the localization to the face, in these cases also with melanomas more than 4 mm thick margins of 1 cm are used.

In recent years, great importance was served to sentinel lymph node biopsy (SLNB) for the detection of lymph node metastases, in fact in adult melanoma therapy, it has become a mandatory procedure in the current AJCC staging system; however its use in the pediatric population has been limited.

Lymph node are the most common site of initial metastases [70], the lack of disease in the sentinel lymph node should indicate the lack of dissemination.

SLNB will select, with a minimally invasive technique, patients who should undergo regional lymph node dissection for clinically occult loco-regional metastases, so as to avoid completion lymph node dissection if the sentinel node is negative.

SLNB was first described by Morton et al. in 1992 [71] The procedure is usually performed concurrent with re-excision of the primary lesion, and is advised for lesions thicker than 1 mm or for those between 0,76 mm and 1 mm with ulceration or reticular dermal invasion.

The procedure involves injection of the primary cutaneous lesion site with technectium-99m sulfur colloid followed by lymphoscintigraphy in the nuclear medicine suite. This is done on the morning of scheduled re-excision, and the patient is brought to the operating room in the afternoon. The lesion is injected with approximately 1 ml of 1% isosulfan blue dye. The dye is allowed to travel through lymphatics for several minutes, and a hand held gamma counter is used to determine the area of maximal radiolabeled tracer intensity for lymph node sampling. An incision is made over the area identified to have the most active uptake of radiolabeled tracer as determined by the handled gamma probe and the preoperative lymphoscintigraphy. Upon examination of the draining lymph node basin, all nodes that are blue, palpable, or show significant activity with the gamma probe are excised and sent fresh to pathology [72].

The incision must be oriented so as to allow an eventual loco-regional lymphadenectomy, the lymph node is identified with the gamma camera and visually with the blue dye; the lymph node is removed after ligation of the afferent and efferent lymphatic vessels, after the removal it is necessary to evaluate "ex vivo" the radioactivity of the lymph node and the possible presence of other involved nodes.

A small lymphocele may result in postoperative period, usually with the possibility of spontaneous regression.

Elective regional lymph node dissection is subsequently performed if the result of the SLNB is positive for metastases [38].

8. Treatment of metastatic disease

8.1. Congenital melanoma and transplacental metastases

Congenital melanoma as a result of placental transmission from a mother with metastatic melanoma is extremely rare, with only a few cases described in literature [73, 74, 75, 76, 77]

To date, metastatic disease transmission from fetus to mother has never been reported. [78, 79]

8.2. Lymph node metastases

8.2.1. Staging

After primary surgery and diagnosis of melanoma, staging of the disease is completed by pathologic detection of lymphatic involvement. Comprehensive staging guidelines for paediatric and adolescent melanoma have not been clearly established.

The American Joint Committee on Cancer (AJCC) provides a reproducible model on the natural history of melanoma and a detailed description of important prognostic variables. For localised disease, ulceration has been recognized as an important predictor of outcome and growing consideration is given to the significance of melanoma thickness. New importance has been recognized to the number of lymph nodes involved, the significance of in-transit or satellite metastases, the description of the sites of metastases and the prognostic value of serum lactic dehydrogenase [23].

Future trials including paediatric and adolescent melanoma patients should incorporate this new staging system to achieve a wider interpretation of results from institutions and patient populations. In addition, the routine use of sentinel node biopsy for the staging of paediatric and adolescent melanoma is mandatory, in order to determine the prognostic and therapeutic value of this procedure in young patients and to compare these results with those reported in the adult literature [80]

Although in adult patients the routine use of chest and abdomen computed tomography is not recommended in literature, in paediatric patients it has been found useful in about 25% of cases to identify clinically undetectable metastases from thick localised melanomas or patients with melanoma arising at an unknown primary site [81, 82]

The routine use of magnetic resonance imaging (MRI) to detect brain metastases is not advocated. For localised lesions under 1.5mm thick, investigations include a complete blood count, serum chemistries including liver function tests, and a chest radiograph.

Positron emission tomography (PET) is a very useful tool in adults, but its use in paediatric patients has not been validated [23]

8.2.2. Sentinel lymph nodes

Early primary excision of melanoma is the mainstay of definitive treatment of the tumour. With the introduction of sentinel lymph node biopsy (SLNB) the treatment of patients with melanoma has been revolutioned.

The adoption of SLNB has led to selection of patients who do not need elective lymph node dissection (ELND) and in which the morbidity linked to this procedure can be avoided. The techniques of preoperative lymphoscintigraphy and sentinel lymph node (SLN) biopsy have become the standard of care for staging adult patients after detection of a primary melanoma. SLNB is particularly important in intermediate-thickness (1.2-3.5 mm) primary melanomas in order to indicate elective lymphadenectomy and has also a prognostic value [83]. SLNB is a very promising technique also in paediatric patients [84, 85, 86]. However, due to paucity of available data, the role of SLNB in paediatric patients is still debated, as concerns both its prognostic [87] and therapeutic implications.

SLN biopsy should be included in the surgical management of children. The indications for SLN biopsy in paediatric and adolescent patients are based on the adult literature and include the presence of lesions thicker than 1 mm, the presence of ulceration or a Clark's level of invasion of IV or V in patients with lesion thickness of less than 1 mm. The technique is the same as in adults. Excision with 2 mm margins of normal skin is performed. After diagnosis of melanoma, the patient undergoes SLNB for tumour thickness ≥ 1 mm followed by wide excision of the tumour site with 2 cm margins and primary closure or skin graft. SLNB is performed using preoperative lymphoscintigraphy, intraoperative blue dye injection around the site of excision and hand-held gamma probe for radio-localization [38,88]. One day before the operation, between 18.5 and 40 MBq of Tc-99m microcolloid is injected intradermally around the scar. The drainage of the colloid is localized by detecting radiation, and the location of the SLN is marked on the skin. The position of the SLN is confirmed with a handheld gamma probe before starting the operation. At the author's center the procedure is performed under epidural anaesthesia and sedation or general anaesthesia. As reported by some authors, subcutaneous infusion anaesthesia (SIA) can be useful [89]. Patent blue is additionally injected intradermally around the scar as standard procedure. Sentinel lymph node biopsy is then accomplished with the help of repeated measurements with the handheld gamma probe. The SLN(s) is (are) removed, and the wound is closed.

A comparison between adults and patients younger than 21 years who underwent either lymph node dissection or SLNB showed a higher rate of lymph node metastasis in the paediatric age (44%) as compared to the adult (23.9%). However this finding had no statistical significance. In this series, paediatric patients either with Stage I or Stage II disease showed a 94.4% 10-year survival, while patients with Stage III melanoma had a 60.1% 10-year survival [90]

Recent data show that although the SLNB positivity rate is higher in paediatric and adolescent melanoma patients than in adults, non SLNB positivity and melanoma specific death rate are low [91]

8.2.3. Regional lymph nodes

In case of positive SLNB many surgeons would proceed to a completion lymph node dissection (CLND),

however survival advantage of this procedure is unclear, and is currently being investigated [92, 93, 94]

In a large series of paediatric melanoma cases 18 patients underwent SNLB, and 7 proceeded to undergo CLND because of findings of metastatic disease to the SLN; two of these had tumour-positive lymph nodes on pathologic analysis of the CLND specimen.

Similarly, the presence of metastases in regional lymph nodes after CLND has been diagnosed in 1 of 3 patients by some authors and in 1 of 4 patients by others [38, 92]

8.2.4. Adjuvant therapy

Consideration of systemic therapy after regional lymph nodes involvement by melanoma cells is under investigation. Treatment plans for children must be extrapolated from adult studies.

Interferon alfa-2b is currently used for adjuvant therapy in high-risk melanoma after surgery in adult patients and can also be used in paediatric melanoma patients with acceptable toxicity [95]

8.3. Distant metastases

The incidence of metastatic melanoma has increased over the last three decades, and the death rate continues to climb faster than that of most other cancers. According to the American Cancer Society, there were approximately 68,000 new cases of melanoma in the United States in 2009, and 8,700 melanoma-related deaths. Melanoma is difficult to treat once it has spread beyond the skin to other parts of the body (metastasized). Very few treatment options exist for people with metastatic melanoma.

8.3.1. Treatment of disseminated disease

Most reports describing the treatment of paediatric melanoma are from single institutions in which diagnostic criteria, staging and pathological evaluation of the primary tumour have varied significantly. Dacarbazine, which is the most active agent in adult melanoma, showed encouraging activity in four children with melanoma treated between 1975 and 1984 [96] Other traditional chemotherapeutic regimens have shown some efficacy in metastatic melanoma [23]. The availability of investigational therapies, such as interleukin-2, interferon alfa-2b and vaccines, has been generally restricted to patients who are older than 18 years of age and no prospective trials in adolescents have been performed. Collaborative efforts, now under discussion between paediatric and adult cooperative groups, should help facilitate the enrollment of younger patients onto trials that use experimental therapies.

8.3.2. Radiotherapy

Radiotherapy is rarely indicated in the management of primary paediatric melanoma. However, it should be considered in patients with head and neck melanomas at high risk for parotid or cervical metastases and in those who develop brain metastases. Brain metastases have been reported to occur during the course of the disease in up to 18% of children with melanoma [23]. Ultimately, as in adults, there is no effective therapy for metastatic melanoma in children. Therefore, the main focus of the parent, the paediatrician, and the dermatologist should be risk reduction and early detection of melanoma. The former consists primarily of avoiding intense sunlight exposure, using protective clothing and broad-spectrum sunblock, and educating children. Early detection requires a high index of clinical suspicion, especially by the paediatrician, who sees children with much more regularity than a dermatologist, of any rapidly growing or otherwise atypical pigmented lesion. In addition, the physician should recognize the elevated risk of any child with a family history of melanoma, GCMN, or dysplastic nevi. Again, prevention and early clinical diagnosis are the only current effective cure for cutaneous melanoma [97].

8.4. Prognosis

The outcome for children and adolescents with melanoma also appears to be similar to that reported for adults and is dependent on the initial stage of the tumour. Patients with localised disease have an excellent outcome, whereas those with nodal and distant metastases have estimated 10-year survivals of only 60 and 25%, respectively. Outcome is also stage-dependent and the thickness of the primary lesion correlates with the risk of nodal involvement and subsequent disease recurrence [23]

Melanomas arising on congenital nevi seem to have a better prognosis if they arise during early infancy than in childhood; moreover, metastatic melanoma associated with giant nevi have a worse prognosis than those associated with other skin lesions [32]

Melanoma has also reported to be more frequently metastatic in young children than in adolescents.This can be due to several causative factors but can also reflect a true biologic difference [98, 99]. There were significant differences in baseline characteristics of young children (age < 10 years) compared with adolescents and young adults: the former were more likely to be non-white, to have metastases, to have nodular or other histology, head, face, or neck primaries, thicker lesions and history of cancer.

Multivariate analysis for melanoma survival in children showed significantly worse survival for males, patients with regional or unstaged disease, nodular histology, increasing thickness of the primary tumor, primary disease in the head, face, neck, eye, orbit, central nervous system, genitals, or overlapping sites, earlier year of diagnosis and previous cancer. Five-year melanoma-specific survival for pediatric cases (age < 20 years) was 100% for in situ disease, 96.1% for localized disease, 77.2% for regional disease and 57.3% for distant disease. Five-year overall survival was 88.9% for young children (age < 10 years), 91.5% for adolescents (age 10 to 19 years) and 90.9% for young adults, but the latter data had not statistical significance [100]. Recent data confirm that paediatric melanoma patients in younger ages have an increased risk of lymph node metastasis and thicker tumors. This suggests that the younger paediatric patients may have a disease that differs biologically from that of the older ones [101].

Author details

Andrea Zangari[1], Federico Zangari[2], Mercedes Romano[2], Elisabetta Cerigioni[2], Maria Giovanna Grella[3], Anna Chiara Contini[3] and Martino Ascanio[2]

1 Pediatric Surgery Department San Camillo Hospital, Roma, Italy

2 Pediatric Surgery Department, University Hospital of Ancona, Italy

3 Catholic University of the Sacred Heart, Roma, Italy

References

[1] Clemmensen, O. J, & Kroon, S. The histology of "congenital features" in early acquired melanocytic nevi. *J Am Acad Dermatol*. Oct (1988). , 19(4), 742-6.

[2] Krengel, S, Hauschild, A, & Schafer, T. Melanoma risk in congenital melanocytic nae-
     vi: a systematic review. *Br J Dermatol*. Jul (2006). , 155(1), 1-8.

[3] Ansarin, H, Soltani-arabshahi, R, Mehregan, D, Shayanfar, N, & Soltanzadeh, P.
     Giant congenital melanocytic nevus with neurofibroma-like changes and spina bifida
     occulta. *Int J Dermatol*. Nov (2006). , 45(11), 1347-50.

[4] Cruz, M. A, Cho, E. S, Schwartz, R. A, & Janniger, C. K. Congenital neurocutaneous
     melanosis. *Cutis*. Oct (1997). , 60(4), 178-81.

[5] Silfen, R, Skoll, P. J, & Hudson, D. A. Congenital giant hairy nevi and neurofibroma-
     tosis: the significance of their common origin. *Plast Reconstr Surg*. Oct (2002). , 110(5),
     1364-5.

[6] Cramer, S. F. The melanocytic differentiation pathway in congenital melanocytic ne-
     vi: theoretical considerations. *Pediatr Pathol*. (1988). , 8(3), 253-65.

[7] Kinsler, V. A, Abu-amero, S, Budd, P, Jackson, I. J, Ring, S. M, Northstone, K, et al.
     Germline Melanocortin-Receptor Genotype Is Associated with Severity of Cutaneous
     Phenotype in Congenital Melanocytic Nevi: A Role for MC1R in Human Fetal Devel-
     opment. *J Invest Dermatol*. May 10 (2012). , 1.

[8] Kadonaga, J. N, & Frieden, I. J. Neurocutaneous melanosis: definition and review of
     the literature. *J Am Acad Dermatol*. May (1991). Pt 1):747-55.

[9] Bousema, M. T, et al. Non-von Recklingausen's resembling a giant pigmented nevus.
     J Am Acad Dermatol 20:358, 1989

[10] Everett, M. A. Histopathology of congenital pigmented nevi. *Am J Dermatopathol*. Feb
     (1989). , 11(1), 11-2.

[11] Fitzpatrick, s, et al. Dermatology in General Medicine. Vol. I: 1028, (1999).

[12] Fitzpatrick, s, et al. Dermatology in General Medicine. Vol. I: 1030, (1999).

[13] Wu, P. A, Mancini, A. J, Marghoob, A. A, & Frieden, I. J. Simultaneous occurrence of
     infantile hemangioma and congenital melanocytic nevus: Coincidence or real associ-
     ation?. *J Am Acad Dermatol*. Feb (2008). Suppl):S , 16-22.

[14] Changchien, L, Dusza, S. W, Agero, A. L, et al. Age- and site-specific variation in the
     dermoscopic patterns of congenital melanocytic nevi: an aid to accurate classification
     and assessment of melanocytic nevi. *Arch Dermatol*. Aug (2007). , 143(8), 1007-14.

[15] Hale, E. K, Stein, J, Ben-porat, L, et al. Association of melanoma and neurocutaneous
     melanocytosis with large congenital melanocytic naevi--results from the NYU-
     LCMN registry. *Br J Dermatol*. Mar (2005). , 152(3), 512-7.

[16] Fitzpatrick, s, et al. Dermatology in General Medicine. Vol. I: 1034, (1999).

[17] Fitzpatrick, s, et al. Dermatology in General Medicine. Vol. I: 1018-1025, (1999).

[18] Fitzpatrick, s, et al. Dermatology in General Medicine. Vol. I: 1037-1041, (1999).

[19] Rigel, D. S, et al. The incidence of malignant melanoma in the United States:Issues As we approach the 21st century. *J Am Acad Dermatol* 34:839, (1996).

[20] Cosary, C. L, et al. SEER Cancer Statistics Review, 1973-1992: National Cancer Institute, NRH Pub. Bethesda, Maryland, (1995). (96-2789), 96-2789.

[21] Ries, L, Eisner, M, Kosary, C, et al. SEER Cancer Statistics Review Bethesda, MD, National Cancer Institute, (2004). http://seer.cancer.gov/csr/1975_2001/ , 1975-2000.

[22] Pappo, A. S. Ries LAG, Herzog C, et al: Malignant melanoma in the first three decades of life: A report from the U.S. Surveillance, Epidemiology and End Results (SEER) program. 23:721, (2004). abstr 7557)

[23] Pappo AS: Melanoma in children and adolescentsEur J Cancer 39:2651-2661, (2003).

[24] Kraemer, K. H, Lee, M. M, Andrews, A. D, et al. The role of sunlight and DNA repair in melanoma and nonmelanoma skin cancer: The xeroderma pigmentosum paradigm. Arch Dermatol 130:1018-1021, (1994).

[25] Tucker, M. A. Goldstein AM: Melanoma etiology: Where are we? Oncogene , 22, 3042-3052.

[26] Whiteman, D. C, Valery, P, Mcwhirter, W, et al. Risk factors for childhood melanoma in Queensland, Australia. Int J Cancer 70:26-31, (1997).

[27] Ahmed I: Malignant Melanoma: Prognostic IndicatorsMayo Clin Proc 72:356-361, (1997).

[28] Kaskel, P, Sander, S, Kron, M, et al. Outdoor activities in childhood: A protective factor for cutaneous melanoma? Results of a case-control study in 271 matched pairs. Br J Dermatol 145:602-609, (2001).

[29] Saenz, N. C, Saenz-badillos, J, Busam, K, et al. Childhood melanoma survival. Cancer 85:750-754, (1999).

[30] Milton, G. W, Shaw, H. M, Thompson, J. F, et al. Cutaneous melanoma in childhood: Incidence and prognosis. Australas J Dermatol 38:SS48, (1997). suppl 1), 44.

[31] Fears, T. R, Bird, C. C, Guerry, D I. V, et al. Average midrange ultraviolet radiation flux and time outdoors predict melanoma risk. Cancer Res , 62, 3992-3996.

[32] Tannous, Z. S. Mihm Jr MC, Sober AJ, et al Congenital melanocitic nevi: clinical and istopathologic features, risk of melanoma, and clinical management. J Am Acad Dermatol (2005). , 52(2), 197-203.

[33] Michel, J. L, Chalencon, F, Gentil-perret, A, et al. Congenital pigmented nevus: prognosis and therapeutic possibilities. Arch Pediatr (1999). , 6(2), 211-7.

[34] Ruiz-maldonado, R, Tamayo, L, Laterza, A. M, et al. Giant pigmented naevi: clinical histopatologic and therapeutic considerations. J Pediatr (1992).

[35] Zaal, L. H, & Mooi, W. J. Sillevis Smith JH, et al. Classification of congenital melanocytic naevi and malignant transformation: a review of the literature. Br J Plast Surg (2004). , 57(8), 707-19.

[36] Yesudian, P. D. Parslew RAG. A guide to the management of pigmented skin naevi in children. Curr Paediatr (2003). , 13, 407-12.

[37] Saenz, N. C, Saenz-badillos, J, Busam, K, et al. Childhood melanoma survival. Cancer (1999). , 85, 750-4.

[38] Zangari, A, Bernardini, M. L, Tallarico, R, Ilari, M, Giangiacomi, M, & Offidani, A. M. Martino A: Indications for excision of nevi and melanoma diagnosed in a pediatric surgical unit. J Pediatr Surg. (2007). Aug; , 42(8), 1412-6.

[39] Gelbard, S. N, Tripp, J. M, Marghoob, A. A, et al. Management of Spitz nevi: a survey of dermatologists in the United States. J Am Acad Dermatol (2002). , 47(2), 224-30.

[40] Dyon GCTMSnels MD, Elysèe TM, et al. Risk of cutaneous malignant melanoma in patients with nonfamilial atypical nevi from a pigmented lesions clinic. Leiden, The Netherlands. J Am Acad Dermatol (1999). , 40, 686-93.

[41] Zaal, L. H, Mooi, W. J, Klip, H, et al. Risk of malignant transformation of congenital melanocytic nevi: a retrospective nationwide study from The Netherlands. *Plast Reconstr Surg*. Dec (2005). , 116(7), 1902-9.

[42] Rhodes, A. R, & Melski, J. W. Small congenital nevocellular nevi and the risk of cutaneous melanoma. *J Pediatr*. Feb (1982). , 100(2), 219-24.

[43] Sahin, S, Levin, L, Kopf, A. W, et al. Risk of melanoma in medium-sized congenital melanocytic nevi: a follow-up study. J Am Acad Dermatol. Sep (1998). , 39(3), 428-33.

[44] Kearney-cooke, A. (2002). Familial influences on body image development. In T. F. Cash & T. Pruzinsky (Eds.), Body image: A handbook of theory, and clinical practice (New York: Guilford., 99-107.

[45] Bradbury, E. (1997). Understanding the problems. In R. Lansdown, N. Rumsey, E. Bradbury, A. Carr, & J. Partridge (Eds.), Visibly different: Coping with disfigurement (Oxford: Butterworth-Heinemann., 180-193.

[46] Turner, S, Thomas, P, Dowell, T, Rumsey, N, & Sandy, J. (1997). Psychological outcomes amongst cleft patients and their families. British Journal of Plastic Surgery, , 50, 1-9.

[47] Gilbert, S, & Thompson, J. (2002). Body shame in childhood & adolescence. In P. Gilbert & J. Miles (Eds.), Body Shame (Hove: Brunner-Routledge., 55-74.

[48] Harter, S. (1999). *The construction of the self: A developmental perspective.* New York: Guilford.

[49] Hearst, D, & Middleton, J. (1997). Psychological intervention and models of current working practice. In R. Lansdown, N. Rumsey, E. Bradbury, A. Carr, & J. Partridge (Eds.), *Visibly different: Coping with disfigurement* (Oxford: Butterworth-Heinemann., 158-171.

[50] Bauer, B. S, & Corcoran, J. Treatment of large and giant nevi. *Clin Plast Surg.* Jan (2005). vii., 32(1), 11-8.

[51] Margulis, A, Bauer, B. S, & Fine, N. A. Large and giant congenital pigmented nevi of the upper extremity: an algorithm to surgical management. *Ann Plast Surg.* Feb (2004). , 52(2), 158-67.

[52] Arneja, J. S, & Gosain, A. K. Giant congenital melanocytic nevi. *Plast Reconstr Surg.* Aug (2007). e-40e.

[53] Bauer, B. S, & Corcoran, J. Treatment of large and giant nevi. *Clin Plast Surg.* Jan (2005). vii., 32(1), 11-8.

[54] Pearson, G. D, Goodman, M, & Sadove, A. M. Congenital nevus: the Indiana University's approach to treatment. *J Craniofac Surg.* Sep (2005). , 16(5), 915-20.

[55] Rumsey, N, & Harcourt, D. Body image and disfigurement: issues and interventions. Body Image (2004). , 1(2004), 83-97.

[56] Vinod K JainMahendra K Singhi, and Rajiv Goyal: Serial Excision of Congenital Melanocytic Nevi. J Cutan Aesthet Surg. (2008). January; , 1(1), 17-18.

[57] Gosain, A. K, Santoro, T. D, & Larson, D. L. Gingrass RP Giant congenital nevi: a 20-year experience and an algorithm for their management. Plast Reconstr Surg. (2001). Sep 1; , 108(3), 622-36.

[58] Pasyk, K. A, Argenta, L. C, & Hassett, C. Quantitative analysis of the thickness of human skin and subcutaneous tissue following controlled expansion with a silicone implant. Plast Reconstr Surg. Apr (1988). , 81(4), 516-23.

[59] Timothy, M. Johnson, Md Lori Lowe, Md Marc D. Brown, Md Michael J. Sullivan, Md Bruce R. Nelson, Md: Histology and Physiology of Tissue Expansion. J Dermatol Surg Oncol (1993). , 19, 1074-1078.

[60] Chao, J. J, Longaker, M. T, & Zide, B. M. Expanding horizons in head and neck expansion. Copyright (1998). by W.B. Saunders Company

[61] Farhad HafeziBijan Naghibzadeh, Mohammad Pegahmehr, Amirhossein Nouhi: Use of overinflated tissue expanders in the surgical repair of head and neck scars Journal of Plastic, Reconstructive & Aesthetic Surgery ((2008). xx, 1e8

[62] BauerBruce S. M.D.; Few, Julius W. M.D.; Chavez, C. D. M.D., and; Galiano, R. D. B.A.: The Role of Tissue Expansion in the Management of Large Congenital Pigment-

ed Nevi of the Forehead in the Pediatric Patient. Plastic & Reconstructive Surgery: March (2001). Articles(3-pp), 668-675.

[63]   Lange, J. R, Palis, B. E, Chang, D. C, Soong, S-J, & Balch, C. M. melanoma in children and teenagers: an analysis of patients from the national cancer data base. J Clin Oncol (2007). , 25(11), 2007-1363.

[64]   Balch, C. M, Buzaid, A. C, Soong, S-J, Atkins, M. B, & Cascinelli, N. et alii Final Version of the American Joint Committee on Cancer Staging System for Cutaneous Melanoma. J Clin Oncol, 19, (16) (2001).

[65]   Huynh, P. M, Grant-kels, J. M, & Grin, C. M. Childhood melanoma: update and treatment. Int J Dermatol (2005).

[66]   Eedy, D. J. Surgical treatment of melanoma. Brit J Dermatol 149, (2003).

[67]   Swanson, N. A. Lee Kl, Gorman A, Lee HN. Biopsy techniques: diagnosis of melanoma. Dermatol Clin 20, (2002).

[68]   NCCNNCCN clinical practice guidelines in oncology: melanoma (Washington, DC: NCCN (2008). , 2

[69]   Swetter, S. M. Malignant melanoma. eMedicine.com, Inc.(2004).

[70]   Faries, M. B, & Morton, D. L. Surgery and sentinel lymph node biopsy. Semin Oncol (2007). December; , 34(6), 498-508.

[71]   Morton, D. L, Wen, D. R, & Wong, J. H. Technical details of intraoperative lymphatic mapping for early stage melanoma. Arch Surg (1992). , 127, 392-399.

[72]   Downard, C. D, Rapkin, L. B, & Gow, K. W. Melanoma in children and adolescents. Surgical Oncol ((2007).

[73]   Wiggins, C. L, Berwick, M, et al. Malignant Melanoma in Pregnancy Newton Bishop Obstet Gynecol Clin N Am (2005). , 32(2005), 559-568.

[74]   Richardson, S. K, & Tannous, Z. S. Mihm Jr MC. Congenital and infantile melanoma: review of theliterature and report of an uncommon variant, pigment-synthesizing melanoma. J Am AcadDermatol (2002). , 47, 77-90.

[75]   Alexander, A, Samlowski, W. E, Grossman, D, et al. Metastatic melanoma in pregnancy: risk oftransplacental metastases in the infant. J Clin Oncol (2003). Baergen RN, Johnson D, Moore T, et al. Maternal melanoma metastatic to the placenta: a case report and review of the literature. Arch Pathol Lab Med 1997;121:508-11;, 21, 2179-86.

[76]   Dildy III GAMoise Jr KJ, Carpenter Jr RJ, et al. Maternal malignancy metastatic to the products of conception: a review. Obstet Gynecol Surv (1989). Dargeon HW, Eversole J, Del Duca V. Malignant melanoma in an infant. Cancer 1950;3:299-306;, 44, 535-40.

[77]   Brodsky, I, Baren, M, & Kahn, S. B. Lewis G Jr, Tellem M. Metastatic malignant melanoma from mother to fetus. Cancer (1965). , 18, 1048-54.

[78] Richardson, S. K, & Tannous, Z. S. Mihm Jr MC. Congenital and infantile melanoma: review of the literature and report of an uncommon variant, pigment-synthesizing melanoma. J Am Acad Dermatol (2002). , 47, 77-90.

[79] Brenn, T. Phillip H McKee P: Melanoma in children and adolescents Diagnostic Histopathology, January (2008). , 14(1), 18-27.

[80] Kogut, K. A, Fleming, M, Pappo, A. S, et al. Sentinel lymph node biopsy for melanoma in young children. J Pediatr Surg (2000). , 35, 965-6.

[81] Buzaid, A. C, Sandler, A. B, Mani, S, et al. Role of computed tomography in the staging of primary melanoma. J Clin Oncol (1993). , 1993(11), 638-643.

[82] Kaste, S. C, & Pappo, A. S. Jenkins III JJ, Pratt CB. Malignant melanoma in children: imaging spectrum. Pediatr Radiol (1996). , 1996(26), 800-805.

[83] Morton, D. L, Thompson, J. F, Cochran, A. J, et al. MSLT Group. Sentinel node biopsy or nodal observation in melanoma. N Engl J Med (2006). , 355, 1307-17.

[84] Roaten, J. B, Partrick, D. A, Pearlman, N, et al. Sentinel lymph node biopsy for melanoma and other melanocytic tumors in adolescents. J Pediatr Surg (2005). , 40, 232-5.

[85] Toro, J, Ranieri, J. M, Havlik, R. J, et al. Sentinel lymph node biopsy in children and adolescents with malignant melanoma. J Pediatr Surg (2003). , 38, 1063-75.

[86] Pacella, S. J, Lowe, L, Bradford, C, et al. The utility of sentinel lymph node biopsy in head and neck melanoma in the pediatric population. Plast Reconstr Surg (2003). , 112, 1257-65.

[87] Roka, F, Kittler, H, Cauzig, P, et al. Sentinel node status in melanoma patients is not predictive for overall survival upon multivariate analysis. Br J Cancer (2005). , 92, 662-7.

[88] Butter AndreanaHuib Tom, Chapdelaine Joyaube, Beaunoyer Mona, Flageole Helene, Bouchard Sarah: Melanoma in children and the use of sentinel lymph node biopsy. Journal of Pediatric Surgery ((2005).

[89] Topar GerdaZelger Bernhard: Assessment of value of the sentinel lymph node biopsy in melanoma in children and adolescents and applicability of subcutaneous infusion anestesia Journal of Pediatric Surgery ((2007).

[90] Livestro, D. P, Kaine, E. M, Michaelson, J. S, et al. Melanoma in the young: differences and similarities with adult melanoma: a case-matched controlled analysis. Cancer (2007). , 110, 614-24.

[91] Robert Howman-GilesMD et Al. Sentinel Lymph Node Biopsy in Pediatric and Adolescent Cutaneous Melanoma Patients. Ann Surg Oncol ((2010).

[92]   Gow, K. W, Rapkin, L. B, Olson, T. A, Durham, M. M, & Wyly, B. Shehata BM: Senti-
       nel lymph node biopsy in the pediatric population. Journal of Pediatric Surgery
       ((2008).

[93]   Sabel, M. S, & Arora, A. The role of the surgeon in the management of melanoma.
       Minerva Chir (2006). , 61, 54-141.

[94]   Mcmasters, K. M, Reintgen, D. S, Ross, M. I, et al. Sentinel lymph node biopsy for
       melanoma: controversy despite widespread agreement. Journal of Clinical Oncology
       (2001). , 19, 2851-5.

[95]   Shah, N. C, Gerstle, J. T, Stuart, M, et al. Use of sentinel lymph node biopsy and high-
       dose interferon in pediatric patients with high-risk melanoma: the Hospital for Sick
       Children experience. J Pediatr Hematol Oncol (2006). , 28, 496-500.

[96]   Boddie AW JrCangir A. Adjuvant and neoadjuvant chemotherapy with dacarbazine
       in high-risk childhood melanoma. Cancer. (1987). Oct 15; , 60(8), 1720-3.

[97]   Fishman, C, & Mihm, M. C. Sober AJ: Diagnosis and Management of Nevi And Cuta-
       neous Melanoma in Infants And Children. Clinics in Dermatology Y (2002). , 20,
       44-50.

[98]   Bressac-de-paillerets, B, Avril, M. F, Chompret, A, & Demenais, F. Genetic and envi-
       ronmental factors in cutaneous malignant melanoma. Biochimie. (2002). , 84, 67-74.

[99]   Brenn, T. McKee PH: Melanoma in children and adolescents Diagnostic Histopathol-
       ogy, January (2008). , 14(1), 18-27.

[100] Strouse, J. J, Fears, T. R, & Tucker, M. A. Wayne AS: Pediatric Melanoma: Risk Factor
       and Survival Analysis of the Surveillance, Epidemiology and End Results Database
       Journal of Clinical Oncology, July 20), (2005). , 23(21), 4735-4741.

[101] Moore-olufemi, S, Herzog, C, & Warneke, C. Gershenwald Jerry E, Mansfield P, Ross
       M, Prieto V, Lally KP and Hayes-Jordan A: Outcomes in Pediatric Melanoma. Com-
       paring Prepubertal to Adolescent Pediatric Patients. Annals of Surgery (2011). ,
       253(6), 1211-15.

Chapter 4

Adoptive Cell Therapy of Melanoma: The Challenges of Targeting the Beating Heart

Jennifer Makalowski and Hinrich Abken

Additional information is available at the end of the chapter

1. Introduction

The identification of melanoma-associated antigens, the isolation of tumor infiltrating T cells from melanoma lesions, and the significant progress in engineering redirected T cells has favored the development of various strategies in the adoptive immunotherapy of melanoma. Recent trials in adoptive cell therapy (ACT) have achieved spectacular results in inducing remission in advanced stages of the disease, although produced on-target off-tumor toxicities, emphasizing the tremendous potential benefit of harnessing the immune system for fighting the disease. Moreover, the identification of so-called melanoma stem cells along with strategies for selectively eliminating subsets of melanoma cells implies that there is a need for redefining therapeutic targets in melanoma. This review discusses current challenges in the rational design of adoptive cell therapy to target "the beating heart" of melanoma.

1.1. Advanced stages of melanoma resist conventional therapeutic regimens

Surgical resection of tumor lesions in early stages of the disease is the curative option for combating melanoma; a 10-year-survival rate of 75 - 85% can be achieved for melanoma in stage I or II. However, melanoma in stage III or IV is still associated with low survival rates of less than 1 year upon diagnosis [1]. Despite the development of novel drugs and major improvements in therapeutic regimens, significant responses were only achieved in predefined groups and of short duration. Treatment with the chemotherapeutic drug dacarbazine (DTIC) and vemurafenib, an inhibitor of mutated BRAF, produced a median progression-free survival of 64% with dacarbazine, respectively 84% with vemurafenib of approximately 6 months [2-4]. The biology of melanoma and the heterogeneity of malignant cells are thought to be responsible for this unsatisfactory situation. First, melanoma cells can persist for long periods of time in a "dormant" stage without any progression in tumor formation [5]. Second, melanoma cells can disseminate early into distant organs including the brain forming micro-metastases, which are small in cell numbers and frequently beyond the detection limit of current imaging procedures [6, 7]. Third, many melanoma cells are notoriously resistant to chemo- and radiation therapy [8-10], making alternative strategies in tumor cell elimination necessary.

Therefore, in more progressed stages of the disease the recruitment of the cellular immune defense to eliminate cancer cells is thought to be an alternative. Administration of high dose interleukin-2 (IL-2) [11] and anti-cytotoxic T-lymphocyte-associated antigen-4 (CTLA-4) antibody [12] as well as interferon (IFN) α-2b prolongs the disease-free survival although at a relatively low response rate and without being curative over time [13, 14]. However, these and other observations imply that activation or modulation of the patient's immune response may be effective in the treatment of melanoma. A number of approaches for enhancing the immune cell response against melanoma are currently explored with some success. In particular, the adoptive transfer of autologous T cells isolated from melanoma lesions and expanded to large numbers ex vivo has produced encouraging phase II results [15, 16]. The administration of patient's blood T cells engineered with defined specificity for melanoma-associated antigens are additionally being explored in a number of trials. In this review, we summarize evidence for the potency of adoptive T cell therapy in the treatment of melanoma and discuss current challenges in achieving long-term remission. Upcoming strategies in selective targeting cancer stem cells are also discussed.

2. Adoptive cell therapy can successfully fight melanoma

Melanoma can trigger a curative immune response; this conclusion is drawn from the clinical observation of spontaneous and complete melanoma regressions and of the higher frequency of melanomas among immune compromised patients [17, 18]. More direct evidence for the immune cell control of melanoma growth was obtained by the treatment with high dose IL-2, which produces an objective response rate of 16%. Indeed, some of the patients receiving thus treatment exhibit a long-term complete response for years [11, 19]. These observations are remarkable in light of the low and short-lived response rates after chemotherapy and currently drive the development of adoptive T cell therapy for treatment of late stage melanoma.

The development of adoptive cell therapy (ACT) was further strengthened by upcoming technologies in isolating tumor infiltrating lymphocytes (TIL's) from melanoma biopsies (Figure 1). First described in 1969 [20], TIL's from melanoma lesions consisted of both effector and helper T cell subsets and can be expanded ex vivo in the presence of IL-2. The expanded cells are then selected for melanoma reactivity. A strong rationale for using these T cells in adoptive therapy is provided by the observation that the infusion of high TIL numbers correlates with better clinical outcome [21, 22] although the prevalence of TIL's in primary melanoma lesions and metastases is not a prognostic factor itself.

Protocols according to GMP standards have been established in several centers to isolate and amplify TIL's to numbers appropriate for adoptive therapy. Melanoma reactive T cells are expanded in the presence of IL-2 by culture on feeder cells expressing melanoma antigens [23]. Subsequent to TIL re-infusions, metastases regressed in the majority of patients and a stable disease phase followed. However, only few patients remained in complete remission [21]. The disappointing therapeutic efficacy, despite high numbers of infused TIL's is thought to be due to low responsiveness of highly expanded T cells which are unable to execute a productive anti-melanoma attack after administration to the patient. Current TIL protocols therefore attempt to administer so-called "young TIL's" (Figure 1), i.e. melanoma infiltrating T cells which underwent short-term culture expansions and therefore passed through fewer cell division cycles prior to re-infusion and thereby exhibit a less differentiated phenotype [24]. Another change in protocols is that TIL's are not selected for melanoma reactivity; the rationale behind this is that re-infusion of *ex vivo* IFN-γ secreting TIL's exhibited no major benefit compared to non-responding TIL's [16]. Early phase I trials showed improved persistence of young TIL's [25] and 50% response rates in a cohort of 20 patients [26], which is just as effective as traditionally grown TIL's [27]. Different non-randomized phase II trials at the NCI and at Sheba Medical Center confirmed these early observations (Table 1) [28, 29]. A roadmap describing critical steps for comparative testing the TIL strategy in a randomized multi-center setting was recently published in a White Paper on adoptive cell therapy [30].

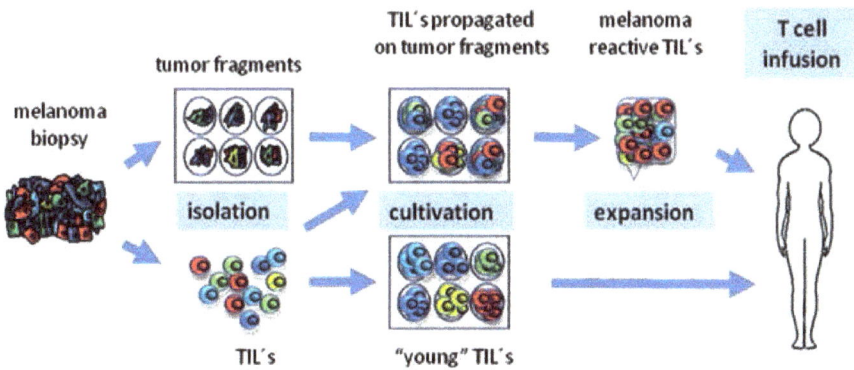

Figure 1. Adoptive cell therapy for metastatic melanoma. Adoptive cell therapy with tumor infiltrating lymphocytes (TIL´s) makes use of melanoma-specific TIL´s which are isolated from a melanoma biopsy, amplified *ex vivo* by stimulation with melanoma biopsy cells and propagated to high numbers in the presence of IL-2. In more recent trials, TIL´s are propagated short-term ex vivo without stimulation by melanoma cells and administered as "young" TIL´s.

Target antigen	Adoptively transferred T cells	NCT ID / Reference	Center
	melanoma specific CD8⁺ T cells	[118]	FHCRC
	melanoma specific T cells	[119]	LUMC
MART-1	MART-1 specific CD8⁺ T cells	[113]	DFCI
MART-1	MART-1 specific CD8⁺ T cells	NCT00512889	DFCI
MART-1	MART-1 specific CD8⁺ T cells	[87]	UR
MART-1	MART-1 specific CD8⁺ T cells	[33]	UNH
MART-1	MART-1 specific CD8⁺ T cells	NCT00324623	CHUV
MART-1	MART-1 specific CD8⁺ T cells	NCT01106235	FHCRC
NY-ESO-1	NY-ESO-1 specific CD8⁺ T cells and anti-CTLA-4 antibody	NCT00871481	FHCRC
	TILs	[114]	NIH
	TIL	[120]	NIH
	TILs	[27]	NIH
	TILs	[29]	NIH
	TILs	[115]	NIH
	TILs	NCT00287131	SMC
	TILs	NCT000604136	HMO
	TILs	NCT01005745	MOFFITT
	TILs and IFN-γ	NCT01082887	NUH
	"young" TILs	[116]	NIH
	"young" TILs	[28]	SMC
	"young" TILs	NCT01118091	NIH
	"young" TILs	NCT01319565	NIH
	"young" TILs	NCT01369888	MIH
	"young" TILs	NCT01468818	NIH
	"young" TILs	NCT00513604	NIH
MART-1	MART-1 specific TILs	NCT00720031	NUH
MART-1	MART-1 specific TILs (DMF5)	NCT00924001	CC
	IL-2 engineered TILs	[117]	NIH
	IL-2 engineered TIL	NCT00062036	NIH
	IL-12 engineered TIL	NCT01236573	NIH
	CXCR2 engineered TIL	[86]	MDACC
NY-ESO-1	anti-NY-ESO-1 TCR	[121]	NIH
NY-ESO-1	anti-NY-ESO-1 TCR	NCT00670748	NIH
MART-1	anti-MART-1 TCR (low-affinity)	[49]	NIH
MART-1	anti-MART-1 TCR	NCT00910650	UC
MART-1	anti-MART-1 TCR (high-affinity)	[38]	NIH
gp-100	anti-gp-100 TCR	[38]	NIH
MART-1	anti-MART-1 TCR	[114]	NIH
gp-100	anti-gp-100 TCR	[114]	NIH
MART-1	anti-MART-1 TCR	NCT00612222	NIH
gp-100	anti-gp-100 TCR	NCT00610311	NIH
MART-1	anti-MART-1 TCR plus MART-1 vaccination	NCT00923195	NIH
gp-100	anti-gp-100 TCR plus gp-100 vaccination	NCT00923195	NIH
p53	anti-p53 TCR	NCT00393029	NIH
VEGFR2	anti-VEGFR2 CAR engineered CD8⁺ T cells	NCT01218867	NIH
Ganglioside GD-3	anti-GD-3 CAR	PI: M. Davies	MDACC

CHUV, Centre Hospitalier Universitaire Vaudois; **DFCI**, Dana-Farber Cancer Institute; **FHCRC**, Fred Hutchinson Cancer Research Center; **HMO**, Hadassah Medical Organization; **LUMC**, Leiden University Medical Center; **MDACC**, M.D. Anderson Cancer Center; **MOFFITT**, H. Lee Moffitt Cancer Center and Research Institute; **NIH**, National Institutes of Health; **NUH**, Nantes University Hospital; **PI**, principal investigator; **SMC**, Sheba Medical Center; **UC**, University of California; **UR**, University of Regensburg

Table 1. Adoptive cell therapy trials in patients with metastatic melanoma

3. Adoptive cell therapy with antigen-specific T cells

The rationale for using melanoma antigen-specific T cells is based on the observation that the success of TIL therapy in some patients correlates with the presence of melanoma-reactive T cells, in particular with those cells specific for Melan-A, MART-1 or gp100 [23, 31]. The median survival of patients treated with Melan-A specific TIL's was 53.5 months compared to 3.5 months for patients who received TIL's without Melan-A specificity [32]. These observations together with a number of technical obstacles in obtaining TIL's from biopsies strengthened efforts to derive melanoma-specific T cell clones from peripheral blood lymphocytes for the use in adoptive cell therapy. The strategy was corroborated by a 50% response rate obtained after transfer of MART-1 or gp100 specific T cell clones isolated and propagated *ex vivo* from peripheral blood lymphocytes (Table 1) [33]. Melanoma reactive T cell clones in peripheral blood are rare, TIL therapy increases the otherwise low magnitude of the tumor-reactive T cell compartment *in vivo*, which matches the reactivity in the TIL product [34]. Interestingly, individual TIL products from different patients contain unique patterns of reactivity against shared melanoma-associated antigens [34]. TIL isolation and expansion *in vitro*, however, is extremely laborious. This limit leads to attempts to engineer patient's blood T cells with pre-defined specificity for more specifically redirecting the cytotoxic response toward melanoma. It is therefore assumed that the clinical efficacy of TIL therapy can be improved by application of T cells with more defined tumor-reactivity.

To engineer specificity for melanoma, T cell receptors (TCR's) were cloned from TIL's of responding melanoma patients and transferred to peripheral blood T cells of the same patient (Figure 2) [35-38]. The gp100 specific TCR was one of the first TCR's, cloned from melanoma TIL's and introduced *ex vivo* by retrovirus-mediated gene transfer into blood T cells, which thus obtained redirected specificity for gp100 positive cells. In contrast to their non-modified counterparts, TCR engineered T cells responded to gp100$^+$ melanoma cells by secreting pro-inflammatory cytokines including IFN-γ and by lysing the target cells [45, 46]. Similarly, blood T cells were engineered with recombinant TCR's with specificity for MART-1 or MAGE-A1. The functional avidity of cloned TCR's was improved and engineered T cells were successfully used in subsequent trials [47, 48]. About 30% of patients receiving ACT with MART-1 specific T cells responded with melanoma regression; 19% of patients treated with gp100 specific TCR T cells exhibited objective response, most responses were persistent [38]. TCR engineered T cells also showed efficacy towards brain metastases, which indicates that patients with otherwise incurable metastatic sites may benefit from ACT (Table 1) [115]. In patients with prolonged clinical remission, engineered T cells were present in the circulation for more than a year after initiation of treatment; this indicates that therapeutic efficacy and long-term anti-melanoma immunity may correlate with T cell persistence [49, 50].

However, the enthusiasm for adoptive cell therapy with TCR modified T cells has been dampened by several limitations. Tumor cells including those of the melanoma undergo clonal evolution, and some of these evolved cells evade T cell recognition, for instance, as a result of repression of their MHC complex [51], of mutations in their β2 microglobulin chain [52], and of deficiencies in their antigen processing machinery [51, 53]. Each of these altera-

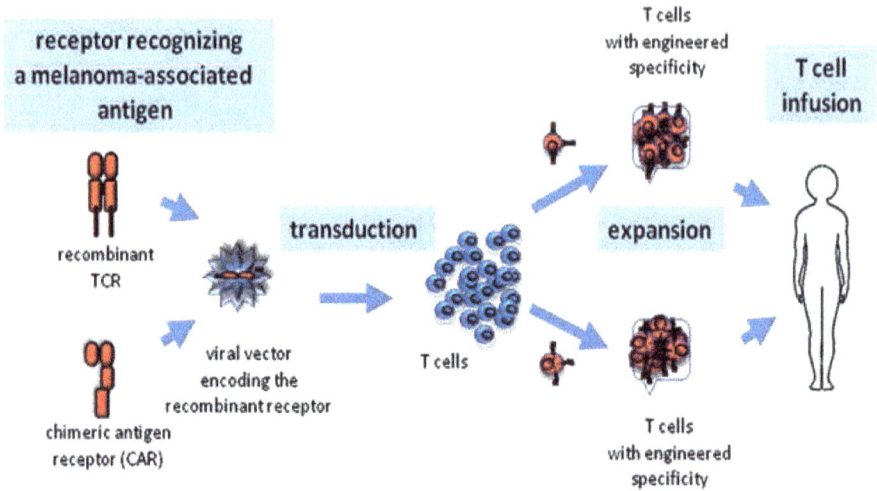

Figure 2. Adoptive cell therapy with redirected T cells. T cells from the peripheral blood of the patient are engineered *ex vivo* by retro- or lentiviral gene transfer with cDNA coding for a T cell receptor (TCR) with specificity for a melanoma-associated antigen. Alternatively, T cells are engineered with a chimeric antigen receptor (CAR) which recognizes a melanoma-associated antigen by an antibody-derived binding domain. Engineered T cells are expanded *ex vivo* prior to administration to the patient.

tions renders the melanoma cell invisible to a TCR-mediated T cell attack. A possible safety hazard moreover became apparent when analyzing in more detail the transgenic TCR, which is co-expressed with the physiological TCR in the same T cell. The transgenic TCR turned out to create new but unpredictable specificities by forming hetero-dimers of the recombinant α and β TCR chains with the respective chains of the physiological TCR. Undesirable mispairing of TCR chains may result in loss of specificity and may induce severe auto-reactivity [54, 55]. Tremendous efforts were subsequently made to solve the problem including replacement of TCR constant moieties by the homologous murine domains [56] and creation of additional cysteine bridges [57] to enforce preferential pairing of the recombinant $\alpha\beta$ TCR chains in the presence of the physiological TCR.

These and other technical difficulties promoted the development of an artificial "one-chain-receptor" molecule to redirect T cells in an antigen-restricted manner (Figure 3). In a seminal paper Zelig Eshhar of the Weizmann Institute of Science described a chimeric antigen receptor (CAR), also named immunoreceptor, which is composed in the extracellular part of a single chain antibody for antigen binding and in the intracellular part of the TCR/CD3ζ endodomain for provision of T cell activation [58]. The CAR modified T cell, also known as "T-body", becomes activated by binding to antigen, and secretes pro-inflammatory cytokines, amplifies and lyses target cells expressing the respective antigen. By using an antibody for binding, the CAR recognizes the target in a MHC-independent fashion and is therefore not affected by loss of HLA molecules, which frequently occurs during neoplastic progression. An additional advantage over transgenic TCR's is that CAR's can be used inde-pendently of the individual HLA subtype. However, the T-body strategy is restricted to an-tigens expressed on the surface of the target cell; intracellular antigens are not visible to CAR's. Due to the broad variety of antibodies available, a nearly unlimited panel of antigens can be targeted with high affinity and specificity, including those which are not classical T cell antigens, e.g. carbohydrates. High affinity CAR's activate engineered T cells even after binding to low amounts of target antigen; this not only makes the approach highly sensitive, but also makes the choice of the appropriate melanoma-selective antigen difficult.

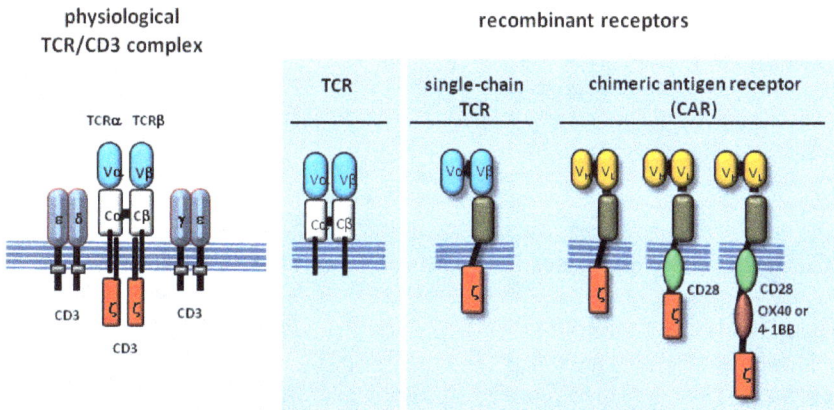

Figure 3. Recombinant receptors to redirect T cells for use in antigen-specific cell therapy. The physiologic T cell receptor (TCR)/CD3 complex consists of the α and β TCR chains, which recognize major histocompatibility complex (MHC)-presented antigen by binding through both variable regions Vα Vβ, and of the CD3 chains. Antigen engage-ment induces clustering of the TCR complex and the primary signal for T cell activation is generated by the intracellu-lar CD3ζ chain. Recombinant TCR α and β chains can be engineered to T cells in order to provide a new specificity. Alternatively, the V regions of the TCR chains can be combined and fused to the intracellular CD3ζ chain to produce a T cell activation signal upon binding to antigen. The chimeric antigen receptor (CAR) makes use of an antibody bind-ing domain for antigen recognition which is enigneered by fusing the variable (V) regions of the immunoglobulin heavy (H) and light (L) chain. The V_H-V_L single chain antibody is linked via a spacer to the intracellular CD3ζ chain to produce the primary T cell activation signal upon antigen binding. Intracellular signaling domains of costimulatory molecules like CD28 can be added to provide appropriate costimulation in addition to the primary CD3ζ signal.

T cells require two signals for full and lasting activation, one provided by the TCR and the other by costimulatory co-receptors; the prototype of which is CD28. The corresponding li-gands are usually not present in the tumor micro-environment. Some effector functions in-cluding IL-2 secretion require CD28 costimulation along with the primary TCR/CD3ζ signal; this provides a rationale for combining the intracellular CD3ζ with the CD28 signaling do-main in one polypeptide chain (Figure 3) [59]. Other costimulatory domains, such as 4-1BB (CD137) and OX40 (CD134), were also linked to CD3ζ; each domain has a different impact on T cell effector functions [60]. Costimulatory domains were furthermore combined in so-called 3rd generation CAR's, and a number of additional modifications have been introduced in the last years to improve T cell persistence and activation [61, 62]. CAR's with a costimulatory domain clearly demonstrated clinical benefit and improved T cell persistence compared to CAR's targeting the same antigen but with only the CD3ζ domain [63-65].

Various CARs were engineered for targeting melanoma-associated antigens, including HMW-MAA, also known as MCSP [67, 68], melanotransferrin [69], the ganglioside GD2 [70] and GD3 [71]. A clinical trial targeting melanoma cells with CAR engineered T cells is currently recruiting participants [66]. Recent phase I trials using CAR redirected T cells in the treatment of lymphoma/leukemia exhibited spectacular efficacy [72, 73]. However, the enthusiasm was dampened by reports on serious adverse events and even fatalities after CAR T cell therapy [74, 75]. Targeting ErbB2 produced a cytokine storm and respiratory failure in one case [76] which is thought to be due to low levels of antigen on a number of healthy cells which can trigger CAR T cell activation. On the one hand, this event points out that ACT with CAR modified T cells may be a powerful therapy; but, on the other hand, emphasizes the necessity for careful T cell dose escalation studies to balance anti-tumor efficacy and auto-immunity[61, 77, 78].

4. Challenges and premises in the adoptive cell therapy of melanoma

To date, approximately half of the melanoma patients treated with TIL ACT benefit from this therapy; genetic modification of T cells may further improve clinical response to melanoma, but this will have to be proven in upcoming trials. However, the strategy has potential challenges which need to be addressed.

A major challenge of redirected T cells is the tumor selectivity for the target antigen itself, which in most cases is not exclusively expressed on tumor cells but also on healthy cells [79], although almost always at lower levels: for instance MART-1, which is also expressed by melanocytes. When targeting these antigens, vitiligo and inner ear toxicity resulting in a certain degree of deafness are frequently observed side effects [38]. From this perspective it is reasonable to assume that off-target toxicities may be adverse reactions for clinical efficacy in an anti-melanoma response [80]. Since nearly all tumor-associated antigens are self-antigens, strategies will have to be developed to ensure that off-target toxicities are kept to a minimum. Whether T cells with low-avidity TCR or CAR are less prone to induce such undesirable side effects is currently under investigation.

Melanoma cells, like other cancer cells, down-regulate components of the MHC and become increasingly deficient in antigen processing. As a consequence, TCR engineered T cells can no longer bind to and destroy those melanoma cells. However, they may be visible to a CAR recognizing surface antigens in a MHC independent manner, because of the antibody-derived binding domain (Figure 3). TCR redirected T cells, on the one hand, may also recognize cross-presented targeted antigen, for instance by stroma cells, but this is not the case for CAR engineered T cells. Cross-presented antigen, on the other hand, may help to destroy stroma, which is required to eliminate large tumor lesions [39, 40].

To avoid mispairing of the recombinant TCR with the physiological TCR chains and the resulting unpredictable auto-immunity, TCR-like single chain antibodies were used as targeting domain in a CAR. Thus combining the MHC-restricted recognition of antigen with the T-body strategy. T cells with TCR-like CAR were redirected towards NY-ESO-1 and MAGE-A1, respectively [41, 42]. The possible advantages of these MHC restricted CAR's compared to the use of recombinant TCR's still has to be determined in trials.

The antibody-derived binding domain of a CAR displays extraordinary high affinity compared to a TCR. However, an increase in affinity, for instance, by affinity maturation, does not necessarily improve CAR redirected T cell activation above threshold [41, 43], which is not additionally modulated by CD28 costimulation [44]. A similar effect is also assumed for TCR mediated T cell activation. The TCR or CAR binding avidity probably affects the persistence of engineered T cells at the targeted tumor site. Strong binding to a target antigen may cause the T cells to be trapped and to become fully activated for a cytolytic attack, whereas low avidity interactions may not provide sufficiently long T cell – melanoma cell contacts. In addition to the binding avidity, the amount of target antigen on the cell surface also impacts on the selectivity of redirected T cell activation. In essence, low affinity binding directs the activity of engineered T cells preferentially toward target cells with abundant antigen levels; high affinity binding is likewise effective against low antigen levels on target cells. The optimized affinity to sustain a more selective T cell trafficking to the tumor and activation while avoiding targeting healthy cells that are expressing low quantities of the same antigen, however, still has to be determined.

A beneficial T cell-to-target cell ratio at the tumor site seems to be required for efficient tumor elimination. Higher numbers of engineered T cells applied per dose will probably increase clinical efficacy; the majority of recent trials have applied up to 10^{10} cells per dose [27]. These and higher numbers of engineered T cells can be generated by extended expansion protocols; however, cells with a "young" phenotype may not be generated for adoptive transfer under these conditions. Short-term amplification protocols are therefore envisioned for both TIL's and engineered blood T cells. However, the majority of recent trials targeting CD19[+] leukemia provided evidence for therapeutic efficacy at numbers less than or equal to 10^5 engineered T cells [73]. This once again raises the question of whether high T cell doses are required for a therapeutic effect.

The clinical outcome of adoptive cell therapy correlates with the persistence of adoptively transferred T cells [81]. As long as T cells engage their cognate antigen, T cells will expand and persist in detectable numbers; but when the antigen is no longer present, the T cell population will contract to potentially undetectable levels and disappear from circulation. To improve survival of CAR T cells, Epstein-Barr virus (EBV)-specific T cells were engineered with a tumor-specific CAR based on the rationale that T cells recognizing the low amounts of EBV antigens by their physiological TCR will be maintained in a sizable population in circulation and in the process providing enough CAR T cells to recognize and kill melanoma cells in the surrounding tissues. A clinical trial with EBV-specific T cells engineered with an anti-GD2 CAR thus showed benefit over non-virus-specific, CAR engineered T cells in the treatment of neuroblastoma [81].

Adoptively transferred CD8+ T cell clones may be less persistent than CD4+ T cell clones due to T cell exhaustion after extensive *ex vivo* amplification and multiple rounds of activation. In addition, CD4+ T cell help is essential for CD8+ T cell persistence *in vivo*; adoptively transferred pure CD8+ T cell clones may fail to persist [82]. T cell therapy may be combined with antibody therapy to prolong the initiated immune response. For instance, CTLA-4 is upregulated on the surface of activated T cells, where it acts as negative regulator to return the T cell to a resting stage. Co-application of the anti-CTLA-4 blocking antibody, ipilimumab, may prolong the anti-tumor activation of transferred T cells, although it would also affect all the other T cells.

Besides maintaining a high number of T cells in circulation, another challenge is to accumulate significant numbers of effector T cells in the tumor lesion. A tightly controlled network of chemokines controls the migration of cells in the body; adoptively transferred T cells use these networks to accumulate at the tumor site. The expression of specific chemokine receptors controls how cells will migrate against the chemokine gradient into the targeted lesion. Melanoma cells secrete a number of chemokines including CXCL1. However, early imaging studies revealed that melanoma-specific T cells massively infiltrate the lungs, spleen and liver with some accumulation at the tumor site, which clearly represents a minority of the transferred cells, before the cells decline to undetectable levels in circulation [83-85]. Since those T cells do not express CXCR2, the receptor for melanoma secreted CXCL1, TIL's were engineered with CXCR2 which generated improved melanoma accumulation and anti-tumor activity in a mouse model [86]. The strategy is currently being explored in an early phase I trial (Table 1) [86].

One of the major hurdles of redirected immunotherapy of cancer in general is the tremendous heterogeneity of cancer cells with respect to the expression of the targeted antigen. Low or lack of antigen expression within the malignant lesions will negatively affect the long-term therapeutic efficacy of the approach. Several reports document relapse of antigen-loss tumor metastases after adoptive therapy with melanoma-reactive T cell clones [87-89] and argue for the use of polyclonal T cells with various melanoma specificities. Melanoma cells expressing the target antigen may successfully be eliminated by redirected T cells, whereas antigen-negative tumor cells will not be recognized. T cell populations modified with different CAR's recognizing different antigens expressed by the same tumor may be able to overcome these limitations. However, pro-inflammatory cytokines secreted by redirected T cells into the tumor micro-environment upon activation may attract a second wave of non-antigen restricted effector cells, which in turn may eradiate antigen-negative tumor cells. At least in an animal model, antigen-negative melanoma cells are indeed eliminated when co-inoculated with antibody-targeted cytokines [90]. Moreover, T cells engineered with induced expression of transgenic IL-12 attract innate immune cells including macrophages into the tumor tissue; they eliminate antigen-negative tumor cells in the same lesion [91].

Highly expanded T cells, such as TIL's, become hypo-responsive to CD28 costimulation and rapidly enter activation induced cell death, in particular upon IL-2 driven expansion [92].

This may be counteracted by expansion in the presence of IL-15 and IL-21 and/or by co-stimulation via 4-1BB by an agonistic antibody [93].

Metastatic melanoma patients with the B-raf activating mutation V600E transiently benefit from a small molecule drug, PLX4032 or vemurafenib, which inhibits the mitogen-activated protein kinase (MAPK) pathway. Treatment with vemurafenib is accompanied by increased T cell infiltrations in the melanoma lesions [94, 95]. Combination of B-raf inhibition with melanoma-specific ACT may provide an option to prolong the clinical response.

Although the TCR downstream signaling machinery is used by the prototype CAR, monocytes, macrophages as well as NK cells can also be redirected by CAR's in an antigen-specific fashion [96, 97]. Whether redirected non-T cells are advantageous in tumor elimination to cancer patients in general and to melanoma patients in particular has to be explored in clinical trials.

5. Does targeting "melanoma stem cells" provide hope for long-term remission from melanoma?

Observations that a number of malignant lesions display a tremendous cellular and phenotypic heterogeneity and contain pluripotent stem cells led to the hypothesis that cancer is initiated and maintained by so-called cancer stem cells (CSC's). Low abundance, induction of tumors upon transplantation under limiting conditions, radiation and chemo-resistance, self-renewal and a-symmetric differentiation into a variety of cell types are properties postulated for CSC's. The concept was sustained by deciphering the hierarchical organization in hematological malignancies [98], and subsequently in solid cancers including mammary, prostate, pancreatic, colon carcinoma and glioma [99-103]. Transplantation of melanoma cell subsets under limiting dilution conditions showed that a subset of cancer cells can induce tumors of the same histological phenotype as the parental tumor [99, 104, 105]. A first study using the limiting dilution transplantation assay identified a melanoma cell subset which exhibits stem-like capacities and expresses CD20 [106]. A conclusion drawn from these and other experiments was that melanoma is organized in a hierarchical manner originating from an initiator cell. In this context, several phenomena in melanoma biology which have been clinically observed but not well understood are described by the CSC model, for instance, metastatic relapse more than a decade after surgical treatment of the primary lesion. Residual CSC's are thought to drive cancer relapse even after years of "dormancy" [107]. Moreover, melanoma initiating cells were identified as expressing either the transporter protein ABCB5 [104] or the nerve growth factor receptor CD271; the latter occurs in melanoma in a frequency of approximately 1/2000 cells [108].

However, transplantation under more rigorous conditions, i.e., ideally of one isolated melanoma cell, revealed that nearly every fourth randomly taken melanoma cell (1/2 - 1/15) can induce tumors and raising the question of the validity the stem cell paradigm for melanoma [109, 110]. From these and subsequent studies, it has been concluded that the potential of melanoma induction is not closely associated with a particular phenotype and that the number of potential CSC's in melanoma may not necessarily be low. This resulted in a further conclusion that nearly every melanoma cell is capable to re-program to a tumor initiating cell under certain experimental conditions of xeno-transplantation irrespectively which particular marker phenotype the cell expressed at the time of isolation from a melanoma lesion.

Once the tumor is established, a minor subset seems to take over control of melanoma progression. Evidence is provided by recent observations from a pre-clinical model [69], which addressed the question of whether specific elimination of defined melanoma cells from an established xeno-transplanted lesion causes tumor regression by adoptive transfer of antigen-specific cytotoxic T cell. The rationale is that, if there is a clearly defined hierarchy of cancer cells in an established tumor, specific ablation of the melanoma sustaining cells from the established tumor tissue must inevitably lead to a decay of the tumor lesion independently of targeting the cancer cell mass. However, the melanoma sustaining cell may, but must not, be identical to CSC's identified by the transplantation assay. Targeted elimination of a minor subset of CD20⁺ melanoma cells completely eradicated transplanted melanoma lesions, whereas targeted elimination of any random melanoma cell population in the same lesion did not. CD20⁺ melanoma cells are rare, i.e. approximately 1-2%, in melanoma, independently of the histological type and the transplanted tumor tissue. A caveat is that in approximately 20% of melanoma samples, no CD20⁺ melanoma cells could be detected by histological screening. When these tumors were transplanted, adoptive transfer of CD20-specific CAR T cells did not induce tumor regression. Interestingly, CD20 re-expression in a random subpopulation of those tumor cells did not render the tumor lesion sensitive for complete eradication with CD20-specific T cells. This indicates that CD20 expression *per se* is not dominant in maintaining melanoma progression. However, the phenotype of CD20⁺ melanoma cells may be flexible and associated with additional capabilities which mediate the dominant effect.

The first clinical evidence confirming this concept was recently provided by a case report [111]. A patient with stage III/IV metastatic melanoma, which harbored CD20⁺ melanoma cells at a frequency of 2%, received intra-lesional injections of the anti-CD20 therapeutic antibody rituximab and concomitant dacarbazine treatment. Dacarbazine as mono-therapy had already proved to be ineffective. This treatment produced lasting complete and partial remission accompanied by a decline of the melanoma serum marker S-100 to physiological levels, a switch of a T helper-2 to a more pro-inflammatory T helper-1 response, all without treatment related grade 3/4 toxicity. Although anecdotic, this data provides the first clinical evidence that targeting the subset of CD20⁺ melanoma sustaining cells can produce regression of chemotherapy-refractory melanoma. Moreover, the report highlights the potency of selective cancer cell targeting in the treatment of melanoma.

These observations although so far based on a pre-clinical model and a clinical observation which will have to be reproduced in larger cohorts have major impact on the future development of melanoma therapy.

First, the melanoma maintaining cells may be more resistant to current therapy regimens than the bulk of melanoma cells. Standard therapy strategies attempt to eliminated all cancer cells in a tumor lesion; elimination of any other cancer cells than the tumor progressing cells will rapidly de-bulk the tumor lesion. The melanoma will inevitably relapse, driven by the remaining melanoma sustaining cells, which are extraordinary resistant to chemotherapeutics. This resistance is probably due to transporter molecules like ABCB5, which are highly expressed by a number of CSC's including melanoma [104] and therefore efficiently counteract chemotherapy. Melanoma maintaining cells like other CSC's are merely in a "dormant" state and replicate less frequently than the majority of cancer cells in the same lesion, which reduces the efficacy of anti-proliferative drugs. Low proliferative capacities together with the efficient export of chemotherapeutics contribute to CSC resistance toward a variety of therapeutic drugs. As a consequence, alternative strategies that specifically induce cell death of those cells are required. Moreover, the situation is exacerbated by the fact that the melanoma maintaining cells in the lesion are rare and unlikely to be eliminated by the random targeting provided by most therapeutic agents. Specific targeting by cytotoxic T cells redirected towards CD20 or by CD20-specific therapeutic antibodies like Rituxan™ (rituximab) or Arzerra™ (ofatumumab), probably as adjunct to a tumor de-bulking strategy, may improve the situation.

Second, whether the prevalence of CD20+ melanoma maintaining cells in a tumor lesion may correlate with clinical progression or relapse has to be addressed. If so, the frequency of CD20+ melanoma cells may serve as a surrogate marker for therapeutic efficacy and/or prognosis. Chemotherapy and/or radiation may induce amplification of these cells thus contributing to their accumulation during tumor progression and metastasis.

Third, melanoma maintaining cells may exhibit an extraordinary functional and phenotypic plasticity. As a consequence, continuous presence of targeting therapeutic agents will be required to eliminate those cells, which exhibit newly acquired melanoma initiating and/or maintaining capacities. In their pre-clinical model, Schmidt and colleagues [69] used CAR engineered T cells which penetrate tissues, scan for targets and persist for long-term acting as an antigen-specific guardian. These T cells are present in the targeted lesion as long as cells expressing the target antigen appear. Repetitive restimulation of these T cells, for instance by engaging their TCR with EBV-specific antigens [63, 81], may sustain persistence of CAR T cells in sufficient numbers over long periods of time. In this constellation, cellular therapy has a major advantage compared to pharmaceutical drugs, which are present in therapeutic levels for short periods; in the case of melanoma the required period for screening for re-appearance of such melanoma initiating cells may be many years. The development of an antigen-specific memory by adoptively transferred CAR T cells, as recently shown in a pre-clinical model [112], may be of benefit to patients in preventing a melanoma relapse.

Acknowledgements

Work in the author's laboratory was supported by the Deutsche Krebshilfe, Bonn and Ziel 2. NRW Programm of the Ministerium für Innovation, Wissenschaft, Forschung und Technologie des Landes Nordrhein-Westfalen and of the European Union.

Abbreviations

ACT, adoptive cell therapy; **CAR**, chimeric antigen receptor; **CTLA-4**, anti-cytotoxic T-lymphocyte-associated antigen-4; **CSC**, cancer stem cell; **EBV**, Epstein-Barr virus; **GMP**, Good Manufacturing Practice; **IFN**, interferon; **IL**, interleukin; **TCR**, T cell receptor; **TIL**, tumor infiltrating lymphocyte

Author details

Jennifer Makalowski[1,2] and Hinrich Abken[1,2*]

*Address all correspondence to: hinrich.abken@uk-koeln.de

1 Center for Molecular Medicine Cologne (CMMC), University of Cologne, Cologne, Germany

2 Dept. I Internal Medicine, University Hospital Cologne, Cologne, Germany

References

[1] Garbe C, Peris K, Hauschild A, Saiag P, Middleton M, Spatz A, Grob J-J, Malvehy J, Newton-Bishop J, Stratigos A, Pehamberger H, Eggermont A. Diagnosis and treatment of melanoma: European consensus-based interdisciplinary guideline. European Journal of Cancer 2010;46(2) 270-283.

[2] Chapman PB, Hauschild A, Robert C, Haanen JB, Ascierto P, Larkin J, Dummer R, Garbe C, Testori A, Maio M, Hogg D, Lorigan P, Lebbe C, Jouary T, Schadendorf D, Ribas A, O'Day SJ, Sosman JA, Kirkwood JM, Eggermont AM, Dreno B, Nolop K, Li J, Nelson B, Hou J, Lee RJ, Flaherty KT. Improved survival with vemurafenib in melanoma with BRAF V600E mutation. The New England Journal of Medicine 2011;364 (26) 2507-2516.

[3] Carter RD, Krementz ET, Hill GJ 2nd, Metter GE, Fletcher WS, Golomb FM, Grage TB, Minton JP, Sparks FC. DTIC (nsc-45388) and combination therapy for melanoma. I. Studies with DTIC, BCNU (NSC-409962), CCNU (NSC-79037), vincristine (NSC-67574), and hydroxyurea (NSC-32065). Cancer Treat Rep. 1976;60(5) 601-609.

[4] Flaherty KT, Puzanov I, Kim KB, Ribas A, McArthur GA, Sosman JA, O'Dwyer PJ, Lee RJ, Grippo JF, Nolop K, Chapman PB. Inhibition of mutated, activated BRAF in metastatic melanoma. The New England Journal of Medicine 2010;363(9) 809-819.

[5] Leiter U, Eigentler TK, Forschner A, Pflugfelder A, Weide B, Held L, Meier F, Garbe C. Excision guidelines and follow-up strategies in cutaneous melanoma: Facts and controversies. Clinics in Dermatology 2010;28(3) 311-315.

[6] Denninghoff VC, Kahn AG, Falco J, Curutchet HP, Elsner B. Sentinel lymph node: detection of micrometastases of melanoma in a molecular study. Molecular Diagnosis 2004;8(4) 253-258.

[7] Bedikian AY, Wei C, Detry M, Kim KB, Papadopoulos NE, Hwu WJ, Homsi J, Davies M, McIntyre S, Hwu P. Predictive Factors for the Development of Brain Metastasis in Advanced Unresectable Metastatic Melanoma. American Journal of Clinical Oncology 2010;34(6) 603-610.

[8] Bradbury PA, Middleton MR. DNA repair pathways in drug resistance in melanoma. Anti-cancer Drugs 2004;15(5) 421-426.

[9] Pak BJ, Chu W, Lu SJ, Kerbel RS, Ben-David Y. Lineage-specific mechanism of drug and radiation resistance in melanoma mediated by tyrosinase-related protein 2. Cancer Metastasis Reviews 2001;20(1-2) 27-32.

[10] Pak BJ, Lee J, Thai BL, Fuchs SY, Shaked Y, Ronai Z, Kerbel RS, Ben-David Y. Radiation resistance of human melanoma analysed by retroviral insertional mutagenesis reveals a possible role for dopachrome tautomerase. Oncogene 2004;23(1) 30-38.

[11] Atkins MB, Lotze MT, Dutcher JP, Fisher RI, Weiss G, Margolin K, Abrams J, Sznol M, Parkinson D, Hawkins M, Paradise C, Kunkel L, Rosenberg SA. High-dose recombinant interleukin 2 therapy for patients with metastatic melanoma: analysis of 270 patients treated between 1985 and 1993. Journal of Clinical Oncology 1999;17(7) 2105-2116.

[12] Hodi FS, O'Day SJ, McDermott DF, Weber RW, Sosman JA, Haanen JB, Gonzalez R, Robert C, Schadendorf D, Hassel JC, Akerley W, van den Eertwegh AJ, Lutzky J, Lorigan P, Vaubel JM, Linette GP, Hogg D, Ottensmeier CH, Lebbé C, Peschel C, Quirt I, Clark JI, Wolchok JD, Weber JS, Tian J, Yellin MJ, Nichol GM, Hoos A, Urba WJ. Improved survival with ipilimumab in patients with metastatic melanoma. The New England Journal of Medicine 2010;363(8) 711-723.

[13] Kirkwood JM, Ibrahim JG, Sondak VK, Richards J, Flaherty LE, Ernstoff MS, Smith TJ, Rao U, Steele M, Blum RH. High- and low-dose interferon alfa-2b in high-risk melanoma: first analysis of intergroup trial E1690/S9111/C9190. Journal of Clinical Oncology 2000;18(12) 2444-2458.

[14] Kirkwood JM, Strawderman MH, Ernstoff MS, Smith TJ, Borden EC, Blum RH. Interferon alfa-2b adjuvant therapy of high-risk resected cutaneous melanoma: the Eastern Cooperative Oncology Group Trial EST 1684. Journal of Clinical Oncology 1996;14(1) 7-17.

[15] Galluzzi L, Vacchelli E, Eggermont A, Fridman WH, Galon J, Sautès-Fridman C, Tartour E, Zitvogel L, Kroemer G. Trial Watch: Adoptive cell transfer immunotherapy. Oncoimmunology 2012;1(3) 306-315.

[16] Bernatchez C, Radvanyi LG, Hwu P. Advances in the treatment of metastatic melanoma: adoptive T-cell therapy. Seminars in Oncology 2012;39(2) 215-226.

[17] Grulich AE, van Leeuwen MT, Falster MO, Vajdic CM. Incidence of cancers in people with HIV/AIDS compared with immunosuppressed transplant recipients: a meta-analysis. Lancet 2007;370(9581) 59-67.

[18] Nathanson. Spontaneous regression of malignant melanoma: a review of the literature on incidence, clinical features, and possible mechanisms. National Cancer Institute Monograph 1976;44 67-76.

[19] Rosenberg SA, Yang JC, Topalian SL, Schwartzentruber DJ, Weber JS, Parkinson DR, Seipp CA, Einhorn JH, White DE. Treatment of 283 consecutive patients with metastatic melanoma or renal cell cancer using high-dose bolus interleukin 2. The journal of the American Medical Association 1994;271(12) 907-913.

[20] Clark WH Jr, From L, Bernardino EA, Mihm MC. The histogenesis and biologic behavior of primary human malignant melanomas of the skin. Cancer Research 1969;29(3) 705-727.

[21] Clemente CG, Mihm MC Jr, Bufalino R, Zurrida S, Collini P, Cascinelli N. Prognostic value of tumor infiltrating lymphocytes in the vertical growth phase of primary cutaneous melanoma. Cancer 1996;77(7) 1303-1310.

[22] Burton AL, Roach BA, Mays MP, Chen AF, Ginter BA, Vierling AM, Scoggins CR, Martin RC, Stromberg AJ, Hagendoorn L, McMasters KM. Prognostic significance of tumor infiltrating lymphocytes in melanoma. The American Surgeon 2011;77(2) 188-192.

[23] Vignard V, Lemercier B, Lim A, Pandolfino MC, Guilloux Y, Khammari A, Rabu C, Echasserieau K, Lang F, Gougeon ML, Dreno B, Jotereau F, Labarriere N. Adoptive transfer of tumor-reactive Melan-A-specific CTL clones in melanoma patients is followed by increased frequencies of additional Melan-A-specific T cells. Journal of Immunology 2005;175(7) 4797-4805.

[24] Itzhaki O, Hovav E, Ziporen Y, Levy D, Kubi A, Zikich D, Hershkovitz L, Treves AJ, Shalmon B, Zippel D, Markel G, Shapira-Frommer R, Schachter J, Besser MJ. Establishment and large-scale expansion of minimally cultured "young" tumor infiltrating lymphocytes for adoptive transfer therapy. Journal of Immunology 2011;34(2) 212-220.

[25] Shen X, Zhou J, Hathcock KS, Robbins P, Powell DJ Jr, Rosenberg SA, Hodes RJ. Persistence of tumor infiltrating lymphocytes in adoptive immunotherapy correlates with telomere length. Journal of Immunology 2007;30(1) 123-129.

[26] Besser MJ, Shapira-Frommer R, Treves AJ, Zippel D, Itzhaki O, Schallmach E, Kubi A, Shalmon B, Hardan I, Catane R, Segal E, Markel G, Apter S, Nun AB, Kuchuk I, Shimoni A, Nagler A, Schachter J. Minimally cultured or selected autologous tumor-infiltrating lymphocytes after a lympho-depleting chemotherapy regimen in metastatic melanoma patients. Journal of Immunotherapy 2009;32(4) 415-423.

[27] Dudley ME, Wunderlich JR, Yang JC, Sherry RM, Topalian SL, Restifo NP, Royal RE, Kammula U, White DE, Mavroukakis SA, Rogers LJ, Gracia GJ, Jones SA, Mangiameli DP, Pelletier MM, Gea-Banacloche J, Robinson MR, Berman DM, Filie AC, Abati A, Rosenberg SA. Adoptive cell transfer therapy following non-myeloablative but lymphodepleting chemotherapy for the treatment of patients with refractory metastatic melanoma. Journal of Clinical Oncology 2005;23(10) 2346-2357.

[28] Besser MJ, Shapira-Frommer R, Treves AJ, Zippel D, Itzhaki O, Hershkovitz L, Levy D, Kubi A, Hovav E, Chermoshniuk N, Shalmon B, Hardan I, Catane R, Markel G, Apter S, Ben-Nun A, Kuchuk I, Shimoni A, Nagler A, Schachter J. Clinical responses in a phase II study using adoptive transfer of short-term cultured tumor infiltration lymphocytes in metastatic melanoma patients. Clinical Cancer Research 2010;16(9) 2646-2655.

[29] Dudley ME, Yang JC, Sherry R, Hughes MS, Royal R, Kammula U, Robbins PF, Huang J, Citrin DE, Leitman SF, Wunderlich J, Restifo NP, Thomasian A, Downey SG, Smith FO, Klapper J, Morton K, Laurencot C, White DE, Rosenberg SA. Adoptive cell therapy for patients with metastatic melanoma: evaluation of intensive myeloablative chemoradiation preparative regimens. Journal of Clinical Oncology 2008;26(32) 5233-5239.

[30] Weber J, Atkins M, Hwu P, Radvanyi L, Sznol M, Yee C; Immunotherapy Task Force of the NCI Investigational Drug Steering Committee.

[31] Kawakami Y, Eliyahu S, Jennings C, Sakaguchi K, Kang X, Southwood S, Robbins PF, Sette A, Appella E, Rosenberg SA. Recognition of multiple epitopes in the human melanoma antigen gp100 by tumor-infiltrating T lymphocytes associated with in vivo tumor regression. Journal of Immunology 1995;154(8) 3961-39618.

[32] Benlalam H, Vignard V, Khammari A, Bonnin A, Godet Y, Pandolfino MC, Jotereau F, Dreno B, Labarrière N. Infusion of Melan-A/Mart-1 specific tumor-infiltrating lymphocytes enhanced relapse-free survival of melanoma patients. Cancer Immunology Immunotherapy 2007;56(4) 515-526.

[33] Khammari A, Labarrière N, Vignard V, Nguyen JM, Pandolfino MC, Knol AC, Quéreux G, Saiagh S, Brocard A, Jotereau F, Dreno B. Treatment of metastatic melanoma with autologous Melan-A/MART-1-specific cytotoxic T lymphocyte clones. The Journal of Investigative Dermatology 2009;129(12) 2835-2842.

[34] Kvistborg P, Shu CJ, Heemskerk B, Fankhauser M, Thrue CA, Toebes M, van Rooij N, Linnemann C, van Buuren MM, Urbanus JH, Beltman JB, Thor Straten P, Li YF, Robbins PF, Besser MJ, Schachter J, Kenter GG, Dudley ME, Rosenberg SA, Haanen JB, Hadrup SR, Schumacher TN. TIL therapy broadens the tumor-reactive CD8(+) T cell compartment in melanoma patients. Oncoimmunology 2012;1(4) 409-418.

[35] Johnson LA, Heemskerk B, Powell DJ Jr, Cohen CJ, Morgan RA, Dudley ME, Robbins PF, Rosenberg SA. Gene transfer of tumor-reactive TCR confers both high avidity

and tumor reactivity to nonreactive peripheral blood mononuclear cells and tumor-infiltrating lymphocytes. Journal of Immunology 2006;177(9) 6548-6559.

[36] Zhao Y, Zheng Z, Khong HT, Rosenberg SA, Morgan RA. Transduction of an HLA-DP4-restricted NY-ESO-1-specific TCR into primary human CD4+ lymphocytes. Journal of Immunology 2006;29(4) 398-406.

[37] Frankel TL, Burns WR, Peng PD, Yu Z, Chinnasamy D, Wargo JA, Zheng Z, Restifo NP, Rosenberg SA, Morgan RA. Both CD4 and CD8 T cells mediate equally effective in vivo tumor treatment when engineered with a highly avid TCR targeting tyrosinase. Journal of Immunology 2010;184(11) 5988-5998.

[38] Johnson LA, Morgan RA, Dudley ME, Cassard L, Yang JC, Hughes MS, Kammula US, Royal RE, Sherry RM, Wunderlich JR, Lee CC, Restifo NP, Schwarz SL, Cogdill AP, Bishop RJ, Kim H, Brewer CC, Rudy SF, VanWaes C, Davis JL, Mathur A, Ripley RT, Nathan DA, Laurencot CM, Rosenberg SA. Gene therapy with human and mouse T-cell receptors mediates cancer regression and targets normal tissues expressing cognate antigen. Blood 2009;114(3) 535-546.

[39] Spiotto MT, Rowley DA, and Schreiber H. "Bystander" elimination of antigen loss variants in established tumors. Nature Medicine 2004; 10(3) 294-298.

[40] Schüler T, Blankenstein T. Cutting edge: CD8+ effector T cells reject tumors by direct antigen recognition but indirect action on host cells. Journal of Immunology 2003;170(9) 4427-4431.

[41] Stewart-Jones G, Wadle A, Hombach A, Shenderov E, Held G, Fischer E, Kleber S, Nuber N, Stenner-Liewen F, Bauer S, McMichael A, Knuth A, Abken H, Hombach AA, Cerundolo V, Jones EY, Renner C. Rational development of high-affinity T-cell receptor-like antibodies. Proceedings of the National Academy of Sciences of the United States of America 2009;106(14) 5784-5788.

[42] Willemsen RA, Debets R, Hart E, Hoogenboom HR, Bolhuis RL, Chames P. A phage display selected fab fragment with MHC class I-restricted specificity for MAGE-A1 allows for retargeting of primary human T lymphocytes. Gene Therapy 2001;8(21) 1601-1608.

[43] Chmielewski M, Hombach A, Heuser C, Adams GP, Abken H.T cell activation by antibody-like immunoreceptors: increase in affinity of the single-chain fragment domain above threshold does not increase T cell activation against antigen-positive target cells but decreases selectivity. Journal of Immunology 2004; 173(12) 7647-7653.

[44] Chmielewski M, Hombach AA, Abken H. CD28 cosignalling does not affect the activation threshold in a chimeric antigen receptor-redirected T-cell attack. Gene Therapy 2011;18(1) 62-72.

[45] Schaft N, Willemsen RA, de Vries J, Lankiewicz B, Essers BW, Gratama JW, Figdor CG, Bolhuis RL, Debets R, Adema GJ. Peptide fine specificity of anti-glycoprotein 100

CTL is preserved following transfer of engineered TCR alpha beta genes into primary human T lymphocytes. Journal of Immunology 2003; 170(4) 2186-2194.

[46] Morgan RA, Dudley ME, Yu YY, Zheng Z, Robbins PF, Theoret MR, Wunderlich JR, Hughes MS, Restifo NP, Rosenberg SA. High efficiency TCR gene transfer into primary human lymphocytes affords avid recognition of melanoma tumor antigen glycoprotein 100 and does not alter the recognition of autologous melanoma antigens," Journal of Immunology 2003 ;171(6) 3287-3295.

[47] Hughes MS, Yu YY, Dudley ME, Zheng Z, Robbins PF, Li Y, Wunderlich J, Hawley RG, Moayeri M, Rosenberg SA, Morgan RA. Transfer of a TCR gene derived from a patient with a marked antitumor response conveys highly active T-cell effector functions. Human Gene Therapy 2005;16(4) 457-472.

[48] Willemsen R, Ronteltap C, Heuveling M, Debets R, Bolhuis R. Redirecting human CD4+ T lymphocytes to the MHC class I-restricted melanoma antigen MAGE-A1 by TCR alphabeta gene transfer requires CD8alpha. Gene Therapy 2005; 12(2) 140-146.

[49] Morgan RA, Dudley ME, Wunderlich JR, Hughes MS, Yang JC, Sherry RM, Royal RE, Topalian SL, Kammula US, Restifo NP, Zheng Z, Nahvi A, de Vries CR, Rogers-Freezer LJ, Mavroukakis SA, Rosenberg SA. Cancer Regression in Patients After Transfer of Genetically Engineered Lymphocytes. Science. 2006;314(5796) 126-129.

[50] Coccoris M, Swart E, de Witte MA, van Heijst JW, Haanen JB, Schepers K, Schumacher TN. Long-term functionality of TCR-transduced T cells in vivo. Journal of Immunology 2008; 180(10) 6536-6543.

[51] Seliger B. Molecular mechanisms of MHC class I abnormalities and APM components in human tumors. Cancer Immunology Immunotherapy 2008;57(11) 1719-1726.

[52] Sigalotti L, Fratta E, Coral S, Tanzarella S, Danielli R, Colizzi F, Fonsatti E, Traversari C, Altomonte M, Maio M. Intratumor heterogeneity of cancer/testis antigens expression in human cutaneous melanoma is methylation-regulated and functionally reverted by 5-aza-2'-deoxycytidine. Cancer Research 2004;64(24) 9167-9171.

[53] Vitale M, Pelusi G, Taroni B, Gobbi G, Micheloni C, Rezzani R, Donato F, Wang X, Ferrone S. HLA class I antigen down-regulation in primary ovary carcinoma lesions: association with disease stage. Clinical Cancer Research 2005;11(1) 67-72.

[54] Coccoris M, Straetemans T, Govers C, Lamers C, Sleijfer S, Debets R. T cell receptor (TCR) gene therapy to treat melanoma: lessons from clinical and preclinical studies. Expert Opinion on Biological Therapy 2010;10(4) 547-562.

[55] Bendle GM, Linnemann C, Hooijkaas AI, Bies L, de Witte MA, Jorritsma A, Kaiser AD, Pouw N, Debets R, Kieback E, Uckert W, Song JY, Haanen JB, Schumacher TN. Lethal graft-versus-host disease in mouse models of T cell receptor gene therapy. Nature Medicine 2010; 16(5) 565-570.

[56] Cohen CJ, Zhao Y, Zheng Z, Rosenberg SA, Morgan RA. Enhanced antitumor activity of murine-human hybrid T-cell receptor (TCR) in human lymphocytes is associat-

ed with improved pairing and TCR/CD3 stability. Cancer Research 2006;66(17) 8878-8886.

[57] Kuball J, Dossett ML, Wolfl M, Ho WY, Voss RH, Fowler C, Greenberg PD. Facilitating matched pairing and expression of TCR chains introduced into human T cells. Blood 2007;109(6) 2331-2338.

[58] Eshhar Z, Waks T, Gross G, Schindler DG. Specific activation and targeting of cytotoxic lymphocytes through chimeric single chains consisting of antibody-binding domains and the gamma or zeta subunits of the immunoglobulin and T-cell receptors. Proceedings of the National Academy of Sciences of the United States of America 1993;90(2) 720-724.

[59] Hombach A, Abken H. Costimulation tunes tumor-specific activation of redirected T cells in adoptive immunotherapy," Cancer Immunology Immunotherapy 2007;56(5) 731-737.

[60] Hombach AA, Abken H. Costimulation by chimeric antigen receptors revisited the T cell antitumor response benefits from combined CD28-OX40 signalling. International Journal of Cancer 2011;129(12) 2935-2944.

[61] Bridgeman JS, Hawkins RE, Hombach AA, Abken H, Gilham DE.Building better chimeric antigen receptors for adoptive T cell therapy. Current Gene Therapy 2010; 10(2) 77-90.

[62] Gilham DE, Debets R, Pule M, Hawkins RE, Abken H. CAR-T cells and solid tumors: tuning T cells to challenge an inveterate foe. Trends in Molecular Medicine 2012;18(7) 377-384.

[63] Savoldo B, Rooney CM, Di Stasi A, Abken H, Hombach A, Foster AE, Zhang L, Heslop HE, Brenner MK, Dotti G. Epstein Barr virus specific cytotoxic T lymphocytes expressing the anti-CD30zeta artificial chimeric T-cell receptor for immunotherapy of Hodgkin disease. Blood. 2007;110(7) 2620-2630.

[64] ClinicalTrials.gov A service of the U.S. National Institutes of Health. Trial ID: NCT00586391 http://clinicaltrials.gov/ct2/results?term=NCT+00586391

[65] ClinicalTrials.gov A service of the U.S. National Institutes of Health. Trial ID: NCT00709033 http://clinicaltrials.gov/ct2/results?term=NCT+00709033

[66] ClinicalTrials.gov A service of the U.S. National Institutes of Health. Trial ID: NCT01218867 http://clinicaltrials.gov/ct2/results?term=NCT01218867

[67] Reinhold U, Liu L, Lüdtke-Handjery HC, Heuser C, Hombach A, Wang X, Tilgen W, Ferrone S, Abken H. Specific lysis of melanoma cells by receptor grafted T cells is enhanced by anti-idiotypic monoclonal antibodies directed to the scFv domain of the receptor. The Journal of Investigative Dermatology 1999;112(5) 744-750.

[68] Burns WR, Zhao Y, Frankel TL, Hinrichs CS, Zheng Z, Xu H, Feldman SA, Ferrone S, Rosenberg SA, Morgan RA. A high molecular weight melanoma-associated antigen-

specific chimeric antigen receptor redirects lymphocytes to target human melanomas. Cancer Research 2010;70(8) 3027-3033.

[69] Schmidt P, Kopecky C, Hombach A, Zigrino P, Mauch C, Abken H. Eradication of melanomas by targeted elimination of a minor subset of tumor cells. Proceedings of the National Academy of Sciences of the United States of America 2011;108(6) 2474-2479.

[70] Yvon E, Del Vecchio M, Savoldo B, Hoyos V, Dutour A, Anichini A, Dotti G, Brenner MK. Immunotherapy of metastatic melanoma using genetically engineered GD2-specific T cells. Clinical Cancer Research 2009;15(18) 5852-5860.

[71] Lo AS, Ma Q, Liu DL, Junghans RP. Anti-GD3 chimeric sFv-CD28/T-cell receptor zeta designer T cells for treatment of metastatic melanoma and other neuroectodermal tumors. Clinical Cancer Research 2010;16(10) 2769-2780.

[72] Kalos M, Levine BL, Porter DL, Katz S, Grupp SA, Bagg A, June CH. T cells with chimeric antigen receptors have potent antitumor effects and can establish memory in patients with advanced leukemia. Science Translational Medicine 2011;3(95) 95ra73.

[73] Porter DL, Levine BL, Kalos M, Bagg A, June CH. Chimeric antigen receptor-modified T cells in chronic lymphoid leukemia. The New England Journal of Medicine 2011;365(8) 725-733.

[74] Lamers CH, Sleijfer S, Vulto AG, Kruit WH, Kliffen M, Debets R, Gratama JW, Stoter G, Oosterwijk E. Treatment of metastatic renal cell carcinoma with autologous T-lymphocytes genetically retargeted against carbonic anhydrase IX: first clinical experience. Journal of Clinical Oncology 2006; 24(3) 20-22.

[75] Brentjens R, Yeh R, Bernal Y, Riviere I, Sadelain M. Treatment of chronic lymphocytic leukemia with genetically targeted autologous T cells: case report of an unforeseen adverse event in a phase I clinical trial. Molecular Therapy 2010;18(4) 666-668.

[76] Morgan RA, Yang JC, Kitano M, Dudley ME, Laurencot CM, Rosenberg SA. Case report of a serious adverse event following the administration of T cells transduced with a chimeric antigen receptor recognizing ERBB2. Molecular Therapy 2010;8(4) 843-851.

[77] Hawkins RE, Gilham DE, Debets R, Eshhar Z, Taylor N, Abken H, Schumacher TN, ATTACK Consortium. Development of adoptive cell therapy for cancer: a clinical perspective. Human Gene Therapy 2010;21(6) 665-672.

[78] Büning H, Uckert W, Cichutek K, Hawkins RE, Abken H. Do CARs need a driver's license? Adoptive cell therapy with chimeric antigen receptor-redirected T cells has caused serious adverse events. Human Gene Therapy 2010;21(9) 1039-1042.

[79] Offringa R. Antigen choice in adoptive T-cell therapy of cancer. Current Opinion in Immunology 2009;21(2) 190-199.

[80] Overwijk WW, Theoret MR, Finkelstein SE, Surman DR, de Jong LA, Vyth-Dreese FA, Dellemijn TA, Antony PA, Spiess PJ, Palmer DC, Heimann DM, Klebanoff CA,

Yu Z, Hwang LN, Feigenbaum L, Kruisbeek AM, Rosenberg SA, Restifo NP. Tumor regression and autoimmunity after reversal of a functionally tolerant state of self-reactive CD8+ T cells. The Journal of Experimental Medicine 2003;198(4) 569-580.

[81] Pule MA, Savoldo B, Myers GD, Rossig C, Russell HV, Dotti G, Huls MH, Liu E, Gee AP, Mei Z, Yvon E, Weiss HL, Liu H, Rooney CM, Heslop HE, Brenner MK. Virus-specific T cells engineered to coexpress tumor-specific receptors: persistence and antitumor activity in individuals with neuroblastoma Nature Medicine 2008;14(11) 1264-1270.

[82] Antony PA, Piccirillo CA, Akpinarli A, Finkelstein SE, Speiss PJ, Surman DR, Palmer DC, Chan CC, Klebanoff CA, Overwijk WW, Rosenberg SA, Restifo NP. CD8+ T cell immunity against a tumor/self-antigen is augmented by CD4+ T helper cells and hindered by naturally occurring T regulatory cells. Journal of Immunology 2005;174(5) 2591-2601.

[83] Meidenbauer N, Marienhagen J, Laumer M, Vogl S, Heymann J, Andreesen R, Mackensen A. Survival and tumor localization of adoptively transferred Melan-A-specific T cells in melanoma patients. Journal of Immunology 2003;170(4) 2161-2169.

[84] Griffith KD, Read EJ, Carrasquillo JA, Carter CS, Yang JC, Fisher B, Aebersold P, Packard BS, Yu MY, Rosenberg SA. In vivo distribution of adoptively transferred indium-111-labeled tumor infiltrating lymphocytes and peripheral blood lymphocytes in patients with metastatic melanoma. Journal of the National Cancer Institute 1989;81(22) 1709-1717.

[85] Fisher B, Packard BS, Read EJ, Carrasquillo JA, Carter CS, Topalian SL, Yang JC, Yolles P, Larson SM, Rosenberg SA. Tumor localization of adoptively transferred indium-111 labeled tumor infiltrating lymphocytes in patients with metastatic melanoma. Journal of Clinical Oncology 1989;7(2) 250-261.

[86] Peng W, Ye Y, Rabinovich BA, Liu C, Lou Y, Zhang M, Whittington M, Yang Y, Overwijk WW, Lizée G, Hwu P. Transduction of tumor-specific T cells with CXCR2 chemokine receptor improves migration to tumor and antitumor immune responses. Clinical Cancer Research 2010;16(22) 5458-5468.

[87] Mackensen A, Meidenbauer N, Vogl S, Laumer M, Berger J, Andreesen R. Phase I study of adoptive T-cell therapy using antigen-specific CD8+ T cells for the treatment of patients with metastatic melanoma. Journal of Clinical Oncology 2006;24(31) 5060-5069.

[88] Yee C, Thompson JA, Byrd D, Riddell SR, Roche P, Celis E, Greenberg PD. Adoptive T cell therapy using antigen-specific CD8+ T cell clones for the treatment of patients with metastatic melanoma: in vivo persistence, migration, and antitumor effect of transferred T cells. Proceedings of the National Academy of Science of the United States of America 2002;99(25) 16168-16173.

[89] Lozupone F, Rivoltini L, Luciani F, Venditti M, Lugini L, Cova A, Squarcina P, Parmiani G, Belardelli F, Fais S. Adoptive transfer of an anti-MART-1(27-35)-specific

CD8+ T cell clone leads to immunoselection of human melanoma antigen-loss variants in SCID mice. European Journal of Immunology 2003;33(2) 556-566.

[90] Becker JC, Varki N, Gillies SD, Furukawa K, Reisfeld RA. An antibody-interleukin 2 fusion protein overcomes tumor heterogeneity by induction of a cellular immune response," Proceedings of the National Academy of Sciences of the United States of America 1996;93(15) 7826-7831.

[91] Chmielewski M, Kopecky C, Hombach AA, Abken H. IL-12 release by engineered T cells expressing chimeric antigen receptors can effectively Muster an antigen-independent macrophage response on tumor cells that have shut down tumor antigen expression. Cancer Research 2011;71(17) 5697-5706.

[92] Li Y, Liu S, Hernandez J, Vence L, Hwu P, Radvanyi L.MART-1-specific melanoma tumor-infiltrating lymphocytes maintaining CD28 expression have improved survival and expansion capability following antigenic restimulation in vitro. Journal of Immunology 2010;184(1) 452-465.

[93] Hernandez-Chacon JA, Li Y, Wu RC, Bernatchez C, Wang Y, Weber JS, Hwu P, Radvanyi LG. Costimulation through the CD137/4-1BB pathway protects human melanoma tumor-infiltrating lymphocytes from activation-induced cell death and enhances antitumor effector function. Journal of Immunology 2011;34(3) 236-250.

[94] Boni A, Cogdill AP, Dang P, Udayakumar D, Njauw CN, Sloss CM, Ferrone CR, Flaherty KT, Lawrence DP, Fisher DE, Tsao H, Wargo JA. Selective BRAFV600E inhibition enhances T-cell recognition of melanoma without affecting lymphocyte function. Cancer Research 2010;70(13) 5213-5219.

[95] Wilmott JS, Long GV, Howle JR, Haydu LE, Sharma RN, Thompson JF, Kefford RF, Hersey P, Scolyer RA. Selective BRAF inhibitors induce marked T-cell infiltration into human metastatic melanoma. Clinical Cancer Research 2012;18(5) 1386-1394.

[96] Pegram HJ, Jackson JT, Smyth MJ, Kershaw MH, Darcy PK. Adoptive transfer of gene-modified primary NK cells can specifically inhibit tumor progression in vivo. Journal of Immunology 2008;181(5) 3449-3455.

[97] Kruschinski A, Moosmann A, Poschke I, Norell H, Chmielewski M, Seliger B, Kiessling R, Blankenstein T, Abken H, Charo J. Engineering antigen-specific primary human NK cells against HER-2 positive carcinomas," Proceedings of the National Academy of Sciences of the United States of America 2008;105(45) 17481-17486.

[98] Bonnet D, Dick JE. Human acute myeloid leukemia is organized as a hierarchy that originates from a primitive hematopoietic cell. Nature Medicine 1997;3(7) 730-737.

[99] Al-Hajj M, Wicha MS, Benito-Hernandez A, Morrison SJ, Clarke MF. Prospective identification of tumorigenic breast cancer cells. Proceedings of the National Academy of Sciences of the United States of America 2003;100(7) 3983-3988.

[100] Dalerba P, Dylla SJ, Park IK, Liu R, Wang X, Cho RW, Hoey T, Gurney A, Huang EH, Simeone DM, Shelton AA, Parmiani G, Castelli C, Clarke MF. Phenotypic characteri-

zation of human colorectal cancer stem cells. Proceedings of the National Academy of Sciences of the United States of America 2007;104(24) 10158-10163.

[101]   Singh SK, Clarke ID, Terasaki M, Bonn VE, Hawkins C, Squire J, Dirks PB. Identification of a cancer stem cell in human brain tumors. Cancer Research 2003;63(18) 5821-5828.

[102]   Ricci-Vitiani L, Lombardi DG, Pilozzi E, Biffoni M, Todaro M, Peschle C, De Maria R. Identification and expansion of human colon-cancer-initiating cells. Nature 2007;445(7123) 111-115.

[103]   Li C, Heidt DG, Dalerba P, Burant CF, Zhang L, Adsay V, Wicha M, Clarke MF, Simeone DM. Identification of pancreatic cancer stem cells. Cancer Research 2007;67(3) 1030-1037.

[104]   Schatton T, Murphy GF, Frank NY, Yamaura K, Waaga-Gasser AM, Gasser M, Zhan Q, Jordan S, Duncan LM, Weishaupt C, Fuhlbrigge RC, Kupper TS, Sayegh MH, Frank MH. Identification of cells initiating human melanomas. Nature. 2008;451(7176) 345-349.

[105]   Zabierowski SE, Herlyn M. Melanoma stem cells: the dark seed of melanoma. Journal of Clinical Oncology 2008;26(17) 2890-2894.

[106]   Fang D, Nguyen TK, Leishear K, Finko R, Kulp AN, Hotz S, Van Belle PA, Xu X, Elder DE, Herlyn M. A tumorigenic subpopulation with stem cell properties in melanomas. Cancer Research 2005;65(20) 9328-9337.

[107]   Zhou BB, Zhang H, Damelin M, Geles KG, Grindley JC, Dirks PB. Tumour-initiating cells: challenges and opportunities for anticancer drug discovery. Nature Reviews Drug Discovery 2009;8(10) 806-823.

[108]   Boiko AD, Razorenova OV, van de Rijn M, Swetter SM, Johnson DL, Ly DP, Butler PD, Yang GP, Joshua B, Kaplan MJ, Longaker MT, Weissman IL. Human melanoma-initiating cells express neural crest nerve growth factor receptor CD271. Nature 2010;466(7302) 133-137.

[109]   Quintana E, Shackleton M, Sabel MS, Fullen DR, Johnson TM, Morrison SJ. Efficient tumour formation by single human melanoma cells. Nature 2008;456(7222) 593-598.

[110]   Quintana E, Shackleton M, Foster HR, Fullen DR, Sabel MS, Johnson TM, Morrison SJ. Phenotypic Heterogeneity among Tumorigenic Melanoma Cells from Patients that Is Reversible and Not Hierarchically Organized. Cancer Cell 2010;18(5) 510-523.

[111]   Schlaak M, Schmidt P, Bangard C, Kurschat P, Mauch C, Abken H. Regression of metastatic melanoma in a patient by antibody targeting of cancer stem cells. Oncotarget 2012;3(1) 22-30.

[112]   Chmielewski M, Rappl G, Hombach AA, Abken H. T cells redirected by a CD3ζ chimeric antigen receptor can establish self-antigen-specific tumour protection in the

long term. Gene therapy 2012;doi: 10.1038/gt.2012.21. http://www.nature.com/gt/journal/vaop/ncurrent/full/gt201221a.html

[113] Butler MO, Friedlander P, Milstein MI, Mooney MM, Metzler G, Murray AP, Tanaka M, Berezovskaya A, Imataki O, Drury L, Brennan L, Flavin M, Neuberg D, Stevenson K, Lawrence D, Hodi FS, Velazquez EF, Jaklitsch MT, Russell SE, Mihm M, Nadler LM, Hirano N. Establishment of antitumor memory in humans using in vitro-educated CD8+ T cells. Science Translational Medicine 2011;3(80) 80ra34.

[114] Hong JJ, Rosenberg SA, Dudley ME, Yang JC, White DE, Butman JA, Sherry RM. Successful treatment of melanoma brain metastases with adoptive cell therapy. Clinical Cancer Research 2010;16(19) 4892–4898.

[115] Rosenberg SA, Yannelli JR, Yang JC, Topalian SL, Schwartzentruber DJ, Weber JS, Parkinson DR, Seipp CA, Einhorn JH, White DE. Treatment of patients with metastatic melanoma with autologous tumor-infiltrating lymphocytes and interleukin 2. Journal of the National Cancer Institute 1994;86(15) 1159–1166.

[116] Dudley ME, Gross CA, Langhan MM, Garcia MR, Sherry RM, Yang JC, Phan GQ, Kammula US, Hughes MS, Citrin DE, Restifo NP, Wunderlich JR, Prieto PA, Hong JJ, Langan RC, Zlott DA, Morton KE, White DE, Laurencot CM, Rosenberg SA. CD8+ enriched "young" tumor infiltrating lymphocytes can mediate regression of metastatic melanoma. Clinical Cancer Research 2010;16(24) 6122-6131.

[117] Heemskerk B, Liu K, Dudley ME, Johnson LA, Kaiser A, Downey S, Zheng Z, Shelton TE, Matsuda K, Robbins PF, Morgan RA, Rosenberg SA. Adoptive cell therapy for patients with melanoma, using tumor-infiltrating lymphocytes genetically engineered to secrete interleukin-2. Human Gene Therapy 2008;19(5) 496-510.

[118] Wallen H, Thompson JA, Reilly JZ, Rodmyre RM, Cao J, Yee C. Fludarabine modulates immune response and extends in vivo survival of adoptively transferred CD8 T cells in patients with metastatic melanoma. PloS One 2009;4(3) e4749. http://www.plosone.org/article/info%3Adoi%2F10.1371%2Fjournal.pone.0004749

[119] Verdegaal EM, Visser M, Ramwadhdoebé TH, van der Minne CE, van Steijn JA, Kapiteijn E, Haanen JB, van der Burg SH, Nortier JW, Osanto S. Successful treatment of metastatic melanoma by adoptive transfer of blood-derived polyclonal tumor-specific CD4+ and CD8+ T cells in combination with low-dose interferon-alpha. Cancer Immunology Immunotherapy 2011;60(7) 953-963.

[120] Rosenberg SA, Yang JC, Sherry RM, Kammula US, Hughes MS, Phan GQ, Citrin DE, Restifo NP, Robbins PF, Wunderlich JR, Morton KE, Laurencot CM, Steinberg SM, White DE, Dudley ME. Durable complete responses in heavily pretreated patients with metastatic melanoma using T-cell transfer immunotherapy. Clinical Cancer Research 2011;17(13) 4550-4557.

[121] Robbins PF, Morgan RA, Feldman SA, Yang JC, Sherry RM, Dudley ME, Wunderlich JR, Nahvi AV, Helman LJ, Mackall CL, Kammula US, Hughes MS, Restifo NP, Raf-

feld M, Lee CC, Levy CL, Li YF, El-Gamil M, Schwarz SL, Laurencot C, Rosenberg SA. Tumor regression in patients with metastatic synovial cell sarcoma and melanoma using genetically engineered lymphocytes reactive with NY-ESO-1. Journal of Clinical Oncology 2011;29(7) 917-924.

Chapter 5

Surgery and the Staging of Melanoma

Z. Al-Hilli, D. Evoy, J.G. Geraghty,
E.W. McDermott and R.S. Prichard

Additional information is available at the end of the chapter

1. Introduction

An estimated 166,900 patients were diagnosed with malignant melanoma in developed countries last year [1]. The reported incidence of malignant melanoma continues to rise despite increasing understanding of its aetiology. In the United States 76,250 new cases are expected in 2012 with melanoma far outstripping other skin cancers in terms of mortality [2]. Similarly, in the UK, 12,818 new cases of malignant melanoma were diagnosed in 2010 [3]. Approximately, 85% percent of patients with cutaneous melanoma are diagnosed at a localized stage, while 10% have associated regional lymph node involvement and 5% of patients will have distant metastatic disease at presentation. The corresponding 5-year overall survival rates are 98.2% for localized disease, 62.4% for regional lymph node involvement and 15.1% for distant melanomas [4, 5].

Advances in the understanding of the molecular mechanisms and immunology of melanoma have lead to the development of promising novel therapeutic agents. Surgery, however, remains the mainstay of treatment and changes in the surgical approach have been guided by the greater understanding of melanoma pathogenesis. The management of the primary tumour has become more conservative, with acceptance of narrower excision margins. In addition, there has been a move away from the routine performance of elective regional lymph node dissection towards sentinel lymph node biopsy which is associated with less morbidity [6].

The new American Joint Committee on Cancer (AJCC) guidelines for the staging of melanoma were introduced into clinical practice in 2010 [7]. The two most important distinctions with previous guidelines are the incorporation of the mitotic rate of the primary tumor and the key role of the sentinel lymph node, including methods of analysis, in accurately staging clinically occult nodal disease [8].

The purpose of this chapter is twofold. Firstly, this chapter describes the appropriate surgical management of the primary tumour, the associated regional lymph node basin and distant metastatic disease. Secondly, the updated and revised AJCC staging system will be discussed and current controversies addressed.

2. Risk factors

The worldwide incidence of melanoma doubles every ten to fifteen years [9]. Risk factors associated with the development of malignant melanoma are varied and include genetic susceptibility, exposure to ultraviolet radiation, and immunologic factors. The most important of these is ultraviolet exposure where intermittent, unaccustomed sun exposure and sunburn were found to have considerable roles as risk factors for melanoma. However, despite the increase in public awareness, the practice of ultraviolet radiation protection behaviour is low. Also worryingly a survey performed in the US in 2005 documented that up to 14% of adults, primarily women and young adults used an indoor tanning device on at least one occasion [10].

Epidemiological studies have found that blue, green or grey eyes, blonde or red hair, light complexion, freckles, sun sensitivity, and an inability to tan, are risk factors for the development of melanoma [11, 12]. Countries with close proximity to the equator with predominantly fair-skinned populations have shown a higher preponderance to developing melanoma. Risk factors for melanoma also include a positive family history or personal history of melanoma/non-melanoma cancer or in-situ skin carcinomas, large numbers of melanocitic naevi in childhood, and xeroderma pigmentosum [13].

It is suggested that minimising radiation, and the adoption of photo-protective measures, can significantly reduce the risk of developing melanoma [13-15].

3. Surgery

3.1. Initial surgical biopsy

Melanoma can develop either in a pre-existing pigmented lesion or de novo. Features raising suspicion of melanoma in a pre-existing pigmented lesion include a change in size, irregular shape, irregular colour, diameter 7 mm or more, inflammation, oozing or a change in sensation [5,16]. The ABCD system of diagnosis (Asymmetry, Border irregularity, Colour change, and a Diameter greater than 6 mm) has also been advocated to assist early clinical diagnosis, to which 'E' (Evolving or Elevation) has been added [5,17,18]. Table 1 illustrates the seven point checklist and ABCDE system for the assessment of pigmented lesions.

Seven point checklist	The ABCDE lesion system
Major features	
Change in size	A Geometrical Asymmetry in 2 axes
Irregular shape	B Irregular Border
Irregular colour	C At least 2 different Colours in lesion
Minor features	D Maximum Diameter >6mm
Largest diameter 7mm or more	E Elevation
Inflammation	
Oozing	
Itch/ change in sensation	

Table 1. Seven point checklist and ABCDE system for assessment of pigmented lesions [19]

An excision biopsy is indicated for lesions suspected of being a melanoma. An excision biopsy is the recommended method for suspected malignant melanoma as it enables diagnosis and staging of the tumour and may determine future treatment and prognosis [20, 21]. The whole lesion should be excised with a 1-3 mm margin of normal skin including sub-dermal fat. It is crucial to plan this excision carefully with a view towards definitive treatment. Knowledge of lymphatic drainage and subsequent need for sentinel node biopsy should lead to narrow margin excision potentially avoiding interference with subsequent lymphatic mapping. In addition, a longitudinal orientation is preferred in the extremities and incision orientation should be along Langer's lines on the trunk. This allows for subsequent closure of a wide local excision and reduces the need for skin grafting if primary closure is to be achieved.

In certain areas (such as the face, palm of hand, sole of foot, ears, digits and subungal lesions) an excision biopsy may not be appropriate. In these cases, an incisional or punch biopsy of the thickest portion of the lesion may be performed [21]. Shave biopsy is avoided as it makes characterising the lesion difficult by underestimating tumour thickness, which is important in determining further treatment [21]. It also risks leaving residual tumour at the radial and deep margins.

Obtaining an adequate biopsy specimen is crucial for histopathological diagnosis and tumour staging. The tumour thickness, which remains the most powerful prognostic parameter, provides a guide to the margin clearance required for delayed wide excision and need for adjuvant therapy [20, 22]. Pathological examination should evaluate macroscopic features of the tumour such as width, symmetry, and circumscription, and microscopic features such as ulceration, microsatellitosis, angiolymphatic invasion and mitotic rate [22].

3.2. Management of the primary tumour

The surgical management of the primary tumour has shifted from extensive surgical resection, which was not only debilitating but also disfiguring, to a more conservative approach. A multidisciplinary team in a tertiary referral centre should ideally manage patients with malignant melanoma. This team should include: a surgeon, dermatologist,,medical oncologist, pathologist, radiologist, counsellor, specialist nurse and palliative care specialist [23].

Pathological assessment of the surgically excised biopsy specimen allows for staging of the tumour while the thickness of the melanoma at initial biopsy serves as a guide to the subsequent resection. The Breslow thickness, which is the most important prognostic indicator of localised disease, is defined as the distance of invasion and is measured from the granular layer of the epidermis to the point of deepest invasion by tumour cells [5, 24, 25].

Large randomised controlled trials have been performed in an attempt to elucidate the optimal resection margin in melanoma of various thickness (thin, intermediate, and thick melanomas) [26-31]. The trials reported data with not only differing lengths of follow-up but also differing margin excision widths. Therefore interpretation of the results is largely restricted to survival outcomes as a result of this heterogeneity.

The management of lentigo maligna and in situ melanoma present unique problems because of the characteristic, yet unpredictable, subclinical extension of atypical junctional melanocytic hyperplasia, which may extend several centimeters beyond the visible margins [33]. There are no randomized trials looking at the optimal resection margin in these lesions. Guidelines from the American Academy of Dermatology in 2011 recommend a resection margin of 0.5 to 1.0 cm for melanoma in situ [34]. The NCCN recommends a margin of 0.5 cm around the visible lesion. For large in-situ lentigo maligna melanoma, it is felt that surgical margins greater than 0.5 cm may be necessary to achieve a histologically negative margin [33]. More recently, topical imiquimod has been used in lentigo melanoma treatment prior to definitive surgical resection. In a study that included 40 patients, 33 of these were found to have a complete clinical response after the use of imiquimod 5% cream. On histological review, 30 of the patients had no evidence of melanoma. While studies have shown a limited role for this treatment, it does not replace surgery [35].

Three main trials (The World Health Organisation Trial, Swedish Melanoma Study and the French Cooperative Group) looked at the optimal resection margin for T1 and T2 melanomas. The World Health Organisation (WHO) trial included 612 patients with melanomas less than 2.0mm with patients being randomly assigned to a wide local excision with a either a 3cm margin or 1cm margin. At 12 years of follow up, similar survival rates between the groups were noted (87% and 85% respectively) with no statistically significant difference in recurrence dependent upon margin width. As a consequence of this trial recommendations were made that a 1cm margin be used for melanomas ≤1mm. Similarly, the Swedish Melanoma Study Group studied 989 patients with melanomas 0.8 to 2mm thick who were randomly assigned to either a 2cm or 5cm resection margin. At a median follow-up of 11 years the local recurrence rate for all groups was less than 1%. Again there was no significant difference noted in the overall or disease-free survival between the two groups. A third trial, the French Cooperative Group, included 362 patients with melanomas ≤2mm in thickness. Patients were randomly assigned to a wide local excision with either a 2cm or 5cm resection margin. No difference was noted between the groups in terms of local recurrence or overall survival. Therefore at present, a resection margin of 1cm is recommended for melanomas <1mm and 2cm for melanomas 1 - 2mm thick [26-28].

Melanomas between 2 - 4mm are considered intermediate thickness melanomas. Once again, there are a number of trials looking specifically at this cohort of patients which failed to show a benefit of greater than a 2cm excision margin. The Melanoma Intergroup Trial included 468 patients with melanomas of 1 to 4mm thickness. Patients were randomly assigned to an excision margin of either 2cm or 4cm. Forty two percent of patients in the group undergoing 2cm excision had a melanoma thickness >2.0mm, while 46% of patients in the 4cm resection group had melanomas >2.0mm. At mean follow up, a 2cm margin was shown to be as effective as a 4cm margin in both the local control and overall survival for patients with intermediate thickness melanomas. Local recurrence however, was primarily determined by the thickness of the primary lesion and the presence or absence of ulceration [29, 30]. A multi-centre European trial was also performed to tease out the need for wider margins in deeper, intermediate thickness melanomas. In total, 936 patients were included who were assigned randomly to have either a 2cm or 4cm resection margin. At a follow-up of almost 7 years there was no statistically significant difference noted for recurrence or survival between the two groups [31]. Finally a British trial was performed which recruited 900 patients with lesions greater than 2mm to a wide local excision with either a 1cm or 3 cm margin Interestingly, this study demonstrated a higher local recurrence rate when a 1cm margin was used. However, there was no statistically significant difference noted in overall survival. The authors therefore concluded that a margin of 1cm should be restricted to patients with a melanoma thickness of less than 2mm [32]. Therefore, at present a 2cm excision margin is recommended for intermediate (2 – 4mm) thickness melanomas.

There is unfortunately limited evidence or published data on the optimal resection margin for melanomas with a thickness of 4mm or greater. The British Trial included 243 patients with melanomas of > 4mm thickness and the results showed a higher local recurrence rate associated with a margin of 1cm [32]. However, the local recurrence rates with a 3cm margin appeared similar to other trials with only a 2cm margin of excision. In a retrospective review from MD Anderson which assessed patients with melanomas of greater than 6mm thickness, excision margins greater than 2 cm were not found to effect overall survival when compared to margins of 2cm or less. The 5-year overall and disease free survival rates were 55% and 30% in node negative compared to node positive patients which were included in the study. Nodal status, thickness, and ulceration were significantly associated with overall survival by multivariate analysis. However, the neither the disease free nor overall survival was effected by the presence of a local recurrence or the original excision margin in this study [36]. The study authors therefore concluded that a 2 cm margin of excision is adequate for patients with thick melanoma [36].However, overall there is insufficient data to support the preferred use of either a 2cm or 3cm margin, and consequently, it may be reasonable to allow the patient to decide, following an informed discussion of surgical options. The use of the larger 3cm margin may be recommended in patients with deep tumours (> 4mm depth), due to the higher risk of loco-regional recurrence [32]. In selected cases, however, margin size may be modified to accommodate individual anatomic or cosmetic considerations [23].

Although radial excision margins remain somewhat controversial, the depth of excision in clinical practice is defined as an excision down to but not including the deep fascia [37]. This definition has been internationally accepted and forms the basis of the current gold-standard management of melanoma. Unfortunately in facial areas where the 'deep fascia' is less clearly defined (for example, on the ear, nose, or eyelid), or other anatomic sites such as over the breast, existing studies provide no clear guidelines for optimal depth of excision [5].

Margins	
Tis	Histologically clear margins are adequate
T1	1cm margin is recommended
T2	1-2cm margin recommended
T3	2-3cm margin recommended

Table 2. Recommended excision margins based on tumor size [23]

Despite all the evidence discussed above, controversy still remains regarding the optimal width of the surgical excision margins in malignant melanoma and current evidence is not sufficient to address the optimal surgical management for all melanomas. Indeed a Cochrane review which has been recently published attempted to address this complex question [5]. Overall, there was no statistically significant difference in overall survival between either a narrow or wide excision, but this meta-analysis was confounded by the fact that excision margins were not standardized between studies within the overall analysis. Therefore the dilemma regarding surgical margin remains. However, guidelines regarding margin width have been published and should be adhered to where feasible. Further studies are required to determine the appropriate local treatment for thick melanoma which has not been comprehensively addressed in trials thus far.

3.3. In-transit metastasis

The treatment of advanced or recurrent melanoma remains controversial. Around 10% of patients develop in-transit or multiple cutaneous metastases but at least half will survive for two years without developing distant disease [38, 39]. Unfortunately, the 5-year survival has been reported as 12% with a median survival of 19 months [39].

In-transit metastases are defined as cutaneous or subcutaneous deposits of melanoma between the site of the primary disease and regional lymph nodes [40]. These deposits may be found localized around the primary tumour or may be widespread throughout the affected limb or on the head and neck or trunk, depending on the primary site [40] (Figure 1). It is thought that these metastases arise from dissemination of melanoma cells via the lymphatics to tissues located between the primary tumor and the regional lymph node basin. Other theories include that of drift metastases within tissue fluid of the limb or the local implantation of circulating haematogenous melanoma cells [41, 42].

The presence of small in-transit metastatic melanoma presents specific surgical problems. Unlike nodal disease, which can be managed by regional lymph node dissection, in-transit disease is often widespread and may necessitate multiple surgeries as the disease progresses and new deposits become apparent. In its most severe form, in-transit metastasis may become severely disabling and may be refractory to treatment. Treatment is therefore, palliative, even if staging investigations fail to show evidence of distant metastatic disease [40]. Recent studies have recommended that treatment should be tailored to the extent of the disease, with treatments associated with significant morbidity being reserved for bulky advanced metastases [40].

Several therapies have been proposed for the management of in-transit metastasis including surgery, radiotherapy, and intra-lesional therapy. In-transit metastasis are sharply circumscribed with a clear line of demarcation from normal dermis and epidermis. This line does not contain any in-situ component. Therefore, wide excision margins are not recommended for these lesions and a complete macroscopic excision and primary closure is sufficient. If lesions are grouped closely together, an en bloc excision is acceptable [40].

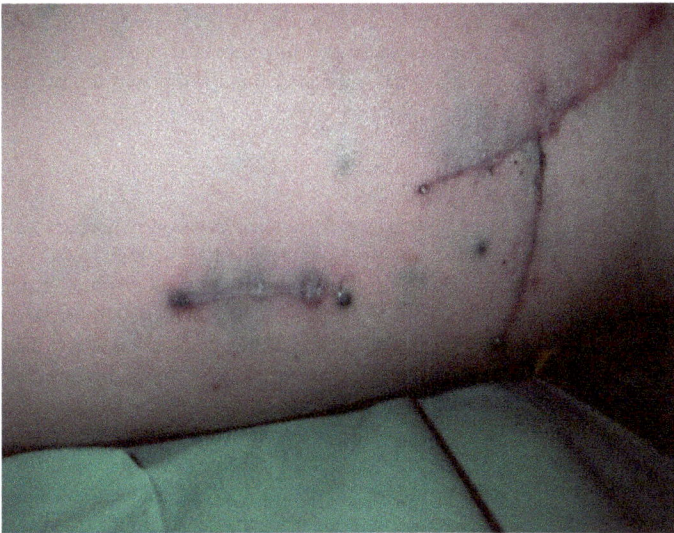

Figure 1. In-transit metastases on the left lower limb

There are numerous treatments available for the management of in-transit metastases that are not suitable for surgical treatment. Carbon dioxide laser therapy has been used in the management of small in-transit metastasis that are not amenable for surgical excision. This is performed as a day case under local anesthetic. Small lesions may be vaporized completely, while larger lesions are first circumscribed with the laser prior to excision of the central core. This well tolerated procedure is more suitable for smaller lesions.

In more advanced diseased, isolated limb perfusion has traditionally been the main method of treatment. This invasive procedure has been replaced by isolated limb infusion, which is simpler, minimally invasive, and a more economical alternative with comparable results [38, 39]. Isolated limb perfusion with chemotherapeutic agents was developed in New Orleans in the mid 1950s by Creech *et al* [38, 39, 43]. It is based on the principle of vascular isolation of the affected limb using a cardiopulmonary bypass circuit through open surgical cannulation of the major limb vessels. This procedure is technically difficult, expensive, and complications are common. Repeated limb perfusions are difficult to perform and morbidity rates increase from 28% to 51% [38]. A simpler alternative, isolated limb infusion was developed by Dr John Thompson in the Sydney Melanoma Unit [44]. It is a less invasive procedure, which involves percutaneous placement of venous and arterial catheters and the infusion of chemotherapeutic agents. This negates the need for a bypass circuit. As opposed to isolated limb perfusion, autologous blood or autologous transfusion of allogenic units is not required. The operating time is reduced from four hours to one hour, and the complication rates are documented to be lower, at only 1% [38, 43].

The presence of in-transit metastases indicates a poor prognosis. The development of in-transit disease may be rapidly followed by distant metastases [40]. The American Committee on Cancer Staging (AJCC) classify it as stage IIIB or IIIC disease, along with regional lymph node metastases. Five year survival rates in patients with stage III disease ranges from 18% to 60%. However, patients with in-transit metastasis have the worst prognosis, with 5 year survival of approximately 25%.

3.4. Reconstruction

The optimal treatment of patients undergoing melanoma excision is primary closure of the wound. Unfortunately, this is not always possible especially in patients with thick melanomas requiring wider excision margins. Therefore, in these cases reconstructive surgery must be considered and where feasible offered to the patient. This will usually depend on the site and extent of the excision to be performed. Skin grafting is the commonest technique employed to ensure skin cover of the anatomical defect. Traditionally, the graft is harvested from the contralateral limb, as melanoma was thought to metastasize primarily via lymphatic routes [15, 45, 46]. However, a recent study looking at the recurrence rates within skin graft donor sites, reported no difference in local recurrence rates when either the ipsilateral or contralateral limbs were used as graft sites. The authors of this study recommended that to improve patient recovery, harvesting the graft from the same limb as the primary tumor is both oncologically safe and technically superior to contralateral skin graft harvest [47]. In certain sites, such as the head and neck, the use of skin grafts may not always be ideal and may result in significant deformity. Local rotation flaps, such as rhomboid flaps, have been found to be safe, versatile, and more aesthetically pleasing when used in these areas [15, 48].

4. Management of the regional lymph node basin

The presence of regional lymph node metastatic disease is a significant predictor of outcome in melanoma and is associated with a 50% reduction in overall survival compared to that of patients without nodal involvement [23]. Indeed the regional lymph node status is thought to be the most powerful prognostic indicator in clinically localised melanoma. The risk of patients developing lymph node metastases increases exponentially with the increasing thickness of the primary melanoma. Melanomas less than 1mm rarely metastasise (less than 10%), while at least 25% of melanomas 1.5- 4.0mm and over 60% of melanomas greater than 4.0mm thick will have lymph node metastasis at presentation[49]. These data form the basis for the current guidelines on which patients should be offered a sentinel lymph node biopsy.

Patients with melanoma can present with either a clinically normal regional lymph node basin or palpable regional lymphadenopathy. Patients with stage III disease commonly have clinically negative lymph nodes but are found to have micro-metastatic disease on their sentinel lymph node biopsy. Such patients have been found to have a more favourable outcome than patients with clinically involved nodes at presentation [8]. The outcome of patients with stage III disease is determined by the number of metastatic nodes and the presence of either microscopic or macroscopic disease. The 5-year survival rate for patients with stage IIIA disease is 67%, and the 10-year survival is 60%. Patients with stage IIIB disease have survival rates estimated at 53%, while stage IIIC disease patients have the worst prognosis with a 5-year survival of approximately 26% [49]. The surgical management of the associated lymph node basin depends on the initial presentation of the patient.

4.1. The sentinel lymph node biopsy

Metastasis to regional lymph nodes is an important prognostic factor in patients with melanoma, upstaging patients to stage III disease and has been shown to occur in about 20% of patients with intermediate thickness melanoma [50]. A sentinel lymph node biopsy (SLNB) is a minimally invasive procedure that aims to identify patients with microscopic lymph node metastasis who would benefit from further lymph node dissection and adjuvant treatment. The sentinel node is defined as any lymph node that receives lymphatic drainage directly from a primary tumour site [51] (Figure 2).

The technical details of sentinel lymph node biopsy can be broken down into a number of steps. First, the patient undergoes preoperative lymphoscintigraphy which identifies the regional nodal basin and estimates the location of the sentinel node. Four intra-dermal injections of 0.1–0.2 ml of 10 MBq radio-colloid are performed around the melanoma or melanoma scar: the injection should raise a small wheal on the skin. The most commonly used radiotracers are 99mTc-labeled albumin (Europe), 99mTc-labeled sulphur colloid and

99mTc-antimony trisulphide colloid. Scintillation cameras are used to obtain dynamic images. These images allow identification of sentinel nodes within the regional nodal basin.
They also allow discrimination of second-tier nodes, which may be falsely interpreted as
sentinel nodes on delayed imaging. The surface location of the sentinel node may be marked
on the skin preoperatively or, alternatively, a gamma probe can be use to locate the node
intra-operatively. Intra-operative lymphatic mapping involves injection of vital blue dye
(Isosulfan blue (Lymphazurin), Methylene Blue or Patent Blue V are used). A combination
of radiotracers and blue dye has been shown to allow sentinel node identification in 99% of
cases. The blue dye is injected intra-dermally in 2-4 locations at the site of the primary lesion, 10-15 minutes before skin incision. The dye is used to visualize the sentinel node intra-
operatively. A gamma probe (covered in a sterile plastic sheath), which detects radiation,
may be used to locate the sentinel node (Figure 3). Counts should be obtained over the skin
before incision, to confirm the location of the sentinel node. A short skin incision is made,
bearing in mind the potential need for complete lymph node dissection. The sentinel nodes
are then identified using the blue dye and gamma probe as a guide, and they are removed
with minimal dissection. An ex-vivo count should be obtained, by measuring the radioactivity of the sentinel node(s) after removal. A bed count is then also obtained following removal of the sentinel node(s), to ensure that no sentinel nodes remain [15, 52].

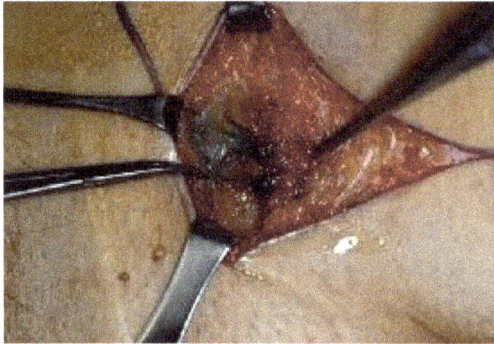

Figure 2. The Sentinel Lymph Node Biopsy

The Multicenter Selective Lymphadenectomy Trial-1 (MSLT-1) is the largest trial to address
the role of lymphatic mapping with SLNB in determining prognosis and its impact on survival [53]. Patients with a primary cutaneous melanoma were randomly assigned to wide
excision and postoperative observation of the regional lymph nodes with lymphadenectomy
being performed only if nodal relapse was confirmed or to wide excision and sentinel-node
biopsy with immediate lymphadenectomy if nodal micro-metastases were detected on biopsy [53]. The MSLT-1 trial confirmed the prognostic importance of SLN status, demonstrating
that SLN status is the most statistically significant predictor of survival for clinically localized (stage I/II) intermediate thickness melanoma (1.2 to 3.5 mm). The 5-year disease-free

survival for patients with positive SLN status was 72.3%, compared to 90.2% in those with negative SLN status [53].

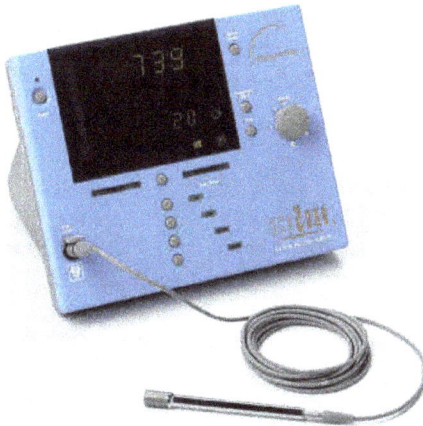

Figure 3. Gamma probe used to locate sentinel lymph node

The AJCC Melanoma Staging Committee recommends that a sentinel lymph node biopsy be performed as a staging procedure in patients for whom the information will be useful in planning subsequent treatments and follow-up regimens. Significant controversy surrounds the use of sentinel lymph node biopsy in thin, early melanomas. There are a number of reasons for this. Firstly, patients with a low-risk of nodal metastases are exposed to the morbidity of a potentially unnecessary procedure. Secondly, the routine use of sentinel lymph node biopsy is expensive: global application of sentinel lymph node biopsy in all patients is estimated to cost between $700,000 and $1,000,000 for every sentinel node metastasis detected [15, 54]. Therefore, for thin melanomas, the routine use of SLNB has not been advocated as the risk of positive nodes is around 5.1% [55]. Indeed, a rate of only 2.7% has been documented with melanomas thinner than 0.75mm [55]. SLNB may be considered, however, in patients with high risk features such as ulceration, a mitotic rate of greater than or equal to $1/mm^2$ especially in patients with melanomas of ≥ 0.76 mm as they are associated with an approximately 10% risk of occult metastases in their sentinel lymph nodes [8]. SLNB is also recommended for patients with intermediate thickness melanoma (2 – 4mm). With regards to thick melanomas, it is expected that around 30% of patients will have evidence of lymph node involvement and the role for SLNB is less clear. It is, however, recommended that SLNB be performed in patients with no clinically evidence positive nodes as it allows for better chances at local disease control [50].

Recent editions of the AJCC melanoma guidelines have altered the criteria for the presence of regional lymph node disease. Originally, the 6th Edition of the AJCC melanoma guidelines recommended histological confirmation of all immunohistochemically (IHC) detected metastasis by routine H&E staining and only after this confirmation could metastatic disease be documented [56]. However, the more recently published guidelines state that positive nodes may be confirmed by either H&E staining or IHC staining with melanoma associated markers [7]. The three most commonly used IHC markers for melanoma are S-100, HMB-45, and Melan A/MART 1. Currently, S-100 remains the most sensitive marker for detection of melanoma, while HMB-45 and Melan A/MART 1 are used for their specificity [57].

More recently, reverse transcriptase polymerase chain reaction (RT-PCR) has been shown to be a promising staging tool used to identify patients with histologically unidentified micrometastatic disease. This technique relies on detection of distinct mRNA expressed by melanoma cells, such as tyrosinase, MAGE-3, MART-1, gp100 and other markers [58, 59]. There has been evidence suggesting the correlation between RT-PCR positive results in blood with stage of melanoma, tumor thickness and known prognostic indicators. The value of RT-PCR in regional lymph nodes is less clear. The number of false positives due to the presence of melanocytic naevi and Schwann cells has limited its use. However, there are results that show that positive results correlate with melanoma thickness [60]. Initial results from 30-month follow-up of the Sunbelt Melanoma Trial did not show any difference in disease-free or overall survival in RT-PCR positive and negative patients [61]. The results were subsequently included in meta-analysis where it has been suggested that RT-PCR may have valuable prognostic use in the prediction of overall and disease free survival [62]. The clinical relevance of the ability to detect micro-metastases by RT-PCR is still under investigation.

4.2. Elective regional lymph node dissection

Completion lymph node dissection (CLND) is recommended for patients with a positive SLN biopsy. It is performed with the intention of halting metastatic spread of melanoma in the early stages of the disease [15, 62, 64]. The five-year survival rate in patients with negative complete lymph node dissection stands at 62.5%, compared with 20.3% in patients with positive non-sentinel nodes [65]. However, the exact role of this and its reflection on overall survival in the setting of positive sentinel nodes has yet to be fully elucidated.

Currently, a complete lymph node dissection is carried out for all patients with a positive sentinel lymph node, irrespective of the type of metastases (micro or macro-metastasis) identified. The value of a complete lymph node dissection in this group of patients has not been extensively investigated and it must constantly be borne in mind that completion lymph node dissection is associated with significant patient morbidity [66]. Indeed, in the MSLT-1, no improvement in OS was seen in the total group randomized to receive SLNB followed by completion lymph node dissection (CLND) if the SLN was positive compared to those randomized to WLE and observation, with nearly identical 5-year melanoma specific-survival of 87.1% versus 86.6% (P = 0.58) [53]. Studies that looked at this difference did not show any statistical significant between the two groups. In addition, it is felt that micro-metastases will become evident if left untreated. Patients with nodal metastases were shown to have a survival advantage with early intervention compared with those who had a delayed lymphadenectomy only when they presented with clinically evident nodal metastasis [15, 53, 67].

However, a significant survival benefit has been noted in patients with a positive sentinel lymph node biopsy, who undergo a complete lymph node dissection, when compared with patients undergoing complete lymph node dissection after nodal metastases become apparent [68]. In a study conducted by Morton et al, a 5-year survival rate of 72% was seen in patients with positive sentinel lymph nodes, followed by immediate lymph node dissection, whereas patients undergoing a delayed lymph node dissection had a 5-year survival rate of only 52% [53]. Further positive non-sentinel lymph nodes are found in a relatively small proportion of patients: previously quoted figures ranged from 17%-24% [15, 69-71]. Interestingly a recent study has shown rates of further positive findings to be as low as 14.8% [15, 53].

Researchers have sought to identify factors which may increase a patient's likelihood of non-sentinel node metastases. Increasing Breslow depth has been associated with increased risk of non-sentinel node metastases, while a depth of less than 1mm has no association with any further positive nodes on completion lymph node dissection [15,65]. Studies have failed to show an association between specific tumour and patient characteristics with an increased rate of non-sentinel nodal metastasis [15, 71], However, a number of histopathological features have been shown to be associated with positive complete lymph node dissections. These include: nodular melanoma, ulceration, melanoma regression, and naevus association [15, 65]. Using a size/ulceration score, Reeves et al. showed ulceration to be an independent predictor of non-sentinel node deposits [72].

Recent studies have examined the association between the size of the sentinel lymph node deposits and the rate of positive complete lymph node dissection. Kunte et al. did not report any patients with micro-metastatic deposits on sentinel lymph node biopsy to have positive findings on complete lymph node dissection [15, 65, 73]. Another study showed a 3-year survival rate in patients with 1mm sentinel lymph node metastasis to be 100%, while 3-year survival in patients with deposits greater than 1mm was 80% [15, 74]. Ollila et al., however, found a significantly higher rate of recurrence in patients with submicrometastatic disease (ie. sentinel lymph node deposits less than 0.1mm), compared with node-negative patients [15, 75].

A significant number of these questions will be address by the publication of the results of The Multicenter Selective Lymphadenectomy Trial-II (MSTL-II) which are currently awaited [76, 77]. This trial aims to address the importance of SLN metastases, the relevance of molecular assessment of the SLN and to evaluate the therapeutic benefit of CLNB after SLNB. Within the trial, all patients with primary melanoma ≥1.2 mm or ≤1.2 mm with Clark level IV / V or ulceration undergo a SLNB. This will be analyzed by both H&E and IHC techniques. Patients with a negative SLNB by H&E and IHC will undergo RT-PCR. All SLN-positive patients identified by H&E/IHC or RT-PCR are randomized to one of two groups: observation of lymph node basin with clinical examination and repeated follow-up ultrasound scanning or to immediate CLND. Patients with negative SLN as determined by RT-PCR are assigned to routine follow-up. The primary endpoint of this study is to determine if

CLND will improve melanoma specific survival in patients with a positive SLNB. Secondary endpoints include assessing the predictive value of immune responses to melanoma- associated antigens, to analyze blood samples from patients for molecular markers of melanoma, both before and after surgery and to assess the quality of life of patients undergoing either CLND or observation after SLNB. Finally the study analyses the predictive value of certain DNA markers of the primary tumor in relation to disease outcome [76, 77].

In conclusion, in the setting of a negative sentinel lymph node biopsy, a completion lymph node dissection is clearly not indicated. The presence of positive nodes warrants consideration of complete lymph node dissection of the involved lymph node basin. Results of the MSLT-II trial are awaited and will give answers to the option of nodal observation.

5. Management of distant metastatic disease

The management of patients with metastatic melanoma remains challenging. Despite improved therapeutic options the prognosis remains poor. A complete surgical resection of metastatic disease in distant sites offers the best chance to improve survival. Patients with in-transit metastasis may be offered further surgical resection of the lesions. Favourable prognostic factors in patients with metastatic disease include a longer disease free survival, single site disease, complete resection and non-visceral metastases [78]. Patients that undergo resection of their non-visceral metastasis have been shown to have a medium survival of between 17 - 50 months, and a 5 - year survival of 9 - 35%. Patients with pulmonary metastasis, who have a complete resection, have a median survival of 8 - 20 months and a 5 year survival of 10 -25%. Brain and gastrointestinal tract metastasis confers a median survival of only 7-10 months [78]. Surgical resection in cases of advanced melanoma has been shown to give good palliation, if all the disease is completely removed. More recently, new systemic biological therapies have been developed, and when combined with surgery may be shown to aid in improved survival. These combinations, however, are still under review [79].

Chemotherapeutic agents have little role to play in the management of metastatic melanoma. Regimens that have previously been utilised include dacarbazine, temozolomide, high dose interleukin-2, paclitaxel and cisplatin or carboplatin. These show a response rate of less than 20% [33]. There is little evidence of its value in metastatic melanoma, however with combination treatments their role is yet to be fully examined.

In 2011, the FDA approved two newer therapies for metastasis melanoma. These include the highly selective BRAF inhibitor, vemurafenib, and ipilimumab, a fully human IgG1 monoclonal antibody. Around 40% to 60% of melanomas are shown to harbor a mutation in the gene encoding for the serine / threonine kinase protein kinase B-raf (BRAF) with 90% of the mutations resulting in a substitution of valine for glutamate at amino acid 600 (V600E) [80]. Mutated BRAF leads to constitutive activation of the mitogen-activated protein kinase pathway (MAPK) that in turn increases cellular proliferation and drives oncogenic activity. Sorafenib, the initial BRAF inhibitor failed to demonstrate significant response rates in melanoma and its use has been largely discontinued. Vemurafenib is a newer highly selective inhibitor with promising results. The main limitation of this novel agent is its limited response with an approximately 40% to 50% response rate in patients with a V600-mutated BRAF gene. Unfortunately, the median duration of response is only 5 to 6 months [33]. GSK2118436 is a newer highly selective inhibitor of BRAF that is still in pre-clinical trials [80].

Melanoma is an immunogenic tumor. Ipilimumab is a monoclonal antibody directed to the cytotoxic T lymphocyte antigen-4 (CTLA-4). Results of two randomized phase III trial of patients with unresectable metastatic disease that progressed during systemic therapy showed an overall improvement in survival in patients randomized to the ipilimumab arm [33,81,82]). In another phase III study looking at the role of ipilumumab and dacarbazine in patients with previously untreated metastatic melanoma, ipilumumab and dacarbazine was shown to have improved patient survival in comparison to the group receiving dacarbazine alone [83[. The limitation of ipilimumab is its association with autoimmune toxicity. In addition, clinical responses may take months to become apparent, and the overall response rate is less than 20% [33]. Research is ongoing in this area. The EORTC18071 trial is ongoing and compares adjuvant treatment with ipilimumab with observation in patients with high risk lymph node positive disease [84].

The role of biochemotherapy has also been studied. This involves using a combination of chemotherapy and biologic agents [33]. The results, however, show no additional survival benefit with this treatment. Finally, palliative radiotherapy may have a role in the setting of metastatic melanoma and has been shown to have good palliation of symptomatic disease [85-87].

6. Staging

An updated Cancer Staging Manual was recently published by the AJCC [7]. Modifications of the melanoma staging guidelines, which have been used since 2002, were based on a multivariate analysis on 38,918 patients [8]. In the revised guidelines melanoma patients have been categorised into 3 groups; those with localised disease with no evidence of metastases (stage I - II), patients with regional disease (stage III), and those with distant metastatic disease (stage IV). Primary tumour thickness remains the factor most associated with prognosis. Tumour thickness is defined in even integers (1.0, 2.0 and 4.0mm) with increasing thickness corresponding with worsening survival. Within each tumour thickness category, the presence of ulceration further upgrades the classification (Table 3).

Mitotic rate is an indicator of tumour proliferation and is measured as the number of mitoses per mm^2. Several studies have shown the mitotic rate to be an independent prognostic factor in patients with melanoma [88-91]. The AJCC guidelines now recommend the "hot spot" technique for calculating the mitotic rate, where the pathologist begins the mitotic count with the most active tumour focus. This is calculated as mitosis/mm^2 [8]. Multiple thresholds of mitotic rate were examined statistically, and the most significant correlation with survival was identified at a threshold of at least 1/mm^2, where a mitotic rate greater than or equal to $1/mm^2$ was found to be independently associated with a poorer disease-specific survival in patients with T1 disease. For non-ulcerated, thin melanomas the 10-year survival was 95% if there were fewer than 1 mitosis per mm^2, compared with 88% 10-year survival if at least one mitosis per mm^2 was present. In addition, the level of invasion, as defined by Wallace Clark, was found to have no statistical significance in staging with the mitotic rate replacing it as an upstaging criterion from stages 1a to 1b [92].

T Classification	Thickness	Ulceration status/mitosis
Tx	Primary tumour cannot be assessed (for example, curettaged or severely regressed melanoma)	
T0	No evidence of primary tumor	
Tis	Melanoma in situ	
T1	Melanoma is 1.0mm or less in thickness	a: without ulceration and mitosis <1/mm2 b: with ulceration or mitoses ≥1/mm2
T2	Melanoma 1.01-2.0mm	a: without ulceration b: with ulceration
T3	Melanoma 2.01- 4.0mm	a: without ulceration b: with ulceration
T4	Melanoma more than 4.0mm	a: without ulceration b: with ulceration

Table 3. T Classification as recommended by the AJCC [7]

Stage III patients have documented lymph node metastasis (microscopic of macroscopic) (Table 4). S-100 is the most sensitive marker for melanocytic lesions while others such as HMB-45, MART-1/Melan-A, tyrosinase, and MITF are very specific but less sensitive [93]. In terms of documenting micro-metastasis, the AJCC accepts immunohistochemical staining of at least one melanoma specific marker to make the diagnosis. Around 5% to 40% of patients will be upstaged to stage III based on the presence of micro-metastatic disease. These patients have a better prognosis than those presenting with macro-metastatic disease as shown in several studies [8, 95]. The new AJCC guidelines reviewed the results of 3307 patients and make a clear distinction between each group. Staging of this group includes defining the number of nodes involved, the presence of microscopic versus macroscopic disease, as well as intra-lymphatic (in-transit or satellite) metastasis, the presence or absence of primary tumour ulceration, and the thickness of the primary melanoma. These factors were found to be predictive of survival on multivariate analysis. In the absence of nodal metastases, patients with intra-lymphatic metastases (N2c) have 5-year and 10-year survival rates of 69% and 52%, respectively while those with combined intra-lymphatic metastases and nodal metastases (N3) have survival rates of 46% and 33%, respectively [8].

N Classification	Nodes involved	Nodal metastatic mass
Nx	Regional nodes cannot be assessed (for example, previously removed for another reason)	
N0	No regional metastasis noted	
N1	1 node	a: micro-metastasis b: macro-metastasis
N2	2-3 nodes	a: micro-metastasis b: macro-metastasis c: in transit mets(s)/ satellite(s) without metastatic nodes
N3	4 or more metastatic nodes, or matted nodes, or in transit met(s)/ satellite(s) with metastatic node(s)	

Table 4. N Classification as recommended by the AJCC [7]

Finally, the database for stage IV patients was expanded to include 7972 patients and the new guidelines now incorporate the serum lactate dehydrogenase as a prognostic marker included in staging (Table 5). An elevated serum LDH was found to be an independent and a highly significant predictor of survival outcome. In a study that looked at the correlation between survival in advanced melanoma from two large trials (Oblimersen GM301 and EORTC 189510), the authors reported an elevated LDH in melanoma patients compared to the normal population. A relationship was found between LD and survival [95]. Patients with elevated serum LDH at diagnosis of melanoma are staged as M1c according to the AJCC guidelines.

M Classification	Site	Serum LDH
M0	No detectable evidence of distant metastases	
M1a	Metastases to skin, subcutaneous, or distant lymph nodes	Normal
M1b	Metastases to lung	Normal
M1c	Metastases to all other visceral sites or distant metastases to any site combined with an elevated serum LDH	Normal- visceral met(s) Elevated- Distant met(s)

Table 5. M Classification as recommended by the AJCC [7]

7. Follow-up

All patients with invasive melanoma should be followed up post-operatively, except for patients with melanoma in-situ. The aim of follow-up is to detect evidence of recurrent disease or a new primary melanoma early [97,98]. The primary site and adjacent skin should be examined for recurrence of new suspicious lesions, as well as the draining lymph node basins [23]. It is estimated that the lifetime risk of developing a second melanoma is around 4 - 6%. Furthermore, around 60 - 80% of recurrences are found at local and/or regional nodal sites. Around two thirds of these will occur within the first three years, 16% after the first five years. Recurrence after more than ten years is also recognised [23].

There is little evidence for the optimum protocol for follow-up. It appears reasonable that all patients with invasive melanoma should be followed up 6-monthly for 2 years. Thereafter, those with melanomas less than 1.0 mm in depth may be discharged from routine follow-up; other patients should be followed up for a further 3 years at 6-monthly intervals. Patients with stage III or IV disease require lifelong follow up [23].

8. Conclusion

The incidence of melanoma continues to rise steadily in the Western World. Despite increased awareness of the disease this does not appear to have a significant impact on its overall poor prognosis. Surgery remains the mainstay of treatment as there is little in the way of adjuvant systemic treatment. Adequate surgical margins with or without local reconstruction can improve local recurrence rates. The utilisation of the sentinel lymph node biopsy has allowed for accurate staging of the disease. The finding of positive sentinel lymph nodes requires patients to undergo further regional lymph node dissection to reduce the risk of loco-regional disease. The impact of this on overall survival has not yet been clearly elucidated. Increased understanding of the melanoma pathogenesis and molecular biology may lead to the development of novel promising therapeutic agents and individualised treatment plans for these patients..

Author details

Z. Al-Hilli, D. Evoy, J.G. Geraghty, E.W. McDermott and R.S. Prichard

St. Vincent's University Hospital, Elm Park, Dublin, Ireland

References

[1] Jemal A, Bray F, Center MM, Ferlay J, Ward E, Forman D. Global cancer statistics. CA: A Cancer Journal for Clinicians 2011; 61(2) 69–90

[2] American Cancer Society: Cancer Facts and Figures 2012. Atlanta, Ga: American Cancer Society, 2012. Last accessed Aug 3rd 2012

[3] Cancer Research UK. http://info.cancerresearchuk.org/cancerstats/types/skin/ (Accessed 6 Aug 2012)

[4] National Cancer Institute. http://seer.cancer.gov/statfacts/html/melan.html (Accessed 3rd Aug 2012)

[5] Sladden MJ, Balch C, Barzilai DA, Berg D, Freiman A, Handiside T, Hollis S, Lens MB, Thompson JF. Surgical excision margins for primary cutaneous melanoma. Cochrane Database of Systematic Reviews 2009, Issue 4. Art. No.: CD004835. DOI: 10.1002/14651858.CD004835.pub2

[6] Stebbins WG, Garibyan, Sober AJ. Sentinel lymph node biopsy and melanoma: 2010 Part I. Journal of the American Academy of Dermatology. 2010; 62(5) 723-734

[7] Edge SB, Byrd DR, Compton CC, Fritz AG, Greene FL, Trotti A (Eds.): AJCC Cancer Staging Manual. New York, NY, Springer, 2009

[8] Balch CM, Gershenwald JE, Soong SJ, Thompson JF, Atkins MB, Byrd DR, Buzaid AC, Cochran AJ, Coit DG, Ding S, Eggermont AM, Flaherty KT, Gimotty PA, Kirkwood JM, McMasters KM, Mihm Jr MC, Morton DL, Ross MI, Sober AJ, Sondak VK. Final Version of 2009 AJCC Melanoma Staging and Classification. Journal of Clinical Oncology. 2009; 27(36) 6199-206

[9] Cascinelli N, Marchesini R. Increasing incidence of cutaneous melanoma, ultraviolet radiation and the clinician. Photochemistry and Photobiology. 1989; 50 497-505

[10] The American Cancer Society. (2010). What are the key statistics about Melanoma?, In : The American Cancer Society, Available from http://www.cancer.org/Cancer/SkinCancerMelanoma/DetailedGuide/melanoma-skin-cancer-key-statistics (Accessed 8 Aug 2012)

[11] Evans RD, Kopf, Lew RA, Rigel DS, Bart RS, Friedman RJ, Rivers JK. Risk factors for the development of malignant melanoma: I. Review of case-control studies. The journal of Detmatologic Surgery and Oncology 1988; 14(4) 292-408

[12] Gellin GA, Kopf AW, Garfinkel L. Malignant melanoma: A controlled study of possibly associated factors. Archives of Dermatology 2008; 99(1) 61-67

[13] Friedman RJ, Rigel DS, Silverman MK, Kopf AW, Vissaert KA. Malignant melanoma in the 1990s: the continued importance of early detection and the role of physician examination and self-examination of the skin. CA A Cancer Journal for Clinicians 1991; 41(4) 201-206

[14] Brozena SJ, Fenske NA, Perez IR. Epidemiology of malignant melanoma, worldwirde incidence and etiologic factors. Seminars in Surgical Oncology 1993; 9(3) 165-167

[15] Joyce DP, Prichard RS, Hill ADK Current controversies in the surgical management of melanoma. Beaumont Hospital, Dublin, Ireland. In: Cao MY (ed.) Curreny management of malignant melanoma. In Tech. 2011 ISBN 978-953-307-264-7

[16] MacKie RM. Clinical recognition of early invasive malignant melanoma. British Medical Journal 1990; 301(6759)1005-1006

[17] Abbasi NR, Shaw HM, Rigel DS, Friedman RJ, McCarthy WH, Osman I, et al. Early diagnosis of cutaneous melanoma: revisiting the ABCD criteria. The Journal of the American Medical Association 2004; 292(22) 2771-6

[18] Friedman RJ, Rigel DS, Kopf AW. Early detection of malignant melanoma: the role of physician examination and self-examination of the skin. CA: A Cancer Journal for Clinicians 1985; 35(3) 130-51

[19] Whited JD, Grichnik JM. The rational clinical examination. Does the patient have a more of a melanoma? The journal of the American Medical Association 1998; 279(9) 696-701

[20] Swanson NA, Lee KK, Gorman A, Lee HN. Biopsy techniques: diagnosis of melanoma. Dermatologic Clinics 2002; 20(4) 677–80

[21] Newton-Bishop JA, Corrie PG, Evans J, Gore ME, Hall PN, Kirkham N, Roberts DL, Anstey AV, Barlow RJ, Cox NH. Melanoma Study Group; British Association of Dermatologists. UK Guidelines for the management of cutaneous melanoma. British Journal of Plastic Surgery 2002; 55(1): 46 - 54

[22] Herd RM, Hunter JAA, McLaren KM, Chetty U, Watson ACH, Gollock JM. Excision biopsy of malignant melanoma by general practitioners in south east Scotland 1982–91. British Medical Journal 1992; 305(6867) 1476–8

[23] Cahill R, Hill ADK, Redmond HP. Royal College of Surgeons in Ireland, Management of Cutaneous Melanoma Clinical Guidelines. 2006

[24] Balch CM, Soong SJ, Atkins MB, Buzaid AC, Cascinelli N, Coit DG, Fleming ID, Gershenwald JE, Houghton A Jr, Kirkwood JM, McMasters KM, Mihm MF, Morton DL, Reintgen DS, Ross MI, Sober A, Thompson JA, Thomson JF. An evidence-based staging system for cutaneous melanoma. CA: A Cancer Journal for Clinicians 2004; 54(3)131-49

[25] Balch CM, Buzaid AC, Soong SJ, Atkins MB, Cascinelli N, Coit DG, Fleming ID, Gershenwald JE, Houghton A Jr, Kirkwood JM, McMasters KM, Mihm MF, Morton DL, Reintgen DS, Ross MI, Sober A, Thompson JA, Thomson JF. New TNM melanoma staging system: linking biology and natural history to clinical outcomes. Seminars in Surgical Oncology 2003; 21(1) 43-52

[26] Cascinelli N, Belli F, Santinami M, Fait V, Testori A, Ruka W, Canaliere R, Mozzillo N, Rossi CR, MacKie RM, Nieweg O, Pace M, Kirov K. Sentinel lymph node biopsy in cutaneous melanoma: the WHO Melanoma Program experience. Annals of Surgical Oncology 2000; 7(6) 469–474

[27] Cohn-Cedermark G, Rutqvist LE, Andersson R, Breivald M, Ingvar C, Johansson H, Jönsson PE, Krysander L, Lindholm C, Ringborg U. Long term results of a random-ized study by the Swedish Melanoma Study Group on 2-cm versus 5-cm resection margins for patients with cutaneous melanoma with a tumor thickness of 0.8-2.0 mm. Cancer. 2000; 89(7) 1495-1501

[28] Khayat D, Rixe O, Martin G, Soubrane C, Banzet M, Bazex JA, Lauret P, Vérola O, Auclerc G, Harper P, Banzet P, French Group of Research on Malignant Melanoma. Surgical margins in cutaneous melanoma (2 cm versus 5 cm for lesions measuring less than 2.1-mm thick).Cancer. 2003; 97(8) 1941-1946

[29] Balch CM, Soong S, Ross MI, Urist MM, Karakousis CP, Temple WJ, Mihm MC, Barnhill RL, Jewell WR, Wanebo HJ, Harrison R. Long-term results of a multi-institu-tional randomized trial comparing prognostic factors and surgical results for inter-mediate thickness melanomas (1.0 to 4.0 mm). Intergroup Melanoma Surgical Trial. Ann Surg Oncol. 2000; 7(2) 87-97

[30] Balch CM, Soong SJ, Smith T, Ross MI, Urist MM, Karakousis CP, Temple WJ, Mihm MC, Barnhill RL, Jewell WR, Wanebo HJ, Desmond R; Investigators from the Inter-group Melanoma Surgical Trial. Long-term results of a prospective surgical trial comparing 2 cm vs. 4 cm excision margins for 740 patients with 1-4 mm melanomas. Annals of Surgical Oncology. 2001 Mar;8(2):101-8

[31] Gillgren P, Drzewiecki KT, Niin M, Gullestad HP, Hellborg H, Månsson-Brahme E, Ingvar C, Ringborg U 2-cm versus 4-cm surgical excision margins for primary cuta-neous melanoma thicker than 2 mm: a randomised, multicentre trial.. Lancet. 2011; 378(9803) 1635-1642

[32] Thomas JM, Newton-Bishop J, A'Hern R, Coombes G, Timmons M, Evans J, Cook M, Theaker J, Fallowfield M, O'Neill T, Ruka W, Bliss JM, United Kingdom Melanoma Study Group, British Association of Plastic Surgeons, Scottish Cancer Therapy Net-work. Excision margins in high-risk malignant melanoma. New England Journal of Medicine. 2004; 350(8) 757-766

[33] Coit DG, Andtbacka R, Anker CJ, Bichakjian CK, Carson WE 3rd, Daud A, Dilawari RA, Dimaio D, Guild V, Halpern AC, Hodi FS Jr, Kelley MC, Khushalani NI, Kud-chadkar RR, Lange JR, Lind A, Martini MC, Olszanski AJ, Pruitt SK, Ross MI, Swetter SM, Tanabe KK, Thompson JA, Trisal V, Urist MM; National Comprehensive Cancer Network. Melanoma. Journal of the Nationall Comprehensive Cancer Network. 2012; 10(3) 366-400

[34] Bichakjian CK, Halpern AC, Johnson TM, Foote Hood A, Grichnik JM, Swetter SM, Tsao H, Barbosa VH, Chuang TY, Duvic M, Ho VC, Sober AJ, Beutner KR, Bhushan R, Smith Begolka W, American Academy of Dermatology Guidelines of care for the management of primary cutaneous melanoma. American Academy of Dermatology. Journal of the American Academy of Dermatology. 2011; 65(5) 1032-1047

[35] Cotter MA, McKenna JK, Bowen GM. Treatment of lentigo maligna with imiquimod before staged excision. Dermatologic Surgery 2008; 34(2) 147–151.

[36] Heaton KM, Sussman JJ, Gershenwald JE, Lee JE, Reintgen DS, Mansfield PF, Ross MI. Surgical margins and prognostic factors in patients with thick (>4mm) primary melanoma. Annals of Surgical Oncology. 1998; 5(4) 322-328

[37] Australian Cancer Network Melanoma Guidelines Revision Working Party. Clinical Practice Guidelines for the Management of Melanoma in Australia and New Zealand. Cancer Council Australia and Australian Cancer Network, Sydney and New Zealand Guidelines Group, Wellington 2008; 73-77

[38] Brady MS, Brown K, Patel A, Fisher C, Marx. A phase II trial of isolated limb infusion with melphalan and dactinomycin for regional melanoma and soft tissue sarcoma of the extremity. Annals of Surgical Oncology 2006; 13(8):1123-9

[39] Mian R, Henderson M, Speakman D, Finkelde D, Ainslie J, McKenzie A. Isolated limb infusion for melanoma: a simple alternative to isolated limb perfusion. Canadian Journal of Surgery. 2001; 44(3) 189-192

[40] Hayes AJ, Clarke MA, Harries M, Thomas JM. Management of in-transit metastases from cutaneous malignant melanoma. British Journal of Surgery. 2004; 91(6) 673-682

[41] McCarthy WH. Melanoma Margins for error-another view. ANZ Journal of Surgery 2002; 72(4) 304-306

[42] Heenan PJ, Ghasnawie M. The pathogenesis of local recurrence of melanoma at the primary excision site. British Journal of Plastic Surgery. 1999; 52(3) 209-213

[43] Al-Hilli Z, Waqar K, Hill ADK. Isolated limb infusion for melanoma. Surgeon. 2007 5(5) 310-312

[44] Thompson JF, Kam PC, Waugh RC, Harman R. Isolated limb infusion with cytotoxic agents: A simple alternative to isolated limb perfusion. Seminars in Surgical Oncology 1998; 14(3) 238-47

[45] Cade S. Malignant melanoma. Annals of the Royal College of Surgeons in England. 1961; 28: 331-366

[46] Roberts DL, Anstey AV, Barlow RJ, et al. U.K. guidelines for the management of cutaneous melanoma. British Journal of Dermatology. 2002; 146 7–17

[47] Schumacher HH, Chia HL, Simcock JW. Ipsilateral skin grafts for lower limb melanoma reconstruction are safe. Plastic and Reconstructive Surgery. 2010; 125(2) 89-91

[48] Lent WM, Ariyan S. Flap reconstruction following wide local excision for primary malignant melanoma of the head and neck region. Annals of Plastic Surgery. 1994; 33(1) 23-27

[49] Balch CM, Soong SJ, Gershenwald JE, et al. Prognostic factors analysis of 17,600 melanoma patients: validation of the American Joint Committee on Cancer melanoma staging system. Journal of Clinical Oncology 2001; 19(16) 3622–3634

[50] Wong SL, Balch CM, Hurley P, Agarwala SS, Akhurst TJ, Cochran A, Cormier JN, Gorman M, Kim TY, McMasters KM, Noyes RD, Schuchter LM, Valsecchi ME, Weaver DL, Lyman GH. Sentinel Lymph Node Biopsy for Melanoma: American Society of Clinical Oncology and Society of Surgical Oncology Joint Clinical Practice Guideline. Annals of Surgical Oncology 2012 July 6 [Epub ahead of print] PMID: 22766987

[51] Uren RF, Howman-Giles R, Thompson JF, Shaw HM, Quinn MJ, O'Brien CJ, McCarthy WH. Lymphoscintigraphy to identify sentinel lymph nodes in patients with melanoma. Melanoma Research 1994; 4(6)395–399

[52] Bagaria SP, Faries MB, Morton DL. Sentinel Node Biopsy in Melanoma: Technical Considerations of the Procedure as Performed at the John Wayne Cancer Institute. Journal Surgical Oncology. 2010; 101(8) 669–676

[53] Morton DL, Thompson JF, Cochran AJ, Mozzillo N, Elashoff R, Essner R, Nieweg OE, Roses DF, Hoekstra HJ, Karakousis CP, Reintgen DS, Coventry BJ, Glass EC, Wang HJ, MSLT Group. Sentinel-node biopsy or nodal observation in melanoma. New England Journal of Medicine. 2006; 355(13) 1307-1317

[54] Agnese DM, Abdessalam SF, Burak WE Jr, Magro CM, Pozderac RV, Walker MJ. Cost-effectiveness of sentinel lymph node biopsy in thin melanomas. Surgery. 2003;134(4):542-548

[55] Andtbacka RH, Gershenwald JE. Role of sentinel lymph node biopsy in patients with thin melanoma. Journal of the National Comprehensive Cancer Network. 2009; 7(3) 208-317

[56] AJCC cancer staging manual. 6th ed. Chicago, IL: Springer; 2002

[57] Spanknebel K, Coit DG, Bieligk SC, Gonen M, Rosai J, Klimst DS. Characterization of micrometastatic disease in melanoma sentinel lymph nodes by enhanced pathology: recommendations for standardizing pathologic analysis. American Journal of Surgical Pathology 2005; 29(3) 305-317

[58] Blaheta HJ, Ellwanger U, Schittek B, Sotlar K, MacZey E, Breuninger H, Thelen MH, Bueltmann B, Rassner G, Garbe C. Examination of regional lymph nodes by sentinel node biopsy and molecular analysis provides new staging facilities in primary cutaneous melanoma. The Journal of Investigative Dermatology 2000; 114(4) 637-642.

[59] Palmieri G, Ascierto PA, Cossu A, Mozzillo N, Motti ML, Satriano SM, Botti G, Caraco Cm Celentano E, Satriano RA, Lissia A, Tanda F, Pirastu M, Castello G; Melanoma Cooperative Group. Detection of occult melanoma cells in paraffin- embedded histologically negative sentinel lymph nodes using a reverse transcriptase polymerase chain reaction assay. Journal of Clinical Oncology 2001; 19(5) 1437-1443

[60] Prichard RS, Dijkstra B, McDermott EW, Hill AD, O'Higgins NJ. The role of molecular staging in malignant melanoma. European Journal of Surgical Oncology. 2003 May; 29(4) 306-14.

[61] Scoggins CR, Ross MI, Reintgen DS, Noyes RD, Goydos JS Beitsch PD, Urist MM, Ariyan S, Davidson BS, Sussman JJ, Edwards MJ, Martin RC, Lewis AM, Stromberg AJ, Conrad AJ, Hagendoorn L, Albrecht J, McMasters KM . Prospective multi-institutional study of reverse transcriptase polymerase chain reaction for molecular staging of melanoma. Journal of Clinical Oncology 2006; 24(18) 2849-2857

[62] Mocellin S, Hoon DS, Pilati P, Rossi CR, Nitti D. Sentinel lymph node molecular ultrastaging in patients with melanoma: a systematic review and meta-analysis of prognosis. Journal of Clinical Oncology 2007; 25(12) 1588-1595

[63] Callery C, Cochran AJ, Roe DJ, Rees W, Nathanson SD, Benedetti JK, Elashoff RM, Morton DL. Factors prognostic for survival in patients with malignant melanoma spread to regional lymph nodes. Annals of Surgery 1982;196:69–75

[64] Roses DF, Provet JA, Harris MN, Gumport SL, Dubin N. Prognosis of patients with pathologic stage II cutaneous malignant melanoma. Annals of Surgery 1985;201:103–7

[65] Kunte C, Geimer T, Baumert J, Konz B, Volkenandt M, Flaig M, Ruzicka T, Berking C, Schmid-Wendtner MH. Analysis of predictive factors for the outcome of complete lymph node dissection in melanoma patients with metastatic sentinel lymph nodes. Journal of the American Academy of Dermatology. 2011 Apr;64(4):655-662

[66] Garbe C, Hauschild A, Volkenandt M, Schadendorf D, Stolz W, Reinhold U, Kettelhack C, Frerich B, Keilholz U, Dummer R, Sebastian G, Tilgan W, Schuler G, Mackensen A, Kaufmann R. Evidence and interdisciplinary consensusbased German guidelines: surgical treatment and radiotherapy of melanoma. Melanoma Resarch 2008;18:61-67

[67] Wong SL, Brady MS, Busam KJ, Coit DG. Results of sentinel lymph node biopsy in patients with thin melanoma. Annals of Surgical Oncology. 2006;13(3) 302-309

[68] Kretschmer L, Hilgers R, Mohrle M, Balda BR, Breuninger H, Konz B, Kunte C, Marsch WC, Neumann C, Starz H. Patients with lymphatic metastasis of cutaneous malignant melanoma benefit from sentinel lymphonodectomy and early excision of their nodal disease. European Journal of Cancer 2004; 40: 212-218

[69] Ghaferi AA, Wong SL, Johnson TM, Lowe L, Chang AE, Cimmino VM, Bradford CR, Rees RS, Sabel MS. Prognostic significance of a positive nonsentinel lymph node in cutaneous melanoma. Annals of Surgical Oncology 2009; 16: 2978-84.

[70] Lee JH, Essner R, Torisu-Itakura H, Wanek L, Wang H, Morton DL. Factors predictive of tumour-positive non-sentinel lymph nodes after tumour-positive sentinel lymph node dissection for melanoma. Journal Clinical Oncology 2004; 22: 3677-84.

[71] Rossi CR, De Salvo GL, Bonandini E, Mocellin S, Foletto M, Pasquali S, Pilati P, Lise M, Nitto D, Rizzo E, Montesco MC. Factors predictive of non-sentinel lymph node involvement and clinical outcome in melanoma patients with metastatic sentinel lymph node. Annals of Surgical Oncology 2008;15 :1202-10

[72] Reeves ME, Delgado R, Busam KJ, Brady MS, Coit DG. Prediction of non-sentinel lymph node status in melanoma. Annals of Surgical Oncology 2003; 10: 27-31

[73] Glumac N, Hocevar M, Zadnik V, Snoj M. Sentinel lymph node micrometastasis may predict non-sentinel involvement in cutaneous melanoma patients. Journal of Surgical Oncology 2008;98 46-49

[74] van der Ploeg IM, Kroon BB, Antonini N, Valdes Olmos RA, Nieweg OE. Is completion lymph node dissection needed in case of minimal melanoma metastasis in the sentinel node? Annals of Surgery 2009;249:1003-7

[75] Ollila DW, Ashburn JH, Amos KD, Yeh JJ, Frank JS, Deal AM, Long P, Thomas ND, Meyers MO. Metastatic melanoma cells in the sentinel node cannot be ignored. Journal of the American College of Surgeons 2009; 208: 924-9, discussion 9-30

[76] Multicenter Selective Lymphadenectomy Trial II (MSLT-II) Clinical-Trials.gov identifier: NCT00297895

[77] Stebbins WG, Garibyan, Sober AJ. Sentinel lymph node biopsy and melanoma: 2010 Part II. Journal of the American Academy of Dermatology. 2010; 62(5) 737-748

[78] Coit DG. Role of Surgery in metastatic malignant melanoma: a review. Seminars in Surgical Oncology. 1993; 9(3) 239-245

[79] Leung AM, Hari DM, Morton DL. Surgery for distant melanoma metastasis. Cancer Journal. 2012; 18(2) 176-178

[80] Finn L, Markovic SN, Joseph RW. Therapy for metastatic melanoma: the past, present, and future. BMC Medicine. 2012; 2; 10: 23

[81] Hodi FS, O'Day SJ, McDermott DF, Weber RW, Sosman JA, Haanen JB, Gonzalez R, Robert C, Schadendorf D, Hassel JC, Akerley W, van den Eertwegh AJ, Lutzky J, Lorigan P, Vaubel JM, Linette GP, Hogg D, Ottensmeier CH, Lebbe C, Peschel C, Quirt I, Clark JI, Wolchock JD, Weber JS, Tian J, Yellin MJ, Nichol GM, Hoos A, Urba WJ. Improved survival with ipilimumab in patients with metastatic melanoma. The New England Journal of Medicine 2010; 363(8) 711-723

[82] Robert C, Thomas L, Bondarenko I, O'Day S, M DJ, Garbe C, Lebbe C, Baurain JF, Testori A, Grob JJ, Davidson N, Richards J, Maio M, Hauschild A, Miller WH Jr, Gascon P, Lotem M, Harmankaya K, Ibrahim R, Francis S, Chenn TTm Humphrey R, Hoos A, Wolchock JD. Ipilimumab plus dacarbazine for previously untreated metastatic melanoma. The New England journal of Medicine 2011; 364(26) 2517-2526

[83] Robert C, Thomas L, Bonderanko I, O'Day S, MD JW, Garbe C, Lebbe C, Baurin JF, Testori A, Grobb JJ, Davidson N, Richards J, Maio M, Hauschild A, Miller WH Jr,

Gascon P, Lotern M, Harmankaya K, Ibrahim R, Francis S, Chenn TT, Humphrey R, Hoos A, Wolchock JD. Ipilumumab plus dacarbazine for previously untreated metastatic melanoma. New England Journal of Medicine. 2011 264(26) 2517-2526

[84] Eggermont AM, Robert C. New drugs in melanoma: it's a whole new world. European Journal of Cancer. 2011 47(14) 2150-2157

[85] Seegenschmiedt MH, Keilholz L, Altendorf-Hofmann A, Urban A, Schell H, Hohenberger W, Sauer R. Palliative radiotherapy for recurrent and metastatic malignant melanoma: prognostic factors for tumor response and long-term outcome: a 20-year experience. International Journal of Radiation Oncology, Biology and Physics 1999; 44(3) 607–618

[86] Overgaard J, von der Maase H, Overgaard M. A randomized study comparing two high-dose per fraction radiation schedules in recurrent or metastatic malignant melanoma. International Journal of Radiation Oncology, Biology and Physics 1985; 11(10) 1837–1839

[87] Olivier KR, Schild SE, Morris CG, Brown PD, Markovic SN. A higher radiotherapy dose is associated with more durable palliation and longer survival in patients with metastatic melanoma. Cancer 2007; 110(8) 1791–1795

[88] Barnhill RL, Katzen J, Spatz A, Fine J, Berwick M. The importance of mitotic rate as a prognostic factor for localized cutaneous melanoma. Journal of Cutaneous Pathology 2005; 32(4) 268–273

[89] Azzola MF, Shaw HM, Thompson JF, Soong SJ, Scolyer RA, Watson GF, Colman MH, Zhang Y. Tumor mitotic rate is a more powerful prognostic indicator than ulceration in patients with primary cutaneous melanoma: an analysis of 3661 patients from a single center. Cancer 2003; 97(6)1488–1498

[90] Francken AB, Shaw HM, Thompson JF, Soong SJ, Accrott NA, Azzola MF, Scoyler RA, Milton GW, McCarthy WH, Colman MHm McGovern VJ. The prognostic importance of tumor mitotic rate confirmed in 1317 patients with primary cutaneous melanoma and long follow-up. Annals of Surgical Oncology 2004; 11(4) 426–433

[91] Gimotty PA, Elder DE, Fraker DL, Botbyl J, Sellers K, Elenitsas R, Ming ME, Schuchter L, Spitz FR, Czerniecki BJ, Geurry D. Identification of high-risk patients among those diagnosed with thin cutaneous melanomas. Journal of Clinical Oncology 2007; 25(9) 1129–1134

[92] Clark WH Jr, From L, Bernardino EA, Mihm MC. The histogenesis and biologic behavior of primary human malignant melanomas of the skin. Cancer Research 1969; 29(3) 705-727

[93] Ohsie SJ, Sarantopoulos GP, Cochran AJ, Binder SW. Immunohistochemical characteristics of melanoma. Journal of Cutaneous Pathology 2008; 35(5) 433–444

[94] Cascinelli N, Belli F, Santinami M, Fait V, Testori A, Ruka W, Canaliere R, Mozzillo N, Rossi CR, MacKie RM, Nieweg O, Pace M, Kirov K. Sentinel lymph node biopsy

in cutaneous melanoma: the WHO Melanoma Program experience. Annals of Surgical Oncology 2000; 7(6) 469–474

[95] Agarwala S, Keilholz U, Gilles E, Bedikian AY, Wu J, Kay R, Stein CA, Itri M, Suciu S, Eggermont AM, LDH correlation with survival in advanced melanoma from two large, randomized trials (Oblimersen GM301 and EORTC 18951). European Journal of Cancer 2009; 45(1) 1807-1814

[96] Martini L, Brandani P, Chiarugi C, Reali UM. First recurrence analysis of 840 cutaneous melanomas: a proposal for a follow-up schedule. Tumori 1994; 80(3) 188-197

[97] Poo-Wwu WJ, Ariyan S, Lambe L, Papac R, Zelterman D, Hu GL, Brown J, Fischer D, Bolognia J, Buzaid AC. Follow-up recommendations for patients with American Joint Committee on Cancer Stages I-III malignant melanoma. Cancer 1999; 86: 2252-2258.

Chapter 6

Cellular and Molecular Mechanisms of Methotrexate Resistance in Melanoma

Luis Sanchez del-Campo, Maria F. Montenegro,
Magali Saez-Ayala, María Piedad Fernández-Pérez,
Juan Cabezas-Herrera and
Jose Neptuno Rodriguez-Lopez

Additional information is available at the end of the chapter

1. Introduction

Melanoma is a cancer that develops in melanocytes, the pigment cells present in the skin. It can be more serious than the other forms of skin cancer because it may spread to other parts of the body (metastasize) and cause serious illness and death. For malignant melanomas standard treatment options have remained remarkably static over the past 30 years [1,2]. At present, the incidence of melanoma continues to increase despite public health initiatives that have promoted protection against the sun. Thus, during the past ten years, the incidence and annual mortality of melanoma has increased more rapidly than any other cancer and according to the American Cancer Society estimate, there will have been approximately 76,250 new cases of invasive melanoma diagnosed in 2012 in the United States, which resulted in approximately 9,180 deaths [3].

Unfortunately, the increase in incidence has not been paralleled by the development of new therapeutic agents with a significant impact on survival. Although many patients with melanoma localized to the skin are cured by surgical excision, increased time to diagnosis is associated with higher stage of disease, and those with regional lymphatic or metastatic disease respond poorly to conventional radiation and chemotherapy with 5-year survival rates ranging from 10 to 50% [4]. Currently, limited therapeutic options exist for patients with metastatic melanomas, and all standard combinations currently used in metastasis therapy have low efficacy and poor response rates. For instance, the only approved chemotherapy for metastatic melanoma, dacarbacine, has a response rate of about 10% and a median survival of 8-9 months.

The other approved agent for advanced melanoma is high dose interleukin-2, which can induce dramatic complete and durable responses [2]. However, only one patient in twenty derives lasting benefit. These data indicate the needed for alternative therapies for this disease and recent results indicated that combined therapies could became an attractive strategy to fight melanoma [2].

Other example of the complications involved in melanoma chemotherapy is the limited effectiveness of antifolates. Although methotrexate (MTX), the most frequently used antifolate, is an efficient drug for several types of cancer, it is not active against melanoma [5-7]. Undoubtedly, unravelling the mechanisms of melanoma resistance to MTX could yield important information on how to circumvent this resistance and could have important pharmacological implications for the design of novel combined therapies. Thus, although an old drug, MTX could become a valuable tool with which to improve melanoma therapy.

2. General mechanisms of resistance to classical antifolates

The antifolate methotrexate was rationally-designed nearly 70 years ago to potently block the folate-dependent enzyme dihydrofolate reductase (DHFR). DHFR (5,6,7,8-tetrahydrofolate: NADP+ oxidoreductase, EC 1.5.1.3) catalyses the reduction of 7,8-dihydrofolate (DHF) to 5,6,7,8-tetrahydrofolate (THF) in the presence of coenzyme NADPH as follows: DHF + NADPH + H+ → THF + NADP+. This enzyme is necessary for maintaining intracellular pools of THF and its derivatives which are essential cofactors in one-carbon metabolism. Coupled with thymidylate synthase (TS) [8], it is directly involved in thymidylate (dTMP) production through a *de novo* pathway. DHFR is therefore pivotal in providing purines and pyrimidine precursors for the biosynthesis of DNA, RNA and amino acids. In addition, it is the target enzyme [9] for antifolate drugs such as the antineoplastic drug MTX and the antibacterial drug trimethoprim (TMP). The mechanisms of resistance to MTX have been extensively studied, mainly in experimental tumours propagated *in vitro* and *in vivo* [5,10,11]; however, the specific basis for the resistance of melanoma cells to MTX is unclear. During decades the mechanism of resistance of melanoma to MTX was associated with general mechanisms of resistance detected in other epithelial cancer cell including reduced cellular uptake of this drug, high intracellular levels of DHFR and/or insufficient rate of MTX polyglutamylation, which diminishes long-chain MTX polyglutamates from being preferentially retained intracellularly [11]. However, recently, a melanoma-specific mechanism of resistance to cytotoxic drugs, including MTX, has been described [6,12,13].

Antifolate resistance in cancer cells is believed to be a multifactorial process in which dysregulation of apoptosis, insufficient rates of MTX polyglutamylation, and enhanced DNA repair play important roles [11,14]. In melanoma, another classical mechanism of resistance to MTX, the upregulation of endogenous dihydrofolate reductase (DHFR) activity, has been described [5]; however, the contribution of this mechanism to the overall resistance of melanoma to MTX as well as its possible impact on DNA damage response pathways in cells is unknown. 'Thymineless' death, which occurs upon the depletion of cellular dTTP pools, has been proposed as a mechanism by which antifolate drugs promote apoptosis in cancer cells [15,16]. Although the mechanism of dTTP depletion-induced apoptosis is yet to be determined, Pardee's group recently postulated that dTTP controls E2F1, which regulates both DNA synthesis and apoptosis. This hypothesis was based on the observation that MTX increased E2F1 levels in sensitive cancer cells, resulting in an increase in the E2F1-mediated apoptotic cascade.

Eukaryotic cells have developed complex checkpoint pathways that monitor DNA for damage or incomplete replication. Checkpoint pathways are amplified upon detection of aberrant DNA structures and lead to a delay in cell cycle progression during which damage can be repaired or replication be completed. Alternatively, in case of heavily damaged or seriously deregulated cells, checkpoint activation can result in apoptosis. As such, checkpoint mechanisms are essential for the maintenance of genomic integrity [17]. When vertebrate cells experience replication arrest or undergo DNA damage by UV irradiation, the ATR kinase [ataxia telangiectasia mutated (ATM)- and Rad3-related kinase] phosphorylates and activates the Chk1 protein kinase. Activated Chk1 inhibits Cdc25 phosphatases, which control inhibitory phosphorylation sites on cyclin-dependent kinases, the latter being critical regulators of cell cycle transitions [18,19]. Because the ability of cells to delay cell cycle progression and halt DNA synthesis represents a defensive mechanism that spares potential toxicity [20], the activation of Chk1 by MTX could constitute a key event in the resistance of melanoma to MTX.

In addition to these cellular mechanisms of resistance to MTX in melanoma, other mechanism that includes liver transformation of the drug has also been reported. A paradoxical response of malignant melanoma to MTX *in vivo* and *in vitro* has been described [21]. The authors observed that MTX showed consistent cytotoxicity for melanoma cells *in vitro* but was ineffective at equivalent concentrations *in vivo*. MTX undergoes oxidation to its primary metabolite 7-hydroxy-MTX (7-OH-MTX) in the liver by the enzyme aldehyde oxidase [11] and therefore, this transformation has been proposed as a novel mechanism of resistance to explain this paradox [11,21]. In contrast to the large body of literature available on the multiple modalities of MTX resistance, very little is known regarding the ability of 7-OH-MTX to provoke antifolate-resistance phenomena that may disrupt MTX activity. Recent studies seem to indicate that 7-OH-MTX which exceeds by far MTX in the plasma of MTX-treated patients can provoke distinct modalities of antifolate-resistance that severely compromise the efficacy of the parent drug MTX [22].

3. Melanoma-specific mechanisms of resistance to MTX

3.1. The critical role of alpha-folate receptor in the resistance of melanoma to MTX

Experiments from our laboratory and others provide evidence that melanosomes contribute to the refractory properties of melanoma cells by sequestering cytotoxic drugs and increasing melanosome-mediated drug export [6,12,13]. Concretely, we have described that folate receptor α (FRα)-endocytotic transport of MTX facilitates drug melanosomal sequestration and cellular exportation in melanoma cells, which ensures reduced accumulation of MTX in intracellular compartments [6]. An important observation in this study was that MTX was a cytostatic agent on melanoma cells. These cells were resistant to MTX-induced apoptosis but responded to the drug by arresting their growth. A similar response was observed when the murine B16/F10 melanoma cell line was grown in low folate. After 3 days in folate-deficient medium the cells had restricted proliferative activity and also increased their metastatic potential [23]. Taking this into consideration, the results indicate that MTX might also induce depletion of intracellular reduced folate coenzymes by reducing their transport though the FRα and/or competing with them for the reduced folate carrier (RFC). Melanoma cells may be highly sensitive to intracellular depletion of folate coenzymes, and in this situation may enter into a "latent" state. This form of melanoma should indeed be highly resistant to MTX, since antifolate drugs are more effective on fast-dividing cells, which require continuous DNA synthesis. Most likely, the high increases of DHFR expression in cells treated with MTX [5] would represent an adaptation mechanism that allows cells to survive with low intracellular concentrations of folate coenzymes. Increasing the recycling of folate molecules the cells would maintain other cellular functions that are dependent on folate coenzymes, such as the synthesis of purines, pyrimidines, amino acids and methylation reactions. The presence of this "latent" form of melanoma should be critical for the resistance to MTX during *in vivo* therapies. Although MTX chemotherapy could initially halt the development of the tumor, after clearance of the drug from the body the melanoma cells may reinitiate their progression, possibly with an increased metastatic potential [23].

A defect in intracellular folate retention is another recognized mechanism of drug resistance [5,10,11,21]. In addition to a decrease in antifolate polyglutamylation, melanoma cells may also export cytotoxic drugs by melanosome sequestration [12]. The results presented in this study indicated that drug exportation was an operative mechanism of resistance to MTX in melanoma cells. Although the mechanism by which cytotoxic drugs are sequestered into melanosomes remains unclear, we demonstrated that MTX-melanosome trapping may be a consequence of its FRα-endosomal transport [6]. To test the importance of this process on the resistance of melanoma to antifolates, we silenced the expression of the melanosomal structural protein gp100/Pmel17, which is known to play a critical role in melanosome biogenesis [24]. Recently, Xie and collaborators [13] provided the first direct evidence that disruption of the process of normal melanosome biogenesis, by mutation of gp100/Pmel17, increased sensitivity to cisplatin. We also observed that effective silencing of gp100/Pmel17 significantly increased the sensitivity of melanoma cells to MTX, favouring MTX-induced apoptosis. This observation strongly supports the hypothesis which indicates that melanosome biogenesis is a specialization of the endocytic pathway [25,26]; however, the exact mechanism by which MTX induces abnormal trafficking of early endosomes in melanoma cells, favoring the exportation of melanosomes, is still unclear. Whether MTX blocks the formation of carrier vesicles operating between early and late endosomes, inhibits the delivery of endocytosed material from endosomes to lysosomes, promoting, thus, the generation of exosomes [26] and/or induces a failure of lysosomal acidification, which is essential for normal endocytosis [27], remains to be determined.

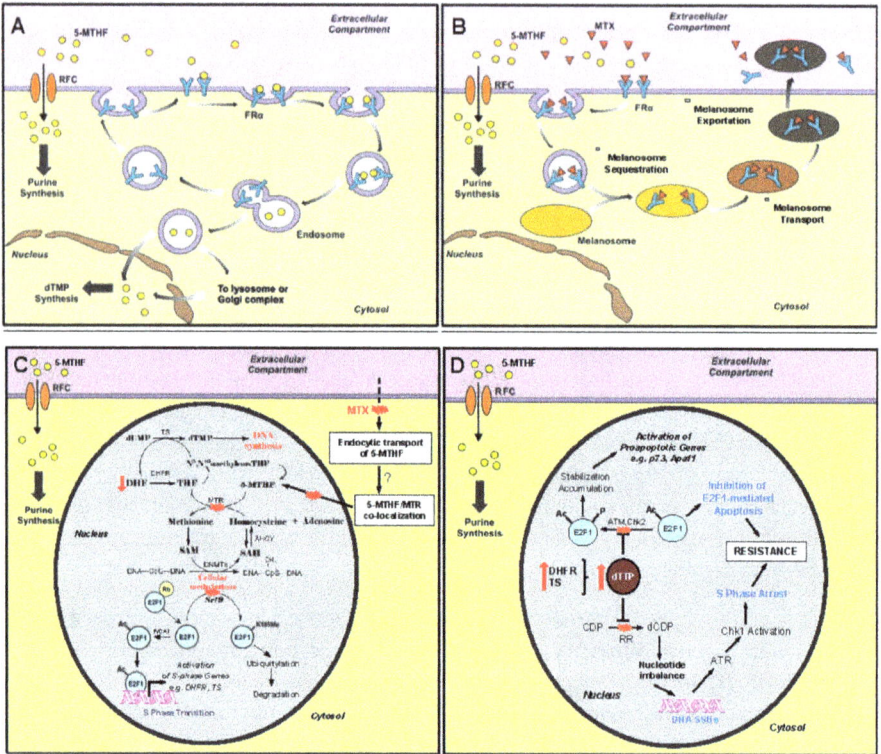

Figure 1. A) Possible mechanisms for transport and trafficking of folates in melanoma cells. (B) Mechanisms to explain the MTX-induced depletion of DHF in melanoma cells. (C) Folate deficiency induces DHF depletion and enhances the transactivational potential of E2F1. (D) Excess of dTTP inhibits E2F1-mediated apoptosis and activates Chk1 in melanoma cells. High levels of DHFR and TS could reactivate *de novo* dTMP biosynthesis impeding depletion of dTTP. Excess of dTTP would prevent apoptosis by several mechanisms. First, dTTP is an allosteric inhibitor of ribonucleotide reductase (RR), the enzyme which reduces cytidine diphosphate (CDP) and uridine diphosphate to dCDP and dUDP.

To explore the relationship between MTX exportation and melanosome trafficking, we studied the possible interaction of MTX with melanin [6]. Such interaction was confirmed by incubating this drug with synthetic 3,4-dihydroxyphenylalanine (DOPA)-melanin. Importantly, folic acid and 5-methyl-THF (5-MTHF), the natural source of cellular folates, did not appear to interact with synthetic DOPA-melanin. A comparison of the interaction of several folates (folic acid and 5-MTHF) and antifolates (MTX and aminopterin) with synthetic DOPA-melanin indicated that the double amino group of the pterin ring is an important molecular requirement for the drug-melanin interaction. Therefore, the physiological importance of the high affinity of melanin for antifolates, such as MTX and aminopterin, for drug melanosomal sequestration is also another important issue that remains to be addressed. Endocytic transport of molecules involves several processes, including the fusion of early and late endosomes and the dissociation of receptor-ligand complexes through the acidic pH of preformed vesicles [28]. After melano-some biogenesis from MTX-loaded endosomes, dissociated MTX could be trapped in the mel-anosomes by its interaction with melanins. In contrast, folate substrates would not be sequestered in melanosomes due to their low affinities for melanin; facilitated by the acidic pH of this organelle, uncharged reduced folates would leave the melanosome by passive dif-fusion and reach the cytosol, where they would become available for cellular functions. There-fore, elucidation of the molecular basis for the (anti)folate interaction with melanins could have important therapeutic implications, and this study might be used as a guide for the synthesis of new antifolates or for using existing antifolates in ways that escape melanin trapping.

3.2. MTX disrupts folate trafficking in melanoma cells

Although MTX is exported within a few hours in contact with cells, in this short time, MTX is capable of inducing important changes in folate metabolism by depleting dihydrofolate (DHF) early on and by inducing the expression of folate-dependent enzymes later on [7]. The in-creased expression of DHFR is a common occurrence in melanoma and other cancer cells in response to MTX treatment; however, the observed depletion of DHF was completely unex-pected. The pathways that comprise folate-mediated one-carbon metabolism have been sug-gested to function in a metabolic network that interconnects the three biosynthetic pathways, namely *de novo* purine biosynthesis, *de novo* dTMP biosynthesis, and homocysteine remethy-lation. Recent studies provide direct evidence for cell cycle–dependent nuclear dTMP biosyn-thesis in the nucleus [29]. However, there are many unanswered questions regarding the role and regulation of nuclear *de novo* dTMP biosynthesis. Nothing is known about the transport, processing, and accumulation of folates into the nucleus, the one-carbon forms of folate present in the nucleus, and the relationship between cell cycle dependency of *de novo* dTMP biosyn-thesis and cell cycle-dependent accumulation of nuclear folate [29]. Although there is no data of how the homocysteine remethylation cycle is compartmentalized, the observation that MTX affected both DHF synthesis and E2F1 methylation (see below) seem to indicate that both the *de novo* dTMP biosynthesis and the homocysteine remethylation cycles might operate simul-taneously in the nucleus.

Using HeLa and MCF-7 cells, Stover and coworkers observed that cytoplasmic serine hydrox-ymethyltransferase (SMTH), TS, and DHFR are all translocated into the nucleus during S and G_2/M phases following their modification by the small ubiquitin-like modifier (SUMO) [30,31]. This finding indicated that the folate cycle may be compartmentalized and that dTMP and DHF synthesis may occur in the nucleus during DNA synthesis. In a recent study, Wollack et al. [32] characterized 5-MTHF uptake and metabolism by primary rat choroid plexus epithelial cells *in vitro*. They distinguish two different processes for 5-MTHF transport, one that was FRα dependent and the other that was independent of this receptor and mediated by the proton couple folate transporter or reduced folate carrier (RFC). This investigation revealed that cel-lular metabolism of 5-MTHF depends on the route of folate entry into the cell. Thus, 5-MTHF taken up via a non-FRα–mediated process was rapidly metabolized to folylpolyglutamates, whereas 5-MTHF that accumulates via FRα remained non-metabolized and associated to en-docytic compartments. The observation that MTX induces the overall depletion of FRα in melanoma cells [6] would suggest that MTX might also induce depletion of reduced folate coenzymes associated to endocytic compartments (Figure 1A and 1B). Therefore, a possible explanation for the depletion of DHF during MTX exposure could be that this drug diminishes the required supply of folates to the nucleus for the maintenance of both dTMP and DHF synthesis; however, how melanoma cells can control endocytic pathways to supply their own nucleus with folates is unknown. Recent studies have indicated that some endocytic proteins are also involved in direct signaling pathways from membranes to the nucleus, and mechanisms for the nuclear translocation of intact or fragmented endosome-localized proteins have been identified [33]. Another possibility is the existence of a late endosome-lysosome transport mechanism for folate [34]. The proximity of lysosomes to the nucleus suggests that folates could be released into the perinuclear region of the cytoplasm, perhaps facilitating their nuclear entry during cell division following the disassembly of the nuclear membrane [29].

Although the uptake of 5-MTHF into mammalian cells is mainly mediated by the RFC, the expression of FRα in several epithelial tissues and especially its overexpression in cancerous cells indicate that this receptor may confer a growth advantage to these cells [35]. The high affinity of FRα for 5-MTHF suggest that this GPI-anchored receptor may play an important role in maintaining nuclear folates even at low extracellular concentrations of this vitamin. This hypothesis is supported by the finding that induction of FRα expression in cells that normally do not express this receptor allows the cells to grow in low nanomolar folate concentrations [36]. On the other hand, the observation that methionine synthase was localized in the nucleus of melanoma cells could explain many of the unanswered questions on the role and regulation of the folate metabolism in the nucleus of these cancer cells. The methionine synthase -mediated catalysis of 5-MTHF would first supply THF and methionine to maintain both dTTP synthesis and the methylation reactions in the nucleus of the cells (Figure 1C) and second would prevent the nuclear accumulation of 5-MTHF, a potent inhibitor of SHMT [29]. Therefore, in melanoma, the existence of a specific folate transport pathway from the plasma membrane to the nucleus, mediated by FRα, is possible [37] and could shed light on the unknown function of overexpressed FRα in cancer cells [38].

4. Melanoma coordinates general and cell-specific mechanisms to promote MTX resistance

4.1. MTX induces E2F1 demethylation and prevents dTTP depletion in melanoma

MTX acts as a cytostatic agent in melanoma cells [6]. To discriminate between the mechanisms by which MTX could induce cell growth arrest without inducing apoptosis, the effect of this drug on the cell cycle of several melanoma cell lines was analysed [7]. The results indicated that, in all the tested melanoma cell lines, MTX conferred an arrest in early S phase; the G_1 peak shifted toward the G_1/S border, and cells were arrested with a minimal increase in their DNA content. Because S phase arrest has been recognized as a major mechanism of resistance in response to non-toxic concentrations of drugs that induce DNA replication stress, these preliminary results suggest that moderate DNA damage could be responsible for the cytostatic effect of MTX on melanoma cells.

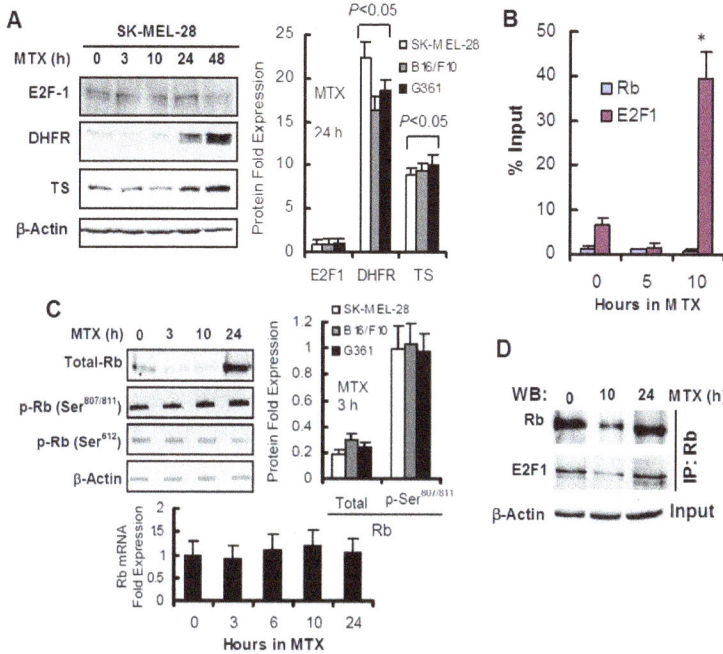

Figure 2. MTX enhances the transactivation potential of E2F1 in melanoma cells. (A) The time-dependent effect of MTX treatment (1 µM) on the expression of E2F1, DHFR, and TS proteins as assayed by western blot (WB). (B) ChIP experiments showing the occupancy of E2F1 and Rb on the DHFR promoter of B16/F10 melanoma cells (*P < 0.05). (C) The upper panels represent the time-dependent effects of MTX (1 µM) treatment on the expression and phosphorylation state of the Rb protein as assayed by WB. The lower panel depicts the Rb mRNA expression as assayed by qRT-PCR. The changes observed after MTX treatment were not statistically significant. (D) Co-immunoprecipitation assays were performed to test the interaction between Rb and E2F1.

To understand the mechanisms involved in G_1 cell cycle progression in MTX-treated melanoma cells, the effect of this drug on several G_1 cell cycle components was analysed. Although the protein levels of E2F1 were not affected by MTX (Figure 2A), this drug significantly increased the protein levels of DHFR and thymidylate synthase (TS), two E2F1-target genes involved in folate metabolism and required for G_1 progression and DNA synthesis (Figure 2A). Chromatin immunoprecipitation (ChIP) experiments that were designed to analyze the occupancy of E2F1 on the DHFR promoter of B16/F10 melanoma cells indicated that MTX stimulated the transcriptional activity of E2F1 (Figure 2B). First, we observed that MTX induced a transient decrease in the hypophosphorylated Rb protein in melanoma cells (Figure 2C) as evidenced by a noticeable lack of Rb co-immunoprecipitation with E2F1 in 10 h MTX-treated SK-MEL-28 cells when compared to untreated controls (Figure 2D). In addition, mass peptide analysis of immunoprecipitated E2F1, after trypsin digestion (Figure 3), indicated that MTX promoted the demethylation of E2F1 at Lys185 (Figures 3B and 3D). A negative crosstalk between methylation and other posttranslational modifications of E2F1, such as acetylation and phosphorylation, has been recently described [39]. We observed that MTX induced the transient co-immunoprecipitation of E2F1 with p300/CBP-associated factor (P/CAF) (Figure 3B), an interaction that has been associated with the transcriptionally active hyperacetylated form of this transcription factor [40]. The hyperacetylated status of E2F1 after MTX treatment was also confirmed by MALDI-TOF mass spectrometry (Figures 3B and 3D). In response to severe DNA damage, the E2F1 protein is stabilized through distinct mechanisms, including direct phosphorylation by Chk2 at Ser^{364} [41] or ATM kinase at Ser^{31} [42]. As we did not observe phosphorylation of E2F1 after MTX treatment (Figures 3C and 3D), these data further suggest that MTX induced moderate DNA damage without inducing double strand breaks (DSBs) [43].

MTX increased E2F1 levels in sensitive cancer cells [16]. However, we did not observe an MTX-mediated increase in E2F1 levels in melanoma cells (Figure 2A) [7], a result that could be explained, at least in part, by the results obtained after determination of dNTP pools in melanoma cells (Figure 4). Contrary to the effects of MTX in most cancer cells [16], this drug increased the levels of dTTP in melanoma. Increased levels of dTTP were accompanied by a decrease in dCTP levels, which resulted in a nucleotide imbalance that favored thymidine excess. The MTX-induced expression of DHFR and TS (Figure 2A) and the low levels of MTX accumulated in melanoma cells [6] could explain this paradoxical response of melanoma cells to a cytotoxic drug that typically depletes dTTP levels.

The data obtained in our study indicate that melanoma cells respond to the lack of folate coenzymes by enhancing the transactivational potential of E2F1. We observed that treatment of melanoma cells with MTX transiently affected the stability of Rb and the posttranslational state of E2F1 [7]. A crosstalk between the methylated and acetylated forms of E2F1 has been suggested [39]. Methylated E2F1 is prone to ubiquitination and degradation, whereas the de-methylation of E2F1 favors its P/CAF-dependent acetylation. Together, the results suggest a model whereby the MTX-induced degradation of Rb and the demethylation of E2F1 would result in the accumulation of E2F1 in its 'free' state, and in the absence of DNA damage, free E2F1 would be acetylated, leading to the transcription of genes required for S phase (Figure 1C). The activation of E2F1 by MTX would allow S phase transition in melanoma cells, and importantly for melanoma survival, cells would recover an operative folate cycle, thereby re-storing the original status of the Rb/E2F1 system. In the absence of exported MTX, high levels of TS and DHFR would impede the lethal depletion of dTTP and in turn, would produce a nucleotide imbalance that would favor a dTTP excess. Contrary to thymidine depletion, excess thymidine stops cells in S phase by blocking synthesis of DNA, an effect known as 'thymidine block' (Figure 1D) [15]. Recently, a mechanism by which dTTP allosterically feedback controls E2F1 has been proposed [15,16]. According to this mechanism, excess of dTTP inhibits E2F1 accumulation acting either upon production of E2F1 or its degradation. Because control of E2F1 is essential for cell survival, this mechanism would prevent E2F1 accumulation, which would result in activation of apoptosis through a process that involves p53 or p73, cytochrome c, and caspases (Figure 1D) [44].

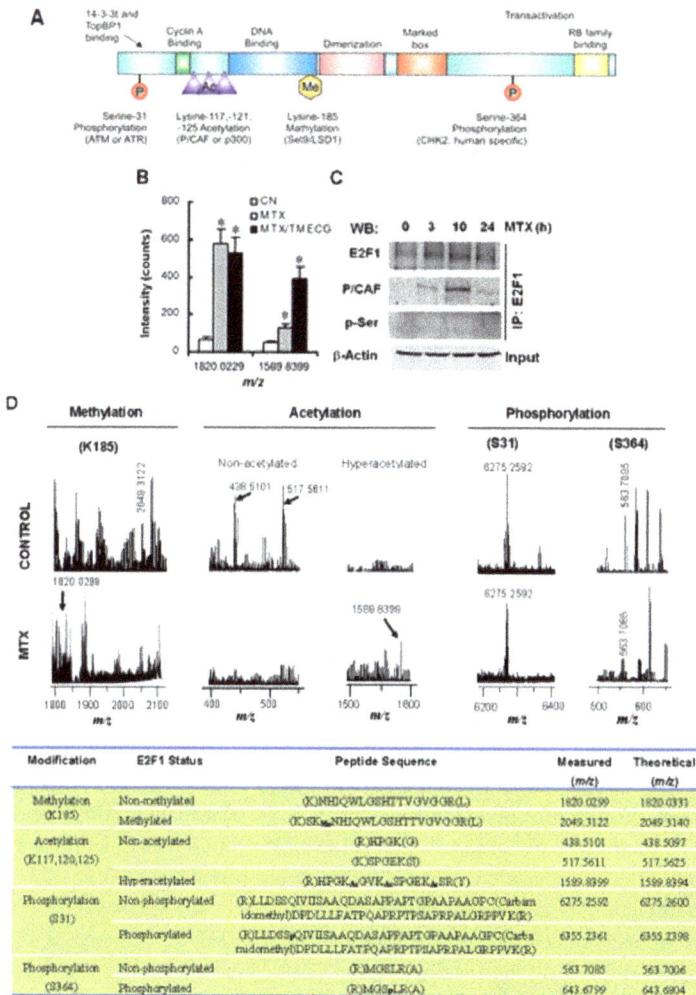

Figure 3. MTX induces demethylation and hyperacetylation of E2F1 in melanoma cells. (A) Schematic representation of the E2F1 protein. Residues susceptible to methylation (K185), acetylation (K117, K120, and K125), and phosphorylation (S31 and S364) are shown. (B) Relative intensity of unmethylated [(K)NHIQWLGSHTTVGVGGR(L); m/z 1820.0229] and hyperacetylated [(R)HPGKAcGVKAcSPGEKAcSR(Y); m/z 1589.8399] peptides in E2F1-trypsin digested samples. Peptides were analyzed in untreated SK-MEL-28 cells (CN) or treated for 10 h with 1 µM MTX (*P < 0.05). Intensities were normalized with respect to an internal matrix control. (C) Cell lysates from SK-MEL-28 cells that had been treated with 1 µM MTX were used for IP assays with E2F1 to test the co-immunoprecipitation of E2F1 with P/CAF and the phosphorylated state of E2F1. (D) MALDI-TOF mass spectra of tryptic digests of immunoprecipitated E2F1. The characteristics peptides involving posttranslational modifications of E2F1 (methylation = Me, acetylation = Ac, and phosphorylation = P), as well as their measured and theoretical m/z are shown.

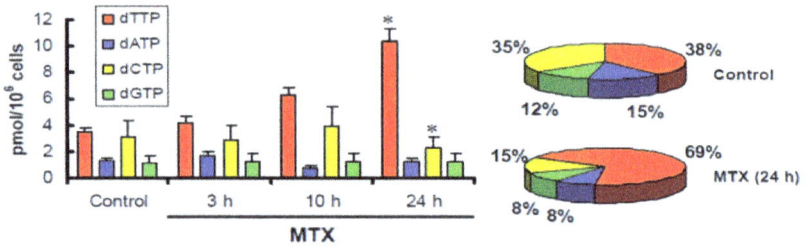

Figure 4. MTX does not deplete dTTP levels in melanoma cells. dNTP quantification in SK-MEL-28 control cells and cells subjected to MTX (1 µM) treatment (*P < 0.05). Data collected from the left panel was used to determine the total amounts of each dNTP at each time point. The percent contribution of each dNTP to the total pool after 24 h of treatment is represented.

4.2. Excess of dTTP favours Chk1 activation in melanoma after MTX treatment

Excess thymidine induces little detectable DNA damage in the form of DSBs. The ATR-mediated response appears to play a more prominent role under these cellular conditions [45]. As it is known that the central mechanism responsible for Chk1 activation upon DNA damage is the distribution of ATR into nuclear foci [46], the effects of MTX on the localization of ATR and the phosphorylation of Chk1 at Ser[345] were analyzed by confocal microscopy and western blot, respectively (Figures 5A and 5B). Time- and dose-dependent experiments clearly indicated that MTX induced Chk1 phosphorylation in melanoma cells. Because Chk1 phosphorylation may not directly correspond to Chk1 activation, we next analyzed the dose-dependent effects of MTX on the stability of Cdc25A (Figure 5B). We found that Chk1 phosphorylation led to a corresponding decrease in Cdc25A abundance, indicating that MTX not only conferred Chk1 phosphorylation, but it also activated Chk1. Conversely, phosphorylation of Chk2 was not observed in melanoma cells that had been treated with MTX for as long as 48 h (Figure 5B), indicating that this drug specifically induced Chk1 activation in response to DNA single strand breaks (SSBs). To determine the extent to which Chk1 activation affected the resistance of melanoma to MTX, we took two independent experimental approaches. First, we silenced the expression of Chk1 in SK-MEL-28 (p53 mutant) cells and studied the sensitivity of the cells to MTX (Figure 5C). The results indicated that the downregulation of Chk1 increased the sensitivity of SK-MEL-28 cells to MTX and led to apoptosis. As a second approach, we evaluated the ability of Chk1 to protect B16/F10 murine cells (p53 wild-type) from MTX-induced apoptosis by first inducing an S phase arrest with MTX and then treating the S-arrested cells with a combination of MTX and 7-hydroxystaurosporine (UCN-01). We observed that B16/F10 S phase-arrested cells were sensitive to MTX treatment after the effective inhibition of Chk1 (Figure 5C).

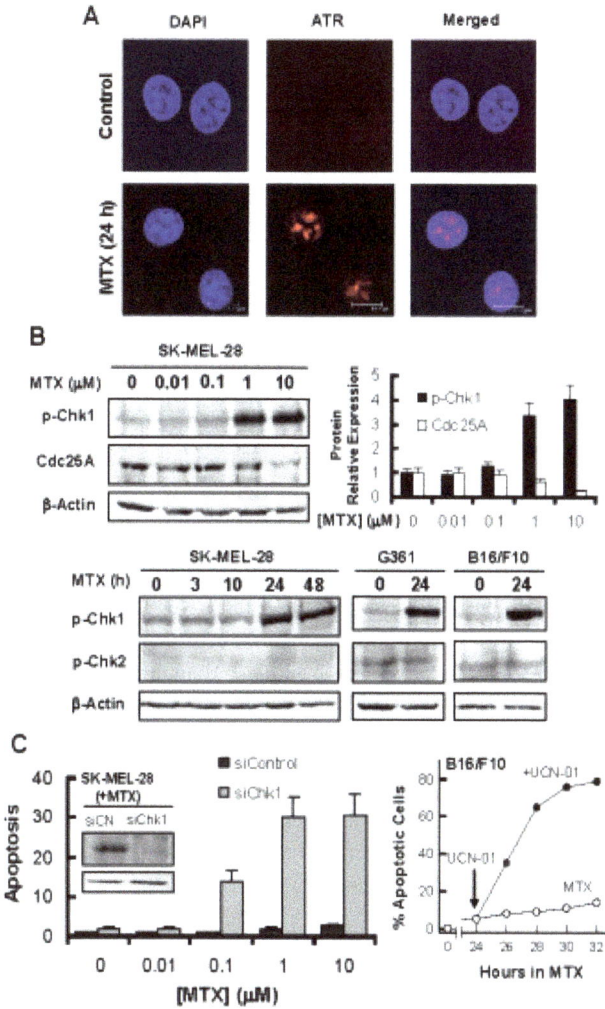

Figure 5. MTX activates Chk1 in melanoma cells. (A) SK-MEL-28 cells were treated with 1 μM MTX for 24 h and then examined for ATR nuclear foci. Nuclei were stained with DAPI. (B) The dose-dependent effects of MTX on Chk1 phosphorylation and Cdc25A degradation in SK-MEL-28 after 24 h of drug exposure (*$P < 0.05$). MTX (1 μM) induced the time-dependent phosphorylation of Chk1, but not Chk2, in different melanoma cell lines. (C) Chk1 siRNA sensitizes SK-MEL-28 cells to MTX-induced toxicity (left panel). siControl (siCN)- and siChk1-transfected cells were treated with increasing doses of MTX for 48 h (*$P < 0.05$). The effective silencing of Chk1 was tested by WB. The induction of the phosphorylated form of Chk1 was analyzed after 24 h of MTX treatment (1 μM). The induction of apoptosis by UCN-01 in MTX-arrested B16/F10 cells is shown in the right-side panel. Cells were incubated with 1 μM MTX continuously for 32 h, and 50 nM UCN-01 was added at 24 h to one group of cells following splitting of the culture. As a control experiment, SK-MEL-28 cells were treated with 50 nM UCN-01 only for 32 h.

Inhibitors of DNA synthesis, such as excess thymidine, hydroxyurea, and camptothecin, are normally poor inducers of apoptosis; however, these agents become potent inducers of death in S phase cells upon the small interfering RNA-mediated depletion of Chk1 [45]. Here, we observed that MTX activated Chk1 and induced an early S phase arrest in melanoma cells lines that were harboring either wild-type or mutant p53. The impact of MTX on the survival of Chk1-silenced melanoma cells and cells co-treated with UCN-01 indicates that MTX provokes a 'thymidine block'-like effect and that S phase arrest, as a result of Chk1 activation, might constitute a major and general p53-independent mechanism that is responsible for the resistance of melanomas to MTX. However, it would be difficult to understand this extreme resistance without taking into account the melanosome-mediated exportation of MTX. The activation of the DNA damage response pathway reflects the magnitude and extent of DNA damage that occurs in response to a specific genotoxic agent, and a dual role of Chk1, depending on the extent of DNA damage, has been proposed [45]. Thus, Chk1 may play an anti-apoptotic role in response to weaker replication fork stresses, whereas more catastrophic damage, such as the accumulation of DNA strand breaks, may result in the activation of apoptosis by Chk1. Together, the results indicate that low intracellular levels of MTX in melanoma induce moderate DNA damage that favors the anti-apoptotic role of Chk1 (Figure 1D).

5. Therapeutical implications

Although melanoma resistance to MTX was initially thought to be due to the classical mechanisms of resistance that have been observed in other epithelial cells, recent discoveries indicate that the resistance of melanoma to MTX might be due to the idiosyncrasies of these cancer cells [6,12] where drug melanosomal sequestration and its subsequent cellular exportation may have a marked protagonist. Unravelling the mechanisms of melanoma resistance to MTX could, therefore, yield important information on how to circumvent this resistance and could have important pharmacological implications for the design of novel combined therapies. Taking into account these observations, uses of combined treatments with MTX, to prevent melanosomal drug sequestration [6,12] or to avoid MTX-induced S phase arrest [19], are rational therapeutical approaches. The observation that MTX induces cellular depletion of DHF in melanoma [7] could generate novel combined therapies to efficiently inhibit DHFR with antifolates transported into the cells by FRα-independent processes. Also, of great interest is the observed effect of MTX on the posttranslational status of E2F1 in melanoma (Figure 3). Various studies have suggested that E2F1 plays dual roles in cell survival/apoptosis [47-50]. Therefore, the MTX-induced demethylation and acetylation of E2F1 could favour melanoma cell death when combined with E2F1-stabilizing drugs. In addition to E2F1 phosphorylation, acetylation has also been recognized to play a role in the activation and stabilization of the E2F1 protein during DNA damage and apoptosis [40]. A possible strategy to favour E2F1 apoptosis in melanoma by the combination of MTX with E2F1-stabilizing drugs is depicted in Figure 6.

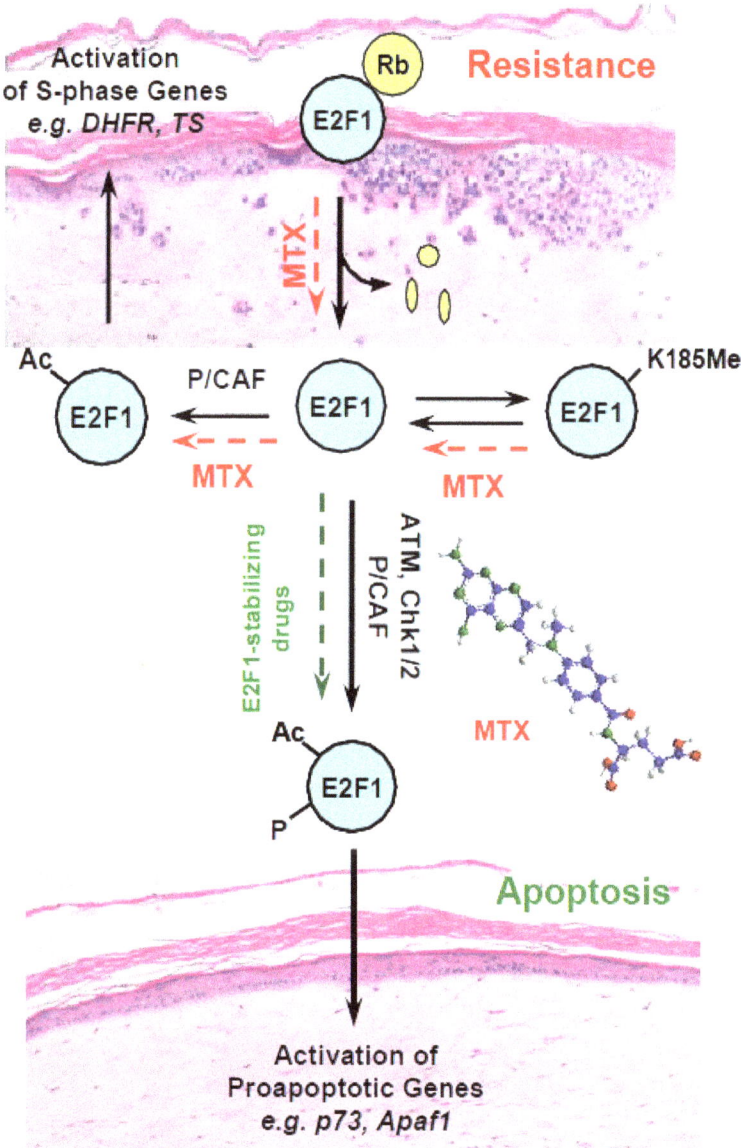

Figure 6. Proposed mechanism for the regulation of E2F1 by MTX. E2F1 is regulated by its interaction with Rb and by several posttranslational modifications, including methylation (Me), acetylation (Ac) and phosphorylation (P) [39]. The effects of MTX (red dashed line) on E2F1 status and that result in melanoma resistance are shown. A possible strategy to stabilize E2F1 (green dashed lines) to induce apoptosis in melanoma cells is also displayed.

6. Conclusions

Melanoma, the most aggressive form of skin cancer, is notoriously resistant to all current modalities of cancer therapy, including to the drug MTX. Melanosomal sequestration and cellular exportation of methotrexate have been proposed to be important melanoma-specific mechanisms that contribute to the resistance of melanoma to methotrexate. In addition, other mechanisms of resistance that are present in most epithelial cancer cells are also operative in melanoma. This chapter reviews how melanoma orchestrates these mechanisms to become extremely resistant to methotrexate, where both E2F1 and Chk1, two molecules with dual roles in survival/apoptosis, play prominent roles. The results indicated that MTX induced the depletion of DHF in melanoma cells, which stimulated the transcriptional activity of E2F1. The elevate expression of DHFR and TS, two E2F1-target genes involved in folate metabolism and required for G_1 progression, favoured dTTP accumulation, which promoted DNA single strand breaks and the subsequent activation of Chk1. Under these conditions, melanoma cells are protected from apoptosis by arresting their cell cycle in S phase. Excess of dTTP could also inhibit E2F1-mediated apoptosis in melanoma cells. In addition, these discoveries could open the way for the development of new combined and directed therapies against this elusive skin pathology.

Acknowledgements

Research described was supported in part by a grant from Ministerio de Ciencia e Innovación (MICINN) (Project SAF2009-12043-C02-01), Fundación Séneca, Región de Murcia (FS-RM) (15230/PI/10) and EU ERA293514. J.C-H is contracted by the Translational Cancer Research Group (Fundación para la Formación e Investigación Sanitarias). MPF-P has a fellowship from Ministerio de Educación, Cultura y Deporte. M.F.M is contracted by an agreement with the Fundación de la Asociación Española contra el Cáncer (FAECC). L.S-d-C has a postdoctoral fellowship from Fundación Séneca (Región de Murcia) for application in the Ludwig Institute for Cancer Research, Nuffield Department of Clinical Medicine, University of Oxford, Headington, Oxford, UK.

Author details

Luis Sanchez del-Campo[1], Maria F. Montenegro[1], Magali Saez-Ayala[1],
María Piedad Fernández-Pérez[1], Juan Cabezas-Herrera[2] and
Jose Neptuno Rodriguez-Lopez[1]

1 Department of Biochemistry & Molecular Biology A, University of Murcia, Spain

2 Research Unit of Clinical Analusis Service, University Hospital Virgen de la Arrixaca, Spain

References

[1] Sullivan, R. J, & Atkins, M. B. Molecular-targeted therapy in malignant melanoma. Expert Review of Anticancer Therapy (2009). , 9(5), 567-581.

[2] Ascierto, P. A, Streicher, H. Z, & Sznol, M. Melanoma: a model for testing new agents in combination therapies. J Transl Med (2010). , 8, 38.

[3] American Cancer SocietyCancer Facts & Figures 2011. Atlanta; 2011.

[4] Tawbi, H. A, & Buch, S. C. Chemotherapy resistance abrogation in metastatic melanoma. Clinical Advances in Hematology & Oncology (2010). , 8(4), 259-266.

[5] Kufe, D. W, Wick, M. M, & Abelson, H. T. Natural resistance to methotrexate in human melanomas. Journal of Investigative Dermatology (1980). , 75(4), 357-359.

[6] Sánchez-del-campo, L, Montenegro, M. F, Cabezas-herrera, J, & Rodríguez-lópez, J. N. The critical role of alpha-folate receptor in the resistance of melanoma to methotrexate. Pigment Cell & Melanoma Research (2009). , 22(5), 588-600.

[7] Saez-ayala, M, Fernandez-perez, M, Montenegro, M. F, Sánchez-del-campo, L, Chazarra, S, Piñero-madrona, A, Cabezas-herrera, J, & Rodríguez-lópez, J. N. Melanoma coordinates general and cell-specific mechanisms to promote methotrexate resistance. Experimental Cell Research (2012). , 318(10), 1146-1159.

[8] Lockshin, A, Moran, R. G, & Danenberg, P. V. Thymidylate synthetase purified to homogeneity from human leukemic cells. Proceedings of the National Academy of Sciences USA (1979). , 76(2), 750-754.

[9] Blakley, R. L. The Biochemistry of Folic Acid and Related Pteridines, Elsevier, New York; (1969).

[10] Zhao, R, & Goldman, I. D. Resistance to antifolates. Oncogene (2003). , 22(47), 7431-7457.

[11] Assaraf, Y. G. Molecular basis of antifolate resistance. Cancer & Metastasis Reviews (2007). , 26(1), 153-181.

[12] Chen, K. G, Valencia, J. C, Lai, B, Zhang, G, Paterson, J. K, Rouzaud, F, Berens, W, Wincovitch, S. M, Garfield, S. H, & Leapman, R. D. Hearing VJ Gottesman MM. Melanosomal sequestration of cytotoxic drugs contributes to the intractability of malignant melanomas. Proceedings of the National Academy of Sciences USA (2006). , 103(26), 9903-9907.

[13] Xie, T, Nguyen, T, Hupe, M, & Wei, M. L. Multidrug resistance decreases with mutations of melanosomal regulatory genes. Cancer Research (2009). , 69(3), 992-999.

[14] De Anta, J. M, Pérez-castro, A. J, Freire, R, & Mayol, X. The DNA damage checkpoint is activated during residual tumour cell survival to methotrexate treatment as an initial step of acquired drug resistance. Anticancer Drugs (2006). , 17(10), 1171-1177.

[15] Pardee, A. B, Li, C. J, & Reddy, G. P. Regulation in S phase by E2F. Cell Cycle (2004). , 3(9), 1091-1094.

[16] Wang, A, Li, C. J, Reddy, P. V, & Pardee, A. B. Cancer chemotherapy by deoxynucleo-tide depletion and E2F-1 elevation. Cancer Research (2005). , 65(17), 7809-7814.

[17] Bartek, J, & Lukas, J. Chk1 and Chk2 kinases in checkpoint control and cancer. Cancer Cell (2003). , 3(5), 421-429.

[18] Xiao, Z, Xue, J, Sowin, T. J, Rosenberg, S. H, & Zhang, H. A novel mechanism of check-point abrogation conferred by Chk1 downregulation. Oncogene (2005). , 24(8), 1403-1411.

[19] Tse, A. N, Carvajal, R, & Schwartz, G. K. Targeting checkpoint kinase 1 in cancer ther-apeutics. Clinical Cancer Research (2007). , 13(7), 1955-1960.

[20] Shi, Z, Azuma, A, Sampath, D, Li, Y. X, & Huang, P. Plunkett W. S-Phase arrest by nucleoside analogues and abrogation of survival without cell cycle progression by 7-hydroxystaurosporine. Cancer Research (2001). , 61(3), 1065-1072.

[21] Gaukroger J, Wilson L, Stewart M, Farid Y, Habeshaw T, Harding N, Mackie R. Para-doxical response of malignant melanoma to methotrexate in vivo and in vitro. British Journal of Cancer, 1983; 47(5) 671-679.

[22] Joerger, M, & Huitema, A. D. van den Bongard HJ, Baas P, Schornagel JH, Schellens JH, Beijnen JH. Determinants of the elimination of methotrexate and 7-hydroxy-me-thotrexate following high-dose infusional therapy to cancer patients. British Journal of Clinical Pharmacology (2006). , 62(1), 71-80.

[23] Branda, R. F, Mccormack, J. J, Perlmutter, C. A, Mathews, L. A, & Robison, S. H. Effects of folate deficiency on the metastatic potential of murine melanoma cells. Cancer Re-search (1988).

[24] Theos, A. C, Truschel, S. T, Raposo, G, & Marks, M. S. The Silver locus product Pmel17/ gp100/ Silv/ME20: controversial in name and in function. Pigment Cell Research (2005). , 18(5), 322-336.

[25] Raposo, G, & Marks, M. S. The dark side of lysosome-related organelles: specialization of the endocytic pathway for melanosome biogenesis. Traffic (2002). , 3(4), 237-248.

[26] Raposo, G, & Marks, M. S. Melanosomes-dark organelles enlighten endosomal mem-brane transport. Nature Reviews Molecular Cell Biology (2007). , 8(10), 786-797.

[27] Branda, R. F, Mccormack, J. J, Perlmutter, C. A, Mathews, L. A, & Robison, S. H. Effects of folate deficiency on the metastatic potential of murine melanoma cells. Cancer Re-search (1988). , 48(16), 4529-4534.

[28] Sabharanjak, S, & Mayor, S. Folate receptor endocytosis and trafficking. Advanced Drug Delivery Reviews (2004). , 56(8), 1099-1109.

[29] Stover, P. J, & Field, M. S. Trafficking of Intracellular Folates. Advances in Nutrition (2011). , 2(4), 325-331.

[30] Anderson, D. D, & Stover, P. J. SHMT1 and SHMT2 are functionally redundant in nuclear de novo thymidylate biosynthesis. PLoS ONE (2009). e5839.

[31] Anderson, D. D, Woeller, C. F, & Stover, P. J. Small ubiquitin-like modifier-1 (SUMO-1) modification of thymidylate synthase and dihydrofolate reductase. Clinical Chemistry and Laboratory Medicine (2007). , 45(12), 1760-1763.

[32] Wollack, J. B, Makori, B, Ahlawat, S, Koneru, R, Picinich, S. C, Smith, A, Goldman, I. D, Qiu, A, Cole, P. D, Glod, J, & Kamen, B. Characterization of folate uptake by choroid plexus epithelial cells in a rat primary culture model. Journal of Neurochemestry (2008). , 104(6), 1494-1503.

[33] Mosesson, Y, Mills, G. B, & Yarden, Y. Derailed endocytosis: an emerging feature of cancer. Nature Reviews Cancer (2008). , 8(11), 835-850.

[34] Wong AW, Scales SJ, Reilly DE. DNA internalized via caveolae requires microtubule-dependent, Rab7-independent transport to the late endocytic pathway for delivery to the nucleus. The Journal of Biological Chemistry 2007; 282(31) 22953-22963.

[35] Antony, A. C. Folate receptors. Annual Review of Nutrition (1996). , 16-501.

[36] Luhrs, C. A, Raskin, C. A, Durbin, R, Wu, B, Sadasivan, E, Mcallister, W, & Rothenberg, S. P. Transfection of a glycosylated phosphatidylinositol-anchored folate-binding protein complementary DNA provides cells with the ability to survive in low folate medium. The Journal of Clinical Investigation (1992). , 90(3), 840-847.

[37] Markert, S, Lassmann, S, Gabriel, B, Klar, M, Werner, M, Gitsch, G, Kratz, F, & Hasenburg, A. Alpha-folate receptor expression in epithelial ovarian carcinoma and non-neoplastic ovarian tissue. Anticancer Research (2008). A) , 3567-3572.

[38] Kelemen, L. E. The role of folate receptor alpha in cancer development, progression and treatment: cause, consequence or innocent bystander? International Journal of Cancer (2006). , 119(2), 243-250.

[39] Kontaki, H, & Talianidis, I. Lysine methylation regulates E2F1-induced cell death. Molecular Cell (2010). , 39(1), 152-160.

[40] Martínez-balbás, M. A, Bauer, U. M, Nielsen, S. J, Brehm, A, & Kouzarides, T. Regulation of E2F1 activity by acetylation. The EMBO Journal (2000). , 19(4), 662-671.

[41] Urist, M, Tanaka, T, Poyurovsky, M. V, & Prives, C. p. induction after DNA damage is regulated by checkpoint kinases Chk1 and Chk2. Genes & Development (2004). , 18(24), 3041-3054.

[42] Lin, W. C, Lin, F. T, & Nevins, J. R. Selective induction of E2F1 in response to DNA damage, mediated by ATM-dependent phosphorylation. Genes & Development (2001). , 15(14), 1833-1844.

[43] Chen, J, Zhu, F, Weaks, R. L, Biswas, A. K, Guo, R, Li, Y, & Johnson, D. G. E. F1 promotes the recruitment of DNA repair factors to sites of DNA double-strand breaks. Cell Cycle (2011). , 10(8), 1287-1294.

[44] Phillips, A. C, & Vousden, K. H. E. F-1 induced apoptosis. Apoptosis (2001). , 6(3), 173-182.

[45] Rodriguez, R, Meuth, M, & Chk, p. cooperate to prevent apoptosis during DNA replication fork stress. Molecular Biology of the Cell (2006). , 17(1), 402-412.

[46] Flynn, R. L, & Zou, L. ATR: a master conductor of cellular responses to DNA replication stress. Trends in Biochemical Sciences (2011). , 36(3), 133-140.

[47] Hallstrom, T. C, Mori, S, Nevins, J. R, & An, E. F1-dependent gene expression program that determines the balance between proliferation and cell death. Cancer Cell (2008). , 13(1), 11-22.

[48] Dynlacht, B. D. Live or let die: E2F1 and PI3K pathways intersect to make life or death decisions. Cancer Cell (2008). , 13(1), 1-2.

[49] Rogoff, H. A, & Kowalik, T. F. Life, death and E2F: linking proliferation control and DNA damage signaling via E2F1. Cell Cycle (2004). , 3(7), 845-846.

[50] Rogoff, H. A, Pickering, M. T, Frame, F. M, Debatis, M. E, Sanchez, Y, Jones, S, & Kowalik, T. F. Apoptosis associated with deregulated E2F activity is dependent on E2F1 and Atm/Nbs1/Chk2. Molecular and Cellular Biology (2004). , 24(7), 2968-2977.

Chapter 7

Melanoma: Treatments and Resistance

Jonathan Castillo Arias and
Miriam Galvonas Jasiulionis

Additional information is available at the end of the chapter

1. Introduction

In the past two decades, it has been observed an increased incidence of skin cancer around the world [1-4]. This increase is particularly important in melanoma [5]. Latin-American data have shown both an increase in incidence rates of skin cancer [6] and in mortality from malignant melanoma [7]. The number of melanoma cases worldwide is increasing faster than any other cancer. Although early detection, appropriate surgery, and adjuvant therapy have improved outcomes, the prognosis of metastatic melanoma remains very poor. Advanced melanoma is still associated with an extremely poor median survival, ranging from 2 to 8 months, with only 5% surviving more than 5 years and remains one of the most treatment-refractory malignancy [8]

2. Treatments

The only way to cure a malignant melanoma is early detection and appropriate surgical treatment, because once it reaches an advanced stage, is highly resistant to conventional radiotherapy and chemotherapy [9]. The median survival for patients with metastatic disease is approximately 8 months [10], and chemotherapy has so far failed to improve survival. Treatment options include radiation therapy, chemotherapy, immunotherapy and biochemotherapy which are summarized below.

2.1. Radiotherapy

The use of adjuvant radiotherapy (RT) in melanomas has been controversial. *In vitro* studies have shown that melanoma cells possess a broad shoulder on the cell survival curve and thus have a large capacity for DNA repair. As a result, hypofractionated RT schedules have been developed to counteract this perceived radioresistance, producing excellent locoregional control rates of 85% and higher [11,12]. Radiation Therapy Oncology Group (RTOG) Trial 83-05 was a prospective randomized study comparing hypofractionation to conventional fractionation. The results showed no difference in partial or complete response rates between the two schedules, and the overall response rates were approximately 70% [13]. The role of adjuvant radiation therapy (RT) following nodal surgery in malignant melanoma remains controversial. Despite the high incidence of distant metastases, loco-regional control remains an important goal in the management of melanoma. Surgery and adjuvant RT provides excellent loco-regional control, although distant metastases remain the major cause of mortality.[14]

2.2. Chemotherapy

Chemotherapeutic agents are cytotoxic anticancer drugs which aim is impair the cell division, resulting in the death of rapidly dividing cells. They are widely used in the treatment of malignancies; however, melanomas are resistant to many forms of traditional chemotherapy.

2.2.1. Chemotherapy with single drugs in melanoma

Several antitumoral drugs have been used to treat the melanoma. One of the most known is dacarbazine. In 1975, dacarbazine (DTIC) became the first US Food and Drug Administration (FDA) approved chemotherapeutic agent for the treatment of metastatic melanoma. The response rates with dacarbazine were 15–25%, with median response ranging from 5 to 6 months, but with less than 5% of complete responses [17-19]. Long-term follow-up of patients treated with DTIC alone shows that less than 2% of the patients could survive for 6 years [15,16]. In a meta-analysis comparing two or three-drugs combination regimens with DTIC alone, Huncharek et al. [20] concluded that there was no advantage for the combination in terms of response or survival. Since survival was not improved by the use of single or combination chemotherapy for metastatic melanoma, treatment decisions remain controversial, and quality of life and toxicity issues from treatment assume greater importance.

An orally analogue of DTIC is temozolomide whose activity has been tested in several clinical studies as single agent in metastatic malignant melanoma [18,21,22]. A randomized phase III trial comparing TMZ to DTIC on patients with advanced melanoma demonstrated a statistically significant increase in progression-free survival (1.9 months vs 1.5 months) when TMZ was administered [18].

Fotemustine (FTMU) is the most active nitrosourea used against the metastatic melanoma. It has been widely tested in Europe and has shown overall response of 20–25% including 5–8% of complete response rates and it was the first drug to show significant efficacy in brain metastases [23,24]. However, at conventional doses, little or no activity was observed against melanoma brain metastases [25].

Platinum-based drugs are widely used in the treatment of cancer. In patients with melanoma, cisplatin was shown to induce a 15% response rate with a short median duration of 3 months. Doses up to 150 mg/m^2 in combination with amifostine produced tumor responses in 53% of patients. However, all of those responses were partial, and the median response duration was only 4 months [26]. Regarding carboplatin, in a study on 26 chemotherapy-naive metastatic melanoma patients, a response rate of 19% with 5 partial responses was reported and thrombocytopenia was the dose-limiting toxicity [27].

The vinca alkaloids, especially vindesine and vinblastine, have induced responses in approximately 14% of melanoma patients and they are usually used in combination with other drugs [28]. Docetaxel or paclitaxel, do not have a significant activity in melanoma [29-32]. The role of tamoxifen (TAM) as single agent at standard or high-doses in the treatment of melanoma is negligible with a response rate ranging between 0% and 10%. Currently all of these drugs are rarely used as single agent therapy in metastatic melanoma.

2.2.2. Chemotheraphy with combined drugs in melanoma

In a phase II study, Lattanzi et al. [33] reported their experience with the addition of TAM to the three-drug combination regimen of cisplatin, carmustine and dacarbazine (the Dartmouth regimen) and showed high response rates (55%) with a 20% complete response. Since then several randomized clinical trials have been conducted to confirm the therapeutic benefit of TAM in combination with chemotherapy.

Cocconi et al. [34] published a small phase III trial demonstrating an improvement of response and survival with the addition of tamoxifen to dacarbazine compared to dacarbazine alone. However, two large randomized trials with low and high-dose tamoxifen in combination with either dacarbazine alone or the Dartmouth regimen failed to demonstrate an advantage to the addition of tamoxifen [35,36].

The efficacy of the combination of paclitaxel and carboplatin in the treatment of metastatic melanoma was reported some years ago. Although originally tested in two small phase II clinical trials and deemed not sufficiently clinically active, this evidence suggests that the combination of paclitaxel and carboplatin may be worth further consideration [37].

2.3. Immunotherapy

Immunotherapy in melanoma consists of various approaches leading to specific or non-specific immunomodulation. Immunotherapies are being used for melanoma patients in stage II–III patients in the adjuvant setting, where only a fraction of patients have widespread (microscopic) disease with the aim to prevent relapse of disease, prolong relapse-free survival and, ideally, prolong overall survival (OS). In patients with stage IV disease, there is a need for adequate systemic therapies as median OS for this patient group is only 6–9 months [38]. However, for the first time in >30 years, prospective randomized trials in patients with distant metastatic melanoma demonstrated an OS benefit [39].

Some agents used in the treatment against the melanoma are ipilimumab and tremelimumab, fully human IgG1 and IgG2 monoclonal antibodies, respectively. They block cytotoxic T-lymphocyte- associated antigen 4 (CTLA-4), a negative regulator of T cells, and thus augment T-cell activation and proliferation [40,41]. A phase-III trial was completed first and its results were reported in 2010 [39]. This trial compared ipilimumab alone or in combination with a gp100-peptide vaccine, compared to the vaccine alone in patients who had failed prior therapy or therapies. Melanoma patients receiving ipilimumab and ipilimumab + vaccination had a significantly better survival outcome than those receiving the vaccine alone. Ipilimumab was combined with high-dose IL-2 in 36 patients in the surgery branch of the NCI, with some remarkable observations. There were six patients (17%) with long-lasting complete response, all over 5 years, and none of the patients relapsed. Moreover, there was no increased toxicity as compared to high-dose IL-2 alone [42]. Other study showing a combination of tremelimumab with high-dose interferon yielded a high overall response rate of 30% in 33 melanoma patients, with three complete responses and seven partial responses, all long-lasting responses. Again, there was no increased toxicity compared to high-dose IFN therapy alone [43].

Interferon-α (IFN-α) has been approved in the adjuvant setting for the treatment of high-risk melanoma based on clinical trials in the early 1990s [44,45]. In a metastatic situation, melanoma patients treated with the single agent IFN-α showed approximately 15% of responses, with less than 5% of complete response rates and median response duration between 6 and 9 months with a maximum of 12 months for the best studies [46]. These response rates, while encouraging, were not significant enough to lead to its widespread use in the treatment of metastatic melanoma. However, observations that patients with non-visceral disease were more likely to respond suggested that the use of IFN-α may demonstrated a grater impact in patients with micrometastasis [46, 47]. Other combination studied was IL-2 with IFN-α. This association did not seem to achieve better results (median response rate of 18% with three complete responses) than if these agents were given alone [48-50]. By contrast, in a small randomized phase III trial comparing continuous infusion IL-2 plus interferon vs. continuous infusion decreasing IL-2 plus interferon, Keilholtz and colleagues [51], demonstrated improved response rates and reduced toxicity with decreasing doses of IL-2.

2.4. Biochemotherapy

Because chemotherapy and cytokines have different and synergistic mechanisms of action and in order to improve response rates and durable remissions, several groups developed in the early 1990s the concept of biochemotherapy, a combination of chemotherapy and biologic response modifiers.

Dacarbazine/IFN-α is one of the most evaluated combinations in metastatic malignant melanoma. In a randomized phase II trial, Falkson et al. [52] reported that the association of IFN-α with dacarbazine resulted in an encouraging response rate (53% vs. 20% for dacarbazine alone) and a higher duration of response (8.9 months vs. 2.5 months) but IFN-α significantly increased the toxicity. However, a follow up of a large randomized trial demonstrated no benefit for the addition of IFN-α to dacarbazine and significantly more severe toxic events occurred with treatments containing IFN-α [36].

The other approaches of biochemotherapy have involved sequential chemotherapy (cisplatin, vinblastine, and dacarbazine, CVD) followed by biologic response modifiers (continuous infusion of 9 MIU/m2 of IL-2 + IFN-α) because of concern of toxicity when drugs were given simultaneously or concurrent with chemo-immunotherapy. Both approaches have produced promising results with overall response rates between 40% and 60% and a long-term remission rate of about 9%. The sequential approach was compared to chemotherapy alone in a randomized trial conducted at the MD Anderson Cancer Center. Although both response rate and time to progression were improved in the sequential biochemotherapy group, the survival difference was at borderline significance and the toxicity was very high [53]. The results of the largest phase III trial (ECOG/Intergroup E3695 trial) and most definitive test for biochemotherapy comparing concurrent CVD-Bio to CVD alone showed that biochemotherapy produced slightly higher response rates and significantly longer median progression-free survival than CVD alone, but once again failed to show any improvement in either overall survival or durable responses. Considering the extra toxicity and complexity, this concurrent biochemotherapy regimen should not be recommended for patients with metastatic melanoma [54].

2.5. Signal transduction inhibitors

In the past decades, no significant impact on survival has been made in spite of increased response rates achieved with combinations of chemotherapeutics or with the combination of chemotherapy and cytokines such as interferon (IFN) or interleukin-2 (IL-2). However, great advances have been made in a very short time, both in terms of targeted drugs that kill melanoma cells.

Sorafenib was designed to inhibit tyrosine kinase activity of CRAF, but this drug inhibits both the wild-type RAF protein as the V600E mutant protein. Subsequently, it was shown that sorafenib is actually a multikinase inhibitor, can inhibit many other molecules such as VEGFR2 and 3, PDGFR, p38 MAPK, FLT3, c-Kit and RET [55]. Although preclinical experiments, both *in vitro* and in animal models, seemed to be encouraging, the results of clinical trials have not confirmed the efficacy of sorafenib for the treatment of disseminated melanoma [56]

After the failure of sorafenib in melanoma, was synthesized a more specific BRAF inhibitors, in particular against the protein with the V600E mutation: PLX4032, a low molecular weight drug, for oral administration. In the first clinical trial published in 2010 [57], the objective response was observed in 81% of the BRAF^{V600E} melanoma patients with 2 complete responses and 24 partial responses. Responses occurred in patients with visceral metastases in locations usually resistant to treatment such as liver, intestine and bone. However, despite having achieved a good response, relapses occur early, usually in a period of 8-12 months after treatment [58].

The possibility that c-Kit was a therapeutic target in melanoma has long since shuffled. In fact, c-Kit is a protein that acts as a receptor for a growth factor essential for epidermal melanocytes and has a role in the differentiation and migration of melanocytic cells during embryonic development [59]. In 2011, a phase-II study from China reported 20–30% response rates and prolongation of progression-free survival with imatinib treatment [60].

From 15 to 30% of melanomas have mutations of NRAS. RAS activation mutations stimulate MAP kinase pathway, but also the route of PI3K/AKT among others. A phase II trial using the RAS inhbitor Tipifarnib was performed; however, it was closed for lack of response. None of the patients was selected based on the presence of mutations of NRAS [61].

MEK is a protein of the MAP kinase pathway, located downstream BRAF. Several MEK inhibitors (PD0325901, AZD6244, GSK1120212, and E6201) have been synthesized. Bases on some results, it appears that these pharmacological agents may be effective as single agents in the treatment of melanoma. However, there are many preclinical studies suggesting that it would be a good alternative to the combined treatments, both to avoid resistance in the use of drugs directed against BRAF/V600E mutation, as for the treatment of BRAF mutations other than V600E or mutations of NRAS, especially if associated with inhibitors of PI3K/AKT pathway [62-65]

Different derivatives of rapamycin (CCI-779 or temsirolimus) have been used as inhibitors of the PI3K/AKT pathway. These inhibitors act on mTOR molecule downstream AKT/PKB. There are also dual inhibitors of PI3K and mTOR, PI3K and AKT [66]. Although clinical outcomes of these drugs in phase II trials have not been good, there are several authors proposing their use in combined therapies especially with drugs that inhibit the MAP kinase pathway [62, 63, 65, 67] or even, simultaneous inhibition via PI3K/AKT [68].

3. Resistance to the treatments in melanoma

Simultaneous resistance to several structurally unrelated drugs that do not necessarily have a common mechanism of action is called multidrug resistance phenomena. An important principle in multidrug resistance is that cancer cells are genetically heterogeneous. Although the process results in uncontrolled cell growth for clonal expansion of cancer, tumor cells exposed to chemotherapeutic agents will be selected by their ability to survive and grow in the presence of cytotoxic drugs. Therefore, in any population of cancer cells that are exposed to chemotherapy, more than one mechanism of multidrug resistance may be present [69]. Different types of multidrug resistance mechanisms have been described in cancer cells. Natural resistance to hydrophobic drugs sometimes known as classical multidrug resistance, usually results in the expression of efflux pumps with an ATP-dependent drug broad specificity. These pumps belong to a family of conveyors called ABC transporters (ATP-binding cassette) that show sequence and structural homology [70]. The resistance is caused by increased output by lowering the intracellular concentration of the drug. Resistance may also occur due to reduced entry of the drug. Water-soluble drugs, which are returned by carriers that are used to carry nutrients into the cell, or agents that enter through endocytosis, could fail without evidencing of increased output. Examples of this kind of drugs include the antifolate methotrexate, nucleotide analogues such as 5-fluorouracil and 8-azaguanine, and alkylating agents such as cisplatin [71,72]. Multidrug resistance can also result from the activation of coordinated systems of detoxification, such as DNA repair systems and cytochrome P-450 [73]. In another hand, resistance can also result from a defective apoptotic pathway. This can occur because of malignant transformation, such as in cancer, or as a result of non-functional mutant p53 [74]. Alternatively, cells may acquire apoptotic pathways changes during exposure to chemotherapy and changes in the levels of ceramides [75] or changes in the cell cycle machinery, which triggers checkpoints and prevent initiation of apoptosis. Below we present several mechanisms of resistance to the treatments that have been described in melanoma.

3.1. Antipoptotic characteristics in melanoma

Melanocytes and their stem cell precursors are activated to secrete melanin and protect neighboring keratinocytes and other epidermal cells from further damage [76]. Thus, melanocytes should be programmed to survive. Keratinocytes promote melanocyte expression of Bcl-2 by secreting neuronal growth factor (NGF) and stem cell grow factor (SCF). NGF binds to its receptors in the melanocyte membrane and increases the levels of Bcl-2 [77]. SCF interacts with its receptor c-KIT on the membrane and leads to the activation of transcription factor Mitf, which induces proliferation and differentiation of melanocyte precursors [78]. Tumorigenic melanoma cells may take advantage of high endogenous Bcl-2 levels to survive under adverse environmental conditions that they may encounter during metastatic progression and, given the connection between apoptosis and drug sensitivity, bypass the effects of chemotherapeutic drugs. Similarly, BclxL and Mcl-1, other anti-apoptotic members of the Bcl-2 family, are strongly expressed in normal melanocytes, benign nevi, primary melanoma and melanoma metastases, and may contribute to melanoma resistance to therapy [79,80]

In melanoma, two members of the IAP family, survivin and ML-IAP, have been associated with tumor progression, as they become detectable in melanocytic nevi and further overexpressed in invasive and metastatic melanomas [81,82]. Survivin is abundantly expressed, and its subcellular localization varies depending upon tumor thickness and invasiveness. Survivin overexpression has been shown in squamous cell carcinoma (SCC), and it is involved in UVB-induced carcinogenesis. The presence of survivin both in the nucleus and in the cytoplasm throughout the epidermal layers of psoriatic lesions suggests the involvement of this protein in the keratinocyte alterations typical of this disease [81]. Similarly, suppression of survivin can increase the sensitivity of melanoma cells to chemotherapeutic agents [83,84]. ML-IAP is also upregulated in melanoma cell lines and absent in normal melanocytes [85]. ML-IAP's effects on the mitochondrial pathways are considered to be related to a direct inhibition of the pro-apoptotic factor Smac/Diablo, and the caspases 9 and 3 [86]. The role of ML-IAP on melanoma chemoresistance has not been proven yet, but the overexpression of ML-IAP in breast cancer cell lines (MCF-7) or in HeLa cells protects against the drug Adriamycin and other apoptotic inducers, including TNF-α, FADD or BAX [86,87].

3.2. p53 pathway

p53 suppresses tumor development through multiple activities including induction of growth arrest, apoptosis, senescence, and autophagy [88,89]. Environmental agents such as UV that induce cellular damage activate the p53 tumor suppressor and p53 activation results in p53-dependent programmed cell death (apoptosis) in many cell types. Melanocytes are resistant to UV-induced apoptosis suggesting that p53 activity is somehow blocked (non-functional p53), a state shared with melanoma cells [90], which are resistant to conventional modes of chemotherapy that aim to stimulate p53-dependent apoptosis.

Melanoma is one of a number of tumor types where p53 is still wild type, indicating that other events are contributing to p53 inactivation, in fact p53 function could be disabled by lesions that disrupt other components of the pathway. Studies using mouse models of melanoma have shown that disruption of the upstream p53 regulator p14 [ARF] can functionally replace p53 loss during melanomagenesis [91]. Analogous to the human situation, tumors arising in these mouse models present wild type p53 [91]. Moreover, the abnormal phosphorylation of p53 by Chk2 kinase may contribute to the resistance of melanoma cells to radiotherapy [92]. Disruption of apoptosis downstream of p53 may alleviate pressure to mutate p53 and simultaneously decrease drug sensitivity [93]. For example, Apaf-1 and caspase 9 can be essential downstream effectors of p53-induced apoptosis and their disruption can facilitate oncogenic transformation of cultured fibroblasts [94]. In melanomas, Apaf-1 protein and mRNA expression are frequently downregulated in metastatic cell lines and tumor specimens [95]. Interestingly, Apaf-1 protein levels can be restored by addition of the methylation inhibitor 5-aza-2′-deoxycytidine (5azaCdR), suggesting that DNA methylation contributes to suppression of Apaf-1 levels. Whether methylation blocks Apaf-1 mRNA expression directly by interfering with the recruitment of transcription factors at the Apaf-1 promoter or by affecting a regulator of Apaf-1 expression remains an open question. In any case, Apaf-1 downregulation compromises the apoptotic response of melanoma cells in response to p53 activation [95] or E2F-1 [96]. Restoring physiological levels of Apaf-1 through gene transfer or 5aza2dC treatment enhances chemosensitivity, alleviating cell death defects associated with reduced Apaf-1 expression [95].

In tumor cells, the selective pressure to delete or inactivate p53 is very high. This primarily occurs through mutations in p53, amplification/overexpression of its inhibitors like Mdm2, Mdm4 (Mdm2 family member) [97]. The key molecule in the p53 regulatory network is Mdm2, an E3 ubiquitin ligase with potentially oncogenic activity. Dynamic fine-tuning of the Mdm2-centered network dictates the proper rapidity, intensity, and duration of a p53 response, resulting in the appropriate biological outcomes [98]. Although p53 is one of the most frequently mutated tumor suppressor genes in cancer, it is mutated in only about 13% of uncultured melanoma specimens [99-101]. The absence of p53 mutations in melanoma has been attributed to the epistatic loss of ARF [101] or amplification of HDM2 [102], both of which lead to a functionally debilitating interaction between HDM2 and p53. Ji et al. have provided important data that HDM2 antagonism can effectively restore p53 function, suppress melanoma growth, and synergize with MEK inhibition [103].

3.3. Signaling pathways in melanoma

In malignant melanoma, the PI3K/AKT signaling pathway is frequently constitutively activated [104]. Several studies indicate that only a combinatorial inhibition of PI3K/AKT and MAPK signalling induces apoptosis in melanoma cells efficiently [105,106]. On the other hand, inappropriate activation of survival signaling pathways such as those mediated by mitogen-activated protein kinase (MEK)/extracellular-regulated kinase (ERK) and phosphoinositide 3-kinase (PI3K)/AKT, either as consequences of genetic alterations or resulting from environmental stimulations, is known to play a central role in the resistance of melanoma to apoptosis [107,108].

One-third of primary melanomas and about 50% of metastatic melanoma cell lines showed reduced expression of PTEN as a result of allelic deletion, mutation or transcriptional silencing [109,110], suggesting that inactivation of PTEN is a late, but frequent, event on melanomagenesis [111,112]. Multiple lines of evidence point to the PI3K/AKT/PTEN pathway as a putative candidate for therapeutic intervention in melanoma because PTEN overexpression can revert the invasive phenotype of human and mouse melanoma cell lines [113,114] and elevated PTEN activity may sensitize cells to chemotherapeutic drugs [115].

Recent progress in the identification of genes relevant for melanomagenesis was made, revealing the importance of several signaling pathways. Sinnberg et al. [116] suggest that the oncogenic transcription factor Y-box binding protein-1 (YB-1) play a pivotal role in melanoma cells. YB-1 could be a key player, activated by the signalling pathways MAPK and PI3K/AKT. Indeed, was demostrated that both signaling pathways are able to increase S102-phosphorylation and nuclear translocation of YB-1. It is known that S102-phosphorylated YB-1 can induce the expression of the catalytic subunit of PI3K and by this increases PI3K activity [117].

In melanoma cells, the NF-kB pathway can be altered by upregulation of the NF-kB subunits p50 and RelA [118,119] and downregulation of the NF-kB inhibitor IkB [120,121]. Consequently, downstream NF-kB targets like c-myc, cyclin D1, the anti-apoptotic factor TRAF2, the invasion-associated proteins Mel-CAM or the pro-angiogenic chemokine GRO are also frequently upregulated in melanoma [122]. Recent studies have highlighted that some components of NF- kB family, such as p50 and p65/ RelA proteins, are overexpressed in the nuclei of dysplastic nevi and melanoma cells compared to those of normal nevi and healthy melanocytes, respectively [123]. Other data show that a hyperactivation of NF-kB can be also caused by an increased expression of other factors involved indirectly in NF-kB pathway. Recent studies on the gene expression profile of melanoma cells have shown an increased expression of Osteopontin (OPN) [124], a secreted glycophosphoprotein that induces NF-kB activation through enhancement of the IKK activity based on phosphorylation and degradation of IkBa [125]. Indeed, OPN induces AKT phosphorylation and, in turn, phosphorylated AKT binds to IKKa/b and activates IKK complex [125]. Mutational activation of BRAF, common in human melanomas, has been also associated with an enhanced IKK activity and a concomitant increase in the rate of IkBa ubiquitination and its subsequent degradation. This process overall entails a constitutive induction of NF-kB activity and an increased survival of melanoma cells [126]. Combination of these data with others reported in literature strongly suggests that the enhanced activation of NF-kB may be due to deregulations occurring in upstream signaling pathways such as RAS/RAF, PI3K/AKT and NIK [121].

Oncogenic mutations on Ras-family members, RAS and B-RAF, have been shown to impinge at multiple levels on AKT/NF-kB, RAF/MAPK and RAL/Rho signaling pathways [127] producing survival signals to disengage cell cycle checkpoint controls, favor metastasis and block pro-apoptotic stimuli. In support of this hypothesis, overexpression of N-RAS in human melanoma cells enhances Bcl-2 expression and contributes to a higher tumorigenicity and drug resistance in mouse xenotransplant models (i.e. subcutaneous injections) [128]. Chin and collaborators have generated melanomas in the context of a specific genetic background (INK4a/ARF deficiency) by conditional overexpression of H-RAS in melanocytes. Once the tumors were formed, downregulation of H-RAS expression led to a marked tumor regression by enhanced apoptosis of the tumor cells and also on the host-derived endothelial cells [129]. High-throughput analyses of genetic alterations in human cancers demonstrate that specifically, B-RAF, a RAS effector, was found to be mutated in 66% of human melanomas. Mutations are restricted to a few single amino-acid changes (primarily on V599) that render a constitutive active kinase with transforming properties in NIH3T3 cells [130]. Interestingly, previous studies indicate that wild-type B-RAF may inhibit programmed cell death downstream of cytocrome C release [131].

Although >50 mutations in BRAF have now been described, the most common BRAF mutation in melanoma, accounting for 80% of all of the BRAF mutations, is a valine to glutamic acid (V600E) substitution [130,132]. Acquisition of a V600E mutation in BRAF destabilizes the inactive kinase conformation switching the equilibrium towards the active form, leading to constitutive activity [132]. Mechanistically, mutated BRAF exerts most of its oncogenic effects through the activation of the MAPK pathway [133]. MAPK activity drives the uncontrolled growth of melanoma cells by upregulating the expression of cyclin D1 and through the suppression of the cyclin dependent kinase inhibitor p27[KIP1]. Pre-clinical studies have shown that introduction of mutated BRAF into immortalized melanocytes leads to anchorage independent growth and tumor formation in immunocompromised mice [133]. Conversely, downregulation of mutated BRAF using RNAi causes cell cycle arrest and apoptosis in both *in vitro* and *in vivo* BRAF[V600E] mutant melanoma models [133]. Although it has been suggested that the acquisition of the BRAF[V600E] mutation is an early event in melanoma development, with 80% of all benign nevi showing to be BRAF mutant, the available evidence indicates that mutant BRAF alone cannot initiate melanoma [134,135].

3.4. DNA Mismatch Repair (MMR) proteins

Late et al. [136] determined that melanoma cells exhibiting resistance to cisplatin, etoposide and vindesine present a reduction of 30 to 70% in the nuclear content of each of the DNA mismatch repair (MMR) proteins hMLH1, hMSH2 and hMSH6. A decreased expression level of up to 80% of mRNAs encoding hMLH1 and hMSH2 was observed in drug-resistant melanoma cells selected for cisplatin, etoposide and fotemustine. In melanoma cells that acquired resistance to fotemustine, the activity of O6-methylguanine-DNA methyltransferase (MGMT) was considerably enhanced. The data of this group indicate that modulation of both MMR components and MGMT expression level may contribute to the drug-resistant phenotype of melanoma cells.

DNA mismatch repair (MMR) deficiency and increased O6-methylguanine-DNA methyltransferase (MGMT) activity have been related to resistance to O6-guanine methylating agents in tumour cell lines. However, the clinical relevance of MMR and MGMT as drug resistance factors is still unclear. In a retrospective study, the expression levels of the MMR proteins, hMSH2, hMSH6 and hMLH1, Ma et al. [137] analysed by immunohisto-chemistry in melanoma metastases from 64 patients, who had received dacarbazine (DTIC) based chemotherapy. All tumours showed positive nuclear staining for hMLH1. The response rates were similar in patients with hMSH2 and/or hMSH6 positive tu-mours to these in patients with negative tumours. In other retrospective study, Ma et al. [138] analysed the levels of the DNA repair protein $O(6)$-methylguanine-DNA methyl-transferase (MGMT) in melanoma metastases from patients receiving dacarbazine (DTIC) either as a single drug or as part of combination chemotherapy regimens, and related the expression levels to the clinical response to treatment. DTIC as single agent was given to 44 patients, while 21 received combination chemotherapy. Objective responses to chemo-therapy were seen in 12 patients, while 53 patients failed to respond to treatment. The expression of MGMT was determined according to the proportion of antibody-stained tu-mor cells, using a cut-off level of 50%. In 12 of the patients, more than one metastasis was analyzed, and in seven of these cases, the MGMT expression differed between tu-mours in the same individual. Among the responders a larger proportion (six out of 12, 50%) had tumors containing less than 50% MGMT-positive tumor cells than among the non-responders (12 out of 53, 23%). These data are consistent with the hypothesis that MGMT contributes to resistance to DTIC-based treatment. The conclusion that can be drawn from the fact that the development of drug resistance in melanoma cells is accom-panied by down modulation of certain components of the MMR system and by an in-crease in MGMT activity when $O6$-alkylating agents are applied has several far-reaching implications regarding primary and acquired clinical resistance to these drugs. Further-more, reduction or deficiency in MMR may increase the mutation rate in affected cells leading subsequently to an increased rate of development of resistance to other drugs having different targets. In addition, an enhanced mutation rate may contribute to in-creased phenotypic variation and therefore the clinical aggressiveness of melanomas and their metastases.

Recently, Li et al. [139] demonstrated the expression of DNA repair genes ERCC1 and XPF is induced by cisplatin in melanoma cells and that this induction is regulated by the MAPK pathway, with the role of DUSP6 phosphatase being particularly important. This induction contributes to increased drug resistance, which is one of the major obstacles to melanoma treatment, suggesting that ERCC1 or XPF inhibitors could be used to enhance the effective-ness of cisplatin treatment.

3.5. Multidrug Resistance Proteins (MRP)

The intrinsic multidrug resistance and sensitivity in melanomas and in pigment-producing cells involves multiple ABC transporters and melanosome biogenesis [140]. Melanoma cells express a group of ABC transporters, including ABCA9, ABCB1, ABCB5, ABCB8, ABCC1, ABCC2, and ABCD1 [140,141].

ABCC1 was shown to cooperate with glutathione S-transferase M1 to help melanoma cells escape the cytotoxicity of vincristine [141]. Have been described too that B16 melanoma

(B16M) cells presenting high ABCC1 and GSH content show high metastatic activity and high multidrug and radiation resistance [142]. Elevated expression of ABCC2 was shown to cause cisplatin resistance by reducing nuclear DNA damage, decreasing cell cycle G2-arrest, and increasing reentry into the cell cycle [4].

Has been reported that ABCB5 and ABCB8 mediate doxorubicin resistance in melanoma cells [143, 144]. ABCB5 shares 73% of sequence homology with the classic and the most studied multidrug resistance protein ABCB1 (P-gp, MDR1) [145,146] and was firstly detected in tissues derived from the neuroectodermal lineage including melanocyte progenitors [145], melanoma cell lines and patient specimens [143,146-148]. In melanoma, ABCB5-expressing cells are endowed with self-renewal, differentiation and tumorigenicity abilities [149,150]. Their abundance in clinical melanoma specimens correlates positively with the neoplasic progression suggesting that ABCB5 expression is associated with tumor aggressiveness. Moreover, the growth of melanoma xenografts in mice was delayed when the animals were treated with a monoclonal anti-ABCB5 antibody [149]. As a member of the ABC transporter family, ABCB5 is thought to play a role in drug efflux. This was supported by experiments measuring the intracellular accumulation of Rhodamine 123 [145]. These data suggest that ABC proteins may be important molecular targets for the reversal of multidrug resistance in melanoma cells.

4. Does oxidative stress contribute to the resistance in melanoma?

Free radicals are implicated in the pathogenesis of a multistage process of carcinogenesis. They can cause DNA base alterations, strand breaks, damage to tumor suppressor genes and enhanced expression of proto-oncogenes. The burst of reactive oxygen species (ROS) and the reactive nitrogen species (RNS) has been implicated in the development of cancer [151,152]. Excessive production of ROS can be harmful to both normal and cancer cells. High levels of ROS cause damage to lipids, DNA and cellular proteins, disrupting their normal function. However, some cancer cells can develop mechanisms that use ROS for purposes such as mitogenic upregulation of the expression of antioxidant enzymes [153-155]. Several studies have investigated the role of antioxidant enzymes in cancer and it has been shown that these enzymes play a significant role in regulating cancer growth and survival [156,157]. The carcinogenic effect of oxidative stress is attributed primarily to the genotoxicity of ROS in various cellular processes [158]. For example, hydroxyl radicals can react with purines andor pyrimidines as well as chromatin proteins, resulting in base modifications and genomic instability which can cause alterations in gene expression [159]. These data have suggested the accumulation of ROS as a common phenomenon in many cancer cells. Such accumulations can cause direct damage to DNA by increasing the cellular mutation and/or promoting and maintaining the tumorigenic phenotype by activating a second messenger in intracellular signaling cascades [160]. In addition, ROS have been determined to cause epigenetic alterations that affect the genome and play a major role in the development of carcinogenesis in humans [161]. More specifically, the production of ROS is associated with alterations in DNA methylation patterns [162, 163]. In particular, hydroxyl radicals that produce DNA lesions, such as 8-hydroxyl-2-deoxyguanosine, 8-hydroxyguanine, 8 -OHdG [164-166], and damage to the single strand of DNA [167] have been shown to decrease DNA methylation by means of interfering with the ability of DNA to function as a substrate for the DNA methyltransferases (DNMTs) and thus resulting in global hypomethylation [168].

Oxidative stress may play different roles in the pathogenesis of melanoma and non-melanoma skin cancer. It is likely that in non-melanoma skin cancers, a diminished antioxidant defense caused by chronic UV exposure contributes to the occurrence of mutations and carcinogenesis, whereas melanoma cells are equipped with a high antioxidant capacity and might use their ability to generate ROS for damaging surrounding tissue and thus supporting tumour progression and metastasis [169]. Gidanian et al. showed that melanosomes derived from melanoma cells in comparison to melanocytes actively produce excessive amounts of ROS [170]. Higher intracellular levels of ROS in melanoma cells were also detected by the studies by Meyskens et al. [171]. They furthermore showed that due to these elevated levels of ROS, melanin itself becomes progressively more oxidized and starts to function as a pro-oxidant [172]. They also showed that oxidation of melanin can be further increased by binding of metals, such as iron. These melanin-metal complexes can be converted by the Fenton reaction thereby producing even more ROS [173]. There is supportive evidence that sustained oxidative stress is related to oxidative DNA damage [174]. Atypical melanocytes have increased levels of oxidative stress and oxidative DNA damage [175, 176]. In line with these observations, Leikam et al. found that ROS production was accompanied by enhanced DNA damage [177].

4.1. Oxidative stress by antitumoral treatments

The cytotoxicity of some antitumoral drugs like actinomycin-D (AMD), adriamycin (ADR), cisplatin (Cis-Pt), vincristine (VCR), cytosine arabinoside (Ara-C) and dacarbazine (DTIC) are, to a greater or lesser extent, linked to the generation of free radicals and/or to the antioxidant defense of the cells. AMD and ADR are xenobiotics, which, in the cell, enter to cycles of oxidation and reduction, generating ROS [178,179]. Cis-Pt does not produce ROS; however, during its detoxification the level of glutathione (GSH) decreases [180]. In the case of DTIC, it has been shown that the resistance of melanoma cells to that drug is also partly linked to changes in the level of GSH [17,181]. ROS generated by mitochondria intensify the apoptosis induced by cytosine arabinoside [182].

Radiotherapy is a cornerstone in the treatment of several cancers. Ionic irradiation exposes all cells to high levels of oxidative stress, thus resulting in the formation of ROS, increasing DNA damage and ultimately leading to cell death. Another mechanism of the action of radiotherapy is to alter cellular homeostasis, thus modifying the signal transduction pathways and predisposing to apoptosis [183]. However, there are conflicting reports on the effect of radiotherapy on oxidative stress. Some studies have reported increased oxidative stress after radiotherapy [184], while others have reported decreased oxidative stress after radiotherapy in cancer patients [185, 186].

4.2. Transcription factors Nrf1 and Nrf2 are regulators of oxidative stress signaling

Nrf1 (NF-E2 related factor-1) and Nrf2 (NF-E2 related factor-2) nowadays are known as two oxidative stress sensitive transcription factors that belong to the CNC/bZIP family of transcription factors consisting of NF-E2, Nrf1, Nrf2, Nrf3, BACH1, and BACH2 [45–48]. Both Nrf1 and Nrf2 are responsible for regulating the expression of many antioxidant genes including peroxiredoxin-1 (Prx-1), thioredoxin-1 (Txn-1), GCLC (Glutamate cysteine ligase catalytic subunit - an enzyme responsible for catalyzing the formation of glutathione), glutathione peroxidase (GPX-1), drug metabolizing enzymes (cytochrome P-450s), and several ATP Binding Cassette (ABC) transporters that are responsible for drug efflux [187-190]. All of these genes are essential for the maintenance of oxidative homeostasis and contain an Electrophile Response Element (EpRE) to which Nrf1 and Nrf2 bind (also known as the Antioxidant Response Element). Both Nrf1 and Nrf2 are essential to the cellular response to oxidative stress and several studies have shown that knockdown of Nrf1 and/or Nrf2 expression sensitizes cells to oxidative stress [191-193]. It has also been suggested that Nrf2 responds to inducible oxidative stimuli and that Nrf1 regulates oxidative stress [194]. Increased oxidative stress has been shown to promote tumor proliferation and survival through deregulation of redox-sensitive pathways [153,195,196]. Nrf2 resides predominantly in the cytoplasm where it interacts with the actin-associated cytosolic protein INrf2, which is also known as Keap1 (Kelch-like ECH-associated protein 1). INrf2 functions as a substrate adaptor protein for a Cul3/Rbx1-dependent E3 ubiquitin ligase complex to ubiquitinate and degrade Nrf2, thus maintaining a steady-state level of Nrf2 [197].

Data from tumor cell lines isolated and profiled from human patients have indicated that many tumors have adapted to exploit the cytoprotective actions of Nrf2 both *in vivo* and *in vitro* through mutations of Keap1 and Nrf2, which lead to the constitutive upregulation and permanent activation of Nrf2-signaling to enhance the tolerance of the cancer cells to toxins and thereby limit the efficacy of chemotherapeutic agents. The loss of INrf2 (Keap1) function is shown to lead to nuclear accumulation of Nrf2, activation of metabolizing enzymes and drug resistance [198]. Studies have reported mutations resulting in dysfunctional Nrf2 in lung, breast and bladder cancers [199-203].

In a study carried out by Matundan et al. [204], they demonstrated the basal Nrf2 expression pattern in human melanoma was increased in 7 of 8 human melanoma cell lines. Immunoblots of Nrf2 showed over-expression in 6 of 8 metastatic melanoma cell lines and they determined that Nrf2's contribution was protective against redox stress in melanoma, and that decreased Nrf2 activation sensitizes melanoma cell lines to existing chemotherapeutics [204].

4.3. NRF2 are related with the expression of multidrug resistance proteins

Ogura and colleagues reported previously that Nrf2 binds within the *ABCB1* promoter's -126 and -102 regions, which contain the ATTCAGTCA motif. They have purified Nrf2 from the nuclear extract of K562/ADM cells, a multidrug-resistant cell line derived from human myelogenous leukemia K562 cells. This group determined that ATTCAGTCA motif is a positive regulatory element of MDR1 gene and that the motif is important for Nrf2 binding.

These results suggest that Nrf2 may be involved in the positive regulation of the *ABCB1* gene transcription [205].

Maher and collaborators examined the possibility that Nrf2 is also involved in the expression levels of ABCC1 in mouse embryo fibroblasts. The constitutive expression levels of Mrp1 mRNA and protein were significantly lower in Nrf2 (-/-) cells compared with those in wild type cells. In addition, significant induction by diethyl maleate was observed in wild type, but not in Nrf2 (-/-) cells, suggesting the involvement of Nrf2 in both the constitutive and inducible mRNA and protein expression of ABCC1. In addition, the uptake of [^{3}H]2,4-dinitrophenyl-S-glutathione, a typical substrate of ABCC1, into isolated membrane vesicles also demonstrated that Nrf2 regulates the transport activity of glutathione conjugates in mouse fibroblasts [206]. In another hand, Maher evaluated whether oxidative conditions (that is, the disruption of hepatic GSH synthesis) or the administration of nuclear factor-E2-related factor-2 (Nrf2) activators (oltipraz and butylated hydroxyanisole) can induce hepatic ABC transporters and whether that induction is through the NRF2 transcriptional pathway. Livers from hepatocyte-specific glutamate-cysteine ligase catalytic subunit-null mice had increased nuclear NRF2 levels, marked gene and protein induction of the Nrf2 target gene NAD(P)H: quinone oxidoreductase 1, as well as ABCC2, ABCC3, and ABCC4 expression. The treatment of wild type and Nrf2-null mice with oltipraz and butylated hydroxyanisole demonstrated that the induction of ABCC2, ABCC3, and ABCC4 is NRF2-dependent. In Hepa1c1c7 cells treated with the Nrf2 activator tert-butyl hydroquinone, chromatin immunoprecipitation with Nrf2 antibodies revealed the binding of NRF2 to antioxidant response elements in the promoter regions of mouse ABCC2 [-185 base pairs (bp)], ABCC3 (-9919 bp), and ABCC4 (-3767 bp). In this way, the activation of the Nrf2 regulatory pathway was shown to stimulate the coordinated induction of hepatic ABCs [190].

4.4. NRF2 represses the p53 pathway

You et al. [207] confirmed that Nrf2 is directly involved in the basal expression of Mdm2 through the antioxidant response element, which is located in the first intron of this gene. This linkage between Nrf2 and Mdm2 appears to cause the accumulation of p53 protein in Nrf2-deficent MEFs. They also showed that ovarian carcinoma A2780 cells silenced for Nrf2 by shRNA displayed higher levels of p53 activation in response to hydrogen peroxide treatment, leading to increased cell death. Collectively, those results suggest novel evidence that the inhibition of Nrf2 can suppress Mdm2 expression, which may result in p53 signaling modulation. Thus, forced inhibition of Nrf2 expression in cancer cells may be lead to activation of apoptosis response through the activation of p53 signaling.

4.5. Nrf2 and signalling pathways

The functional interaction between the Keap1-Nrf2 pathway and PTEN-PI3K-AKT pathway has been reported in several studies using cell lines. The pharmacological inhibition of the PI3K-AKT pathway represses the nuclear translocation of Nrf2 [208, 209]. In another hand, Beyer et al. showed that AKT phosphorylation was robustly augmented in the P/K-Alb mice in Nrf2-dependent manner, which is consistent with the previous report that Nrf2 positively regulates the activation of AKT [210]. Recently, Mitsuishi et al. [211] demonstrated a contribution of Nrf2 to cellular metabolic activities in proliferating cells, and the positive feedback loop between the PTEN-PI3K-AKT and Keap1-Nrf2 pathways, which appears to be one of the most substantial mechanisms for promoting the malignant evolution of cancers. It should be noted that Nrf2 accumulation, which is achieved by the functional impairment of Keap1 combined with the sustained activation of PI3K-AKT pathway, allows Nrf2 to get involved in the modulation of metabolism under pathological conditions. In contrast, temporary accumulation of Nrf2 at a low level is sufficient for Nrf2 to exert the cytoprotective function under physiological conditions [211].

Su et al. [212] reported the first evidence that Nrf2 is phosphorylated by MAPKs *in vivo*, however the nuclear accumulation of Nrf2 was slightly enhanced by its phosphorylation. This group concluded that direct phosphorylation of Nrf2 by MAPKs has a limited contribution in regulating the Nrf2-dependent antioxidant responses.

4.6. Nrf2 and anti-apoptotic features

Nrf2 resides predominantly in the cytoplasm where it interacts with the actin-associated cytosolic protein INrf2, which is also known as Keap1 (Kelch-like ECH-associated protein 1). INrf2 functions as a substrate adaptor protein for a Cul3/Rbx1-dependent E3 ubiquitin ligase complex to ubiquitinate and degrade Nrf2, thus maintaining a steady-state level of Nrf2 [197]. A study conducted by Niture et al. demonstrated that INrf2, in association with Cul3/Rbx1, ubiquitinates and degrades Bcl-2 [213]. However they recently demonstrated that Nrf2 binds to Bcl-2 ARE and regulates expression and induction of the Bcl-2 gene. Nrf2 mediated the up-regulation of Bcl-2, down regulated the activity of pro-apoptotic Bax protein and caspases 3/7, and protected cells from etoposide/radiation-mediated apoptosis that leads to drug resistance. Thus, they demonstrate that Nrf2-mediated up-regulation of Bcl-2 plays a significant role in preventing apoptosis, increasing cell survival, and drug resistance [214].

5. Conclusion

Melanoma continues to increase in incidence in many parts of the world, but there is currently no curative treatment once the disease has spread beyond the primary site because of the absence of effective therapies. This is believed to be largely due to the resistance of melanoma cells to induction of apoptosis by available chemotherapeutic drugs and biological reagents. Drug resistance is likely not only a primary consequence of acquired genetic alterations selected during or after therapy, but rather inherent to the malignant behavior of melanoma cells at diagnosis. Data support the existing hypothesis that talks about melanoma cells are "born to survive". Their aggressive behavior stems from intrinsic survival features of their paternal melanocytes nourished by additional alterations acquired during tumor progression. These inherent survival mechanisms may be partly caused by the oxidative stress to which melanoma cells are exposed. Nrf2 is a transcription factor that is considered a double-edged sword because it participates in the regulation of oxidative stress, however has been shown that overexpression of Nrf2 is a common phenomenon in several cancer types, participating in chemoresistance and tumor survival. We assume that this phenomenon also overlaps in melanoma, thus the intrinsic or extrinsic resistance produced in melanoma cells is partly due to overexpression of Nrf2, which can promote cell survival through mechanisms already reviewed in this chapter. Although these mechanisms presented in the last part of this chapter were not studied in melanoma, we believe that future studies endorse our theory. The knowledge about melanoma treatment has been widespread in recent years, but still is not enough, hence we must deepen in this area in order to improve the existing treatments and create effective targeted therapeutic target against this disease.

Acknowledgements

This work was supported by FAPESP (2011/12306-1).

Author details

Jonathan Castillo Arias[1] and Miriam Galvonas Jasiulionis[2]

*Address all correspondence to: mjasiulionis@gmail.com

1 Pharmacological Biochemistry Laboratory, Institute of Biochemistry, Faculty of Sciences, Universidad Austral de Chile, Valdivia, Chile

2 Pharmacology Department, Universidade Federal de São Paulo, São Paulo, Brazil

References

[1] Karagas MR, Greenberg ER, Spencer SK, Stukel TA, Mott LA. Increase in incidence rates of basal cell and squamous cell skin cancer in New Hampshire, USA. New Hampshire Skin Cancer Study Group. International journal of cancer Journal international du cancer. 1999;81(4):555-9. Epub 1999/05/04.

[2] Gloster HM, Jr., Brodland DG. The epidemiology of skin cancer. Dermatologic surgery : official publication for American Society for Dermatologic Surgery [et al]. 1996;22(3):217-26. Epub 1996/03/01.

[3] Plesko I, Severi G, Obsitnikova A, Boyle P. Trends in the incidence of non-melanoma skin cancer in Slovakia, 1978-1995. Neoplasma. 2000;47(3):137-42. Epub 2000/10/24.

[4] Liedert B, Materna V, Schadendorf D, Thomale J, Lage H. Overexpression of cMOAT (MRP2/ABCC2) is associated with decreased formation of platinum-DNA adducts

and decreased G2-arrest in melanoma cells resistant to cisplatin. The Journal of investigative dermatology. 2003;121(1):172-6. Epub 2003/07/04.

[5] Hughes BR, Altman DG, Newton JA. Melanoma and skin cancer: evaluation of a health education programme for secondary schools. The British journal of dermatology. 1993;128(4):412-7. Epub 1993/04/01.

[6] Zemelman V, Roa J, Tagle SR, Valenzuela CY. Malignant melanoma in Chile: an unusual distribution of primary sites in men from low socioeconomic strata. Clinical and experimental dermatology. 2006;31(3):335-8. Epub 2006/05/10.

[7] Zemelman V, Garmendia ML, Kirschbaum A. Malignant melanoma mortality rates in Chile (1988-98). International journal of dermatology. 2002;41(2):99-103. Epub 2002/05/02.

[8] Jemal A, Siegel R, Ward E, Hao Y, Xu J, Murray T, et al. Cancer statistics, 2008. CA: a cancer journal for clinicians. 2008;58(2):71-96. Epub 2008/02/22.

[9] Pawlik TM, Sondak VK. Malignant melanoma: current state of primary and adjuvant treatment. Critical reviews in oncology/hematology. 2003;45(3):245-64. Epub 2003/03/14.

[10] Lee ML, Tomsu K, Von Eschen KB. Duration of survival for disseminated malignant melanoma: results of a meta-analysis. Melanoma research. 2000;10(1):81-92. Epub 2000/03/11.

[11] Ang KK, Peters LJ, Weber RS, Morrison WH, Frankenthaler RA, Garden AS, et al. Postoperative radiotherapy for cutaneous melanoma of the head and neck region. International journal of radiation oncology, biology, physics. 1994;30(4):795-8. Epub 1994/11/15.

[12] Stevens G, Thompson JF, Firth I, O'Brien CJ, McCarthy WH, Quinn MJ. Locally advanced melanoma: results of postoperative hypofractionated radiation therapy. Cancer. 2000;88(1):88-94. Epub 2000/01/05.

[13] Sause WT, Cooper JS, Rush S, Ago CT, Cosmatos D, Coughlin CT, et al. Fraction size in external beam radiation therapy in the treatment of melanoma. International journal of radiation oncology, biology, physics. 1991;20(3):429-32. Epub 1991/03/01.

[14] Conill C, Valduvieco I, Domingo-Domenech J, Arguis P, Vidal-Sicart S, Vilalta A. Loco-regional control after postoperative radiotherapy for patients with regional nodal metastases from melanoma. Clinical & translational oncology : official publication of the Federation of Spanish Oncology Societies and of the National Cancer Institute of Mexico. 2009;11(10):688-93. Epub 2009/10/16.

[15] Comis RL. DTIC (NSC-45388) in malignant melanoma: a perspective. Cancer treatment reports. 1976;60(2):165-76. Epub 1976/02/01.

[16] Hill GJ, 2nd, Metter GE, Krementz ET, Fletcher WS, Golomb FM, Ramirez G, et al. DTIC and combination therapy for melanoma. II. Escalating schedules of DTIC with

BCNU, CCNU, and vincristine. Cancer treatment reports. 1979;63(11-12):1989-92. Epub 1979/11/01.

[17] Bedikian AY, Millward M, Pehamberger H, Conry R, Gore M, Trefzer U, et al. Bcl-2 antisense (oblimersen sodium) plus dacarbazine in patients with advanced melanoma: the Oblimersen Melanoma Study Group. Journal of clinical oncology : official journal of the American Society of Clinical Oncology. 2006;24(29):4738-45. Epub 2006/09/13.

[18] Middleton MR, Grob JJ, Aaronson N, Fierlbeck G, Tilgen W, Seiter S, et al. Randomized phase III study of temozolomide versus dacarbazine in the treatment of patients with advanced metastatic malignant melanoma. Journal of clinical oncology : official journal of the American Society of Clinical Oncology. 2000;18(1):158-66. Epub 2000/01/07.

[19] Chapman PB, Einhorn LH, Meyers ML, Saxman S, Destro AN, Panageas KS, et al. Phase III multicenter randomized trial of the Dartmouth regimen versus dacarbazine in patients with metastatic melanoma. Journal of clinical oncology : official journal of the American Society of Clinical Oncology. 1999;17(9):2745-51. Epub 1999/11/24.

[20] Huncharek M, Caubet JF, McGarry R. Single-agent DTIC versus combination chemotherapy with or without immunotherapy in metastatic melanoma: a meta-analysis of 3273 patients from 20 randomized trials. Melanoma research. 2001;11(1):75-81. Epub 2001/03/20.

[21] Bleehen NM, Newlands ES, Lee SM, Thatcher N, Selby P, Calvert AH, et al. Cancer Research Campaign phase II trial of temozolomide in metastatic melanoma. Journal of clinical oncology : official journal of the American Society of Clinical Oncology. 1995;13(4):910-3. Epub 1995/04/01.

[22] Newlands ES, Blackledge GR, Slack JA, Rustin GJ, Smith DB, Stuart NS, et al. Phase I trial of temozolomide (CCRG 81045: M&B 39831: NSC 362856). British journal of cancer. 1992;65(2):287-91. Epub 1992/02/01.

[23] Jacquillat C, Khayat D, Banzet P, Weil M, Fumoleau P, Avril MF, et al. Final report of the French multicenter phase II study of the nitrosourea fotemustine in 153 evaluable patients with disseminated malignant melanoma including patients with cerebral metastases. Cancer. 1990;66(9):1873-8. Epub 1990/11/01.

[24] Khayat D, Giroux B, Berille J, Cour V, Gerard B, Sarkany M, et al. Fotemustine in the treatment of brain primary tumors and metastases. Cancer investigation. 1994;12(4):414-20. Epub 1994/01/01.

[25] Ahmann DL. Nitrosoureas in the management of disseminated malignant melanoma. Cancer treatment reports. 1976;60(6):747-51. Epub 1976/06/01.

[26] Glover D, Glick JH, Weiler C, Fox K, Guerry D. WR-2721 and high-dose cisplatin: an active combination in the treatment of metastatic melanoma. Journal of clinical oncol-

ogy : official journal of the American Society of Clinical Oncology. 1987;5(4):574-8. Epub 1987/04/01.

[27] Evans LM, Casper ES, Rosenbluth R. Phase II trial of carboplatin in advanced malignant melanoma. Cancer treatment reports. 1987;71(2):171-2. Epub 1987/02/01.

[28] Quagliana JM, Stephens RL, Baker LH, Costanzi JJ. Vindesine in patients with metastatic malignant melanoma: a Southwest Oncology Group study. Journal of clinical oncology : official journal of the American Society of Clinical Oncology. 1984;2(4): 316-9. Epub 1984/04/01.

[29] Aamdal S, Wolff I, Kaplan S, Paridaens R, Kerger J, Schachter J, et al. Docetaxel (Taxotere) in advanced malignant melanoma: a phase II study of the EORTC Early Clinical Trials Group. Eur J Cancer. 1994;30A(8):1061-4. Epub 1994/01/01.

[30] Bedikian AY, Weiss GR, Legha SS, Burris HA, 3rd, Eckardt JR, Jenkins J, et al. Phase II trial of docetaxel in patients with advanced cutaneous malignant melanoma previously untreated with chemotherapy. Journal of clinical oncology : official journal of the American Society of Clinical Oncology. 1995;13(12):2895-9. Epub 1995/12/01.

[31] Einzig AI, Hochster H, Wiernik PH, Trump DL, Dutcher JP, Garowski E, et al. A phase II study of taxol in patients with malignant melanoma. Investigational new drugs. 1991;9(1):59-64. Epub 1991/02/01.

[32] Agarwala SS, Glaspy J, O'Day SJ, Mitchell M, Gutheil J, Whitman E, et al. Results from a randomized phase III study comparing combined treatment with histamine dihydrochloride plus interleukin-2 versus interleukin-2 alone in patients with metastatic melanoma. Journal of clinical oncology : official journal of the American Society of Clinical Oncology. 2002;20(1):125-33. Epub 2002/01/05.

[33] Lattanzi SC, Tosteson T, Chertoff J, Maurer LH, O'Donnell J, LeMarbre PJ, et al. Dacarbazine, cisplatin and carmustine, with or without tamoxifen, for metastatic melanoma: 5-year follow-up. Melanoma research. 1995;5(5):365-9. Epub 1995/10/01.

[34] Cocconi G, Bella M, Calabresi F, Tonato M, Canaletti R, Boni C, et al. Treatment of metastatic malignant melanoma with dacarbazine plus tamoxifen. The New England journal of medicine. 1992;327(8):516-23. Epub 1992/08/20.

[35] Rusthoven JJ, Quirt IC, Iscoe NA, McCulloch PB, James KW, Lohmann RC, et al. Randomized, double-blind, placebo-controlled trial comparing the response rates of carmustine, dacarbazine, and cisplatin with and without tamoxifen in patients with metastatic melanoma. National Cancer Institute of Canada Clinical Trials Group. Journal of clinical oncology : official journal of the American Society of Clinical Oncology. 1996;14(7):2083-90. Epub 1996/07/01.

[36] Falkson CI, Ibrahim J, Kirkwood JM, Coates AS, Atkins MB, Blum RH. Phase III trial of dacarbazine versus dacarbazine with interferon alpha-2b versus dacarbazine with tamoxifen versus dacarbazine with interferon alpha-2b and tamoxifen in patients with metastatic malignant melanoma: an Eastern Cooperative Oncology Group

study. Journal of clinical oncology : official journal of the American Society of Clinical Oncology. 1998;16(5):1743-51. Epub 1998/05/20.

[37]   Rao RD, Holtan SG, Ingle JN, Croghan GA, Kottschade LA, Creagan ET, et al. Combination of paclitaxel and carboplatin as second-line therapy for patients with metastatic melanoma. Cancer. 2006;106(2):375-82. Epub 2005/12/13.

[38]   Garbe C, Eigentler TK, Keilholz U, Hauschild A, Kirkwood JM. Systematic review of medical treatment in melanoma: current status and future prospects. The oncologist. 2011;16(1):5-24. Epub 2011/01/08.

[39]   Hodi FS, O'Day SJ, McDermott DF, Weber RW, Sosman JA, Haanen JB, et al. Improved survival with ipilimumab in patients with metastatic melanoma. The New England journal of medicine. 2010;363(8):711-23. Epub 2010/06/08.

[40]   O'Day SJ, Hamid O, Urba WJ. Targeting cytotoxic T-lymphocyte antigen-4 (CTLA-4): a novel strategy for the treatment of melanoma and other malignancies. Cancer. 2007;110(12):2614-27. Epub 2007/11/16.

[41]   Robert C, Ghiringhelli F. What is the role of cytotoxic T lymphocyte-associated antigen 4 blockade in patients with metastatic melanoma? The oncologist. 2009;14(8): 848-61. Epub 2009/08/04.

[42]   Nancey S, Boschetti G, Cotte E, Ruel K, Almeras T, Chauvenet M, et al. Blockade of cytotoxic T-lymphocyte antigen-4 by ipilimumab is associated with a profound longlasting depletion of Foxp3(+) regulatory T cells: A mechanistic explanation for ipilimumab-induced severe enterocolitis? Inflammatory bowel diseases. 2012;18(8):E1598-600. Epub 2011/11/10.

[43]   Tarhini A, Lo E, Minor DR. Releasing the brake on the immune system: ipilimumab in melanoma and other tumors. Cancer biotherapy & radiopharmaceuticals. 2010;25(6):601-13. Epub 2011/01/06.

[44]   Pehamberger H, Soyer HP, Steiner A, Kofler R, Binder M, Mischer P, et al. Adjuvant interferon alfa-2a treatment in resected primary stage II cutaneous melanoma. Austrian Malignant Melanoma Cooperative Group. Journal of clinical oncology : official journal of the American Society of Clinical Oncology. 1998;16(4):1425-9. Epub 1998/04/29.

[45]   Grob JJ, Dreno B, de la Salmoniere P, Delaunay M, Cupissol D, Guillot B, et al. Randomised trial of interferon alpha-2a as adjuvant therapy in resected primary melanoma thicker than 1.5 mm without clinically detectable node metastases. French Cooperative Group on Melanoma. Lancet. 1998;351(9120):1905-10. Epub 1998/07/08.

[46]   Agarwala SS, Kirkwood JM. Interferons in melanoma. Current opinion in oncology. 1996;8(2):167-74. Epub 1996/03/01.

[47]   Agarwala SS, Kirkwood JM. Potential uses of interferon alpha 2 as adjuvant therapy in cancer. Annals of surgical oncology. 1995;2(4):365-71. Epub 1995/07/01.

[48] Rosenberg SA, Lotze MT, Yang JC, Linehan WM, Seipp C, Calabro S, et al. Combina-
      tion therapy with interleukin-2 and alpha-interferon for the treatment of patients
      with advanced cancer. Journal of clinical oncology : official journal of the American
      Society of Clinical Oncology. 1989;7(12):1863-74. Epub 1989/12/01.

[49] Sparano JA, Fisher RI, Sunderland M, Margolin K, Ernest ML, Sznol M, et al.
      Randomized phase III trial of treatment with high-dose interleukin-2 either alone or
      in combination with interferon alfa-2a in patients with advanced melanoma. Journal
      of clinical oncology : official journal of the American Society of Clinical Oncology.
      1993;11(10):1969-77. Epub 1993/10/01.

[50] Whitehead RP, Figlin R, Citron ML, Pfile J, Moldawer N, Patel D, et al. A phase II
      trial of concomitant human interleukin-2 and interferon-alpha-2a in patients with
      disseminated malignant melanoma. Journal of immunotherapy with emphasis on tu-
      mor immunology : official journal of the Society for Biological Therapy. 1993;13(2):
      117-21. Epub 1993/02/01.

[51] Keilholz U, Goey SH, Punt CJ, Proebstle TM, Salzmann R, Scheibenbogen C, et al. In-
      terferon alfa-2a and interleukin-2 with or without cisplatin in metastatic melanoma: a
      randomized trial of the European Organization for Research and Treatment of Can-
      cer Melanoma Cooperative Group. Journal of clinical oncology : official journal of the
      American Society of Clinical Oncology. 1997;15(7):2579-88. Epub 1997/07/01.

[52] Falkson CI, Falkson G, Falkson HC. Improved results with the addition of interferon
      alfa-2b to dacarbazine in the treatment of patients with metastatic malignant melano-
      ma. Journal of clinical oncology : official journal of the American Society of Clinical
      Oncology. 1991;9(8):1403-8. Epub 1991/08/01.

[53] Eton O, Legha SS, Bedikian AY, Lee JJ, Buzaid AC, Hodges C, et al. Sequential bio-
      chemotherapy versus chemotherapy for metastatic melanoma: results from a phase
      III randomized trial. Journal of clinical oncology : official journal of the American So-
      ciety of Clinical Oncology. 2002;20(8):2045-52. Epub 2002/04/17.

[54] Atkins MB, Hsu J, Lee S, Cohen GI, Flaherty LE, Sosman JA, et al. Phase III trial com-
      paring concurrent biochemotherapy with cisplatin, vinblastine, dacarbazine, inter-
      leukin-2, and interferon alfa-2b with cisplatin, vinblastine, and dacarbazine alone in
      patients with metastatic malignant melanoma (E3695): a trial coordinated by the
      Eastern Cooperative Oncology Group. Journal of clinical oncology : official journal of
      the American Society of Clinical Oncology. 2008;26(35):5748-54. Epub 2008/11/13.

[55] Wilhelm S, Carter C, Lynch M, Lowinger T, Dumas J, Smith RA, et al. Discovery and
      development of sorafenib: a multikinase inhibitor for treating cancer. Nature reviews
      Drug discovery. 2006;5(10):835-44. Epub 2006/10/04.

[56] Wellbrock C, Hurlstone A. BRAF as therapeutic target in melanoma. Biochemical
      pharmacology. 2010;80(5):561-7. Epub 2010/03/31.

[57] Flaherty KT, Puzanov I, Kim KB, Ribas A, McArthur GA, Sosman JA, et al. Inhibition of mutated, activated BRAF in metastatic melanoma. The New England journal of medicine. 2010;363(9):809-19. Epub 2010/09/08.

[58] Solit D, Sawyers CL. Drug discovery: How melanomas bypass new therapy. Nature. 2010;468(7326):902-3. Epub 2010/12/18.

[59] Yoshida H, Kunisada T, Grimm T, Nishimura EK, Nishioka E, Nishikawa SI. Review: melanocyte migration and survival controlled by SCF/c-kit expression. The journal of investigative dermatology Symposium proceedings / the Society for Investigative Dermatology, Inc [and] European Society for Dermatological Research. 2001;6(1):1-5. Epub 2002/01/05.

[60] Guo J, Si L, Kong Y, Flaherty KT, Xu X, Zhu Y, et al. Phase II, open-label, single-arm trial of imatinib mesylate in patients with metastatic melanoma harboring c-Kit mutation or amplification. Journal of clinical oncology : official journal of the American Society of Clinical Oncology. 2011;29(21):2904-9. Epub 2011/06/22.

[61] Flaherty KT, Hodi FS, Bastian BC. Mutation-driven drug development in melanoma. Current opinion in oncology. 2010;22(3):178-83. Epub 2010/04/20.

[62] Ko JM, Fisher DE. A new era: melanoma genetics and therapeutics. The Journal of pathology. 2011;223(2):241-50. Epub 2010/12/03.

[63] Davies MA, Samuels Y. Analysis of the genome to personalize therapy for melanoma. Oncogene. 2010;29(41):5545-55. Epub 2010/08/11.

[64] Friedlander P, Hodi FS. Advances in targeted therapy for melanoma. Clinical advances in hematology & oncology : H&O. 2010;8(9):619-27. Epub 2010/12/16.

[65] Tawbi H, Nimmagadda N. Targeted therapy in melanoma. Biologics : targets & therapy. 2009;3:475-84. Epub 2010/01/08.

[66] Courtney KD, Corcoran RB, Engelman JA. The PI3K pathway as drug target in human cancer. Journal of clinical oncology : official journal of the American Society of Clinical Oncology. 2010;28(6):1075-83. Epub 2010/01/21.

[67] Rother J, Jones D. Molecular markers of tumor progression in melanoma. Current genomics. 2009;10(4):231-9. Epub 2009/12/02.

[68] Werzowa J, Koehrer S, Strommer S, Cejka D, Fuereder T, Zebedin E, et al. Vertical inhibition of the mTORC1/mTORC2/PI3K pathway shows synergistic effects against melanoma in vitro and in vivo. The Journal of investigative dermatology. 2011;131(2):495-503. Epub 2010/11/05.

[69] Dean M, Fojo T, Bates S. Tumour stem cells and drug resistance. Nature reviews Cancer. 2005;5(4):275-84. Epub 2005/04/02.

[70] Dean M, Rzhetsky A, Allikmets R. The human ATP-binding cassette (ABC) transporter superfamily. Genome Res. 2001;11(7):1156-66. Epub 2001/07/04.

[71] Shen DW, Goldenberg S, Pastan I, Gottesman MM. Decreased accumulation of [14C]carboplatin in human cisplatin-resistant cells results from reduced energy-dependent uptake. Journal of cellular physiology. 2000;183(1):108-16. Epub 2000/03/04.

[72] Shen D, Pastan I, Gottesman MM. Cross-resistance to methotrexate and metals in human cisplatin-resistant cell lines results from a pleiotropic defect in accumulation of these compounds associated with reduced plasma membrane binding proteins. Cancer research. 1998;58(2):268-75. Epub 1998/01/27.

[73] Schuetz EG, Beck WT, Schuetz JD. Modulators and substrates of P-glycoprotein and cytochrome P4503A coordinately up-regulate these proteins in human colon carcinoma cells. Molecular pharmacology. 1996;49(2):311-8. Epub 1996/02/01.

[74] Lowe SW, Ruley HE, Jacks T, Housman DE. p53-dependent apoptosis modulates the cytotoxicity of anticancer agents. Cell. 1993;74(6):957-67. Epub 1993/09/24.

[75] Liu YY, Han TY, Giuliano AE, Cabot MC. Ceramide glycosylation potentiates cellular multidrug resistance. FASEB journal : official publication of the Federation of American Societies for Experimental Biology. 2001;15(3):719-30. Epub 2001/03/22.

[76] Matsumura Y, Ananthaswamy HN. Molecular mechanisms of photocarcinogenesis. Frontiers in bioscience : a journal and virtual library. 2002;7:d765-83. Epub 2002/03/19.

[77] Zhai S, Yaar M, Doyle SM, Gilchrest BA. Nerve growth factor rescues pigment cells from ultraviolet-induced apoptosis by upregulating BCL-2 levels. Experimental cell research. 1996;224(2):335-43. Epub 1996/05/01.

[78] Kawaguchi Y, Mori N, Nakayama A. Kit(+) melanocytes seem to contribute to melanocyte proliferation after UV exposure as precursor cells. The Journal of investigative dermatology. 2001;116(6):920-5. Epub 2001/06/16.

[79] Leiter U, Schmid RM, Kaskel P, Peter RU, Krahn G. Antiapoptotic bcl-2 and bcl-xL in advanced malignant melanoma. Archives of dermatological research. 2000;292(5): 225-32. Epub 2000/06/27.

[80] Tron VA, Krajewski S, Klein-Parker H, Li G, Ho VC, Reed JC. Immunohistochemical analysis of Bcl-2 protein regulation in cutaneous melanoma. The American journal of pathology. 1995;146(3):643-50. Epub 1995/03/01.

[81] Dallaglio K, Marconi A, Pincelli C. Survivin: a dual player in healthy and diseased skin. The Journal of investigative dermatology. 2012;132(1):18-27. Epub 2011/09/09.

[82] Oberoi-Khanuja TK, Karreman C, Larisch S, Rapp UR, Rajalingam K. Role of melanoma inhibitor of apoptosis (ML-IAP), a member of baculoviral IAP repeat (BIR) domain family in the regulation of C-RAF kinase and cell migration. The Journal of biological chemistry. 2012. Epub 2012/06/20.

[83] Pennati M, Colella G, Folini M, Citti L, Daidone MG, Zaffaroni N. Ribozyme-mediated attenuation of survivin expression sensitizes human melanoma cells to cisplatin-

induced apoptosis. The Journal of clinical investigation. 2002;109(2):285-6. Epub 2002/01/24.

[84] Mesri M, Wall NR, Li J, Kim RW, Altieri DC. Cancer gene therapy using a survivin mutant adenovirus. The Journal of clinical investigation. 2001;108(7):981-90. Epub 2001/10/03.

[85] Vucic D, Stennicke HR, Pisabarro MT, Salvesen GS, Dixit VM. ML-IAP, a novel inhibitor of apoptosis that is preferentially expressed in human melanomas. Current biology : CB. 2000;10(21):1359-66. Epub 2000/11/21.

[86] Vucic D, Deshayes K, Ackerly H, Pisabarro MT, Kadkhodayan S, Fairbrother WJ, et al. SMAC negatively regulates the anti-apoptotic activity of melanoma inhibitor of apoptosis (ML-IAP). The Journal of biological chemistry. 2002;277(14):12275-9. Epub 2002/01/22.

[87] Kasof GM, Gomes BC. Livin, a novel inhibitor of apoptosis protein family member. The Journal of biological chemistry. 2001;276(5):3238-46. Epub 2000/10/12.

[88] Vousden KH, Prives C. Blinded by the Light: The Growing Complexity of p53. Cell. 2009;137(3):413-31. Epub 2009/05/05.

[89] Donehower LA, Lozano G. 20 years studying p53 functions in genetically engineered mice. Nature reviews Cancer. 2009;9(11):831-41. Epub 2009/09/25.

[90] Perlis C, Herlyn M. Recent advances in melanoma biology. The oncologist. 2004;9(2): 182-7. Epub 2004/03/30.

[91] Chin L, Pomerantz J, Polsky D, Jacobson M, Cohen C, Cordon-Cardo C, et al. Cooperative effects of INK4a and ras in melanoma susceptibility in vivo. Genes & development. 1997;11(21):2822-34. Epub 1997/11/14.

[92] Satyamoorthy K, Chehab NH, Waterman MJ, Lien MC, El-Deiry WS, Herlyn M, et al. Aberrant regulation and function of wild-type p53 in radioresistant melanoma cells. Cell growth & differentiation : the molecular biology journal of the American Association for Cancer Research. 2000;11(9):467-74. Epub 2000/09/28.

[93] Schmitt CA, Fridman JS, Yang M, Baranov E, Hoffman RM, Lowe SW. Dissecting p53 tumor suppressor functions in vivo. Cancer cell. 2002;1(3):289-98. Epub 2002/06/28.

[94] Soengas MS, Alarcon RM, Yoshida H, Giaccia AJ, Hakem R, Mak TW, et al. Apaf-1 and caspase-9 in p53-dependent apoptosis and tumor inhibition. Science. 1999;284(5411):156-9. Epub 1999/04/02.

[95] Soengas MS, Capodieci P, Polsky D, Mora J, Esteller M, Opitz-Araya X, et al. Inactivation of the apoptosis effector Apaf-1 in malignant melanoma. Nature. 2001;409(6817):207-11. Epub 2001/02/24.

[96] Furukawa Y, Nishimura N, Furukawa Y, Satoh M, Endo H, Iwase S, et al. Apaf-1 is a mediator of E2F-1-induced apoptosis. The Journal of biological chemistry. 2002;277(42):39760-8. Epub 2002/08/01.

[97]   Toledo F, Wahl GM. Regulating the p53 pathway: in vitro hypotheses, in vivo veritas. Nature reviews Cancer. 2006;6(12):909-23. Epub 2006/11/28.

[98]   Wang X. p53 regulation: teamwork between RING domains of Mdm2 and MdmX. Cell Cycle. 2011;10(24):4225-9. Epub 2011/12/03.

[99]   Castresana JS, Rubio MP, Vazquez JJ, Idoate M, Sober AJ, Seizinger BR, et al. Lack of allelic deletion and point mutation as mechanisms of p53 activation in human malignant melanoma. International journal of cancer Journal international du cancer. 1993;55(4):562-5. Epub 1993/10/21.

[100] Albino AP, Vidal MJ, McNutt NS, Shea CR, Prieto VG, Nanus DM, et al. Mutation and expression of the p53 gene in human malignant melanoma. Melanoma research. 1994;4(1):35-45. Epub 1994/02/01.

[101] Hocker T, Tsao H. Ultraviolet radiation and melanoma: a systematic review and analysis of reported sequence variants. Human mutation. 2007;28(6):578-88. Epub 2007/02/14.

[102] Muthusamy V, Hobbs C, Nogueira C, Cordon-Cardo C, McKee PH, Chin L, et al. Amplification of CDK4 and MDM2 in malignant melanoma. Genes, chromosomes & cancer. 2006;45(5):447-54. Epub 2006/01/19.

[103] Ji Z, Njauw CN, Taylor M, Neel V, Flaherty KT, Tsao H. p53 rescue through HDM2 antagonism suppresses melanoma growth and potentiates MEK inhibition. The Journal of investigative dermatology. 2012;132(2):356-64. Epub 2011/10/14.

[104] Meier F, Busch S, Lasithiotakis K, Kulms D, Garbe C, Maczey E, et al. Combined targeting of MAPK and AKT signalling pathways is a promising strategy for melanoma treatment. The British journal of dermatology. 2007;156(6):1204-13. Epub 2007/03/29.

[105] Lasithiotakis KG, Sinnberg TW, Schittek B, Flaherty KT, Kulms D, Maczey E, et al. Combined inhibition of MAPK and mTOR signaling inhibits growth, induces cell death, and abrogates invasive growth of melanoma cells. The Journal of investigative dermatology. 2008;128(8):2013-23. Epub 2008/03/08.

[106] Smalley KS, Haass NK, Brafford PA, Lioni M, Flaherty KT, Herlyn M. Multiple signaling pathways must be targeted to overcome drug resistance in cell lines derived from melanoma metastases. Molecular cancer therapeutics. 2006;5(5):1136-44. Epub 2006/05/30.

[107] Soengas MS, Lowe SW. Apoptosis and melanoma chemoresistance. Oncogene. 2003;22(20):3138-51. Epub 2003/06/06.

[108] Hersey P, Zhuang L, Zhang XD. Current strategies in overcoming resistance of cancer cells to apoptosis melanoma as a model. International review of cytology. 2006;251:131-58. Epub 2006/08/31.

[109] Birck A, Ahrenkiel V, Zeuthen J, Hou-Jensen K, Guldberg P. Mutation and allelic loss of the PTEN/MMAC1 gene in primary and metastatic melanoma biopsies. The Journal of investigative dermatology. 2000;114(2):277-80. Epub 2000/01/29.

[110] Zhou XP, Gimm O, Hampel H, Niemann T, Walker MJ, Eng C. Epigenetic PTEN silencing in malignant melanomas without PTEN mutation. The American journal of pathology. 2000;157(4):1123-8. Epub 2000/10/06.

[111] Poetsch M, Dittberner T, Woenckhaus C. PTEN/MMAC1 in malignant melanoma and its importance for tumor progression. Cancer genetics and cytogenetics. 2001;125(1):21-6. Epub 2001/04/12.

[112] Whiteman DC, Zhou XP, Cummings MC, Pavey S, Hayward NK, Eng C. Nuclear PTEN expression and clinicopathologic features in a population-based series of primary cutaneous melanoma. International journal of cancer Journal international du cancer. 2002;99(1):63-7. Epub 2002/04/12.

[113] Hwang PH, Yi HK, Kim DS, Nam SY, Kim JS, Lee DY. Suppression of tumorigenicity and metastasis in B16F10 cells by PTEN/MMAC1/TEP1 gene. Cancer letters. 2001;172(1):83-91. Epub 2001/10/12.

[114] Kotelevets L, van Hengel J, Bruyneel E, Mareel M, van Roy F, Chastre E. The lipid phosphatase activity of PTEN is critical for stabilizing intercellular junctions and reverting invasiveness. The Journal of cell biology. 2001;155(7):1129-35. Epub 2002/01/05.

[115] Mayo LD, Dixon JE, Durden DL, Tonks NK, Donner DB. PTEN protects p53 from Mdm2 and sensitizes cancer cells to chemotherapy. The Journal of biological chemistry. 2002;277(7):5484-9. Epub 2001/12/01.

[116] Sinnberg T, Sauer B, Holm P, Spangler B, Kuphal S, Bosserhoff A, et al. MAPK and PI3K/AKT mediated YB-1 activation promotes melanoma cell proliferation which is counteracted by an autoregulatory loop. Experimental dermatology. 2012;21(4): 265-70. Epub 2012/03/16.

[117] Astanehe A, Finkbeiner MR, Hojabrpour P, To K, Fotovati A, Shadeo A, et al. The transcriptional induction of PIK3CA in tumor cells is dependent on the oncoprotein Y-box binding protein-1. Oncogene. 2009;28(25):2406-18. Epub 2009/05/12.

[118] Meyskens FL, Jr., Buckmeier JA, McNulty SE, Tohidian NB. Activation of nuclear factor-kappa B in human metastatic melanomacells and the effect of oxidative stress. Clinical cancer research : an official journal of the American Association for Cancer Research. 1999;5(5):1197-202. Epub 1999/06/03.

[119] McNulty SE, Tohidian NB, Meyskens FL, Jr. RelA, p50 and inhibitor of kappa B alpha are elevated in human metastatic melanoma cells and respond aberrantly to ultraviolet light B. Pigment cell research / sponsored by the European Society for Pigment Cell Research and the International Pigment Cell Society. 2001;14(6):456-65. Epub 2002/01/05.

[120] Yang J, Richmond A. Constitutive IkappaB kinase activity correlates with nuclear factor-kappaB activation in human melanoma cells. Cancer research. 2001;61(12): 4901-9. Epub 2001/06/19.

[121] Dhawan P, Richmond A. A novel NF-kappa B-inducing kinase-MAPK signaling pathway up-regulates NF-kappa B activity in melanoma cells. The Journal of biological chemistry. 2002;277(10):7920-8. Epub 2002/01/05.

[122] Baldwin AS. Control of oncogenesis and cancer therapy resistance by the transcription factor NF-kappaB. The Journal of clinical investigation. 2001;107(3):241-6. Epub 2001/02/13.

[123] McNulty SE, del Rosario R, Cen D, Meyskens FL, Jr., Yang S. Comparative expression of NFkappaB proteins in melanocytes of normal skin vs. benign intradermal naevus and human metastatic melanoma biopsies. Pigment cell research / sponsored by the European Society for Pigment Cell Research and the International Pigment Cell Society. 2004;17(2):173-80. Epub 2004/03/16.

[124] Shattuck-Brandt RL, Richmond A. Enhanced degradation of I-kappaB alpha contributes to endogenous activation of NF-kappaB in Hs294T melanoma cells. Cancer research. 1997;57(14):3032-9. Epub 1997/07/15.

[125] Das R, Philip S, Mahabeleshwar GH, Bulbule A, Kundu GC. Osteopontin: it's role in regulation of cell motility and nuclear factor kappa B-mediated urokinase type plasminogen activator expression. IUBMB life. 2005;57(6):441-7. Epub 2005/07/14.

[126] Liu J, Suresh Kumar KG, Yu D, Molton SA, McMahon M, Herlyn M, et al. Oncogenic BRAF regulates beta-Trcp expression and NF-kappaB activity in human melanoma cells. Oncogene. 2007;26(13):1954-8. Epub 2006/09/27.

[127] Malumbres M, Pellicer A. RAS pathways to cell cycle control and cell transformation. Frontiers in bioscience : a journal and virtual library. 1998;3:d887-912. Epub 1998/08/11.

[128] Borner C, Schlagbauer Wadl H, Fellay I, Selzer E, Polterauer P, Jansen B. Mutated N-ras upregulates Bcl-2 in human melanoma in vitro and in SCID mice. Melanoma research. 1999;9(4):347-50. Epub 1999/09/30.

[129] Chin L, Merlino G, DePinho RA. Malignant melanoma: modern black plague and genetic black box. Genes & development. 1998;12(22):3467-81. Epub 1998/12/01.

[130] Davies H, Bignell GR, Cox C, Stephens P, Edkins S, Clegg S, et al. Mutations of the BRAF gene in human cancer. Nature. 2002;417(6892):949-54. Epub 2002/06/18.

[131] Erhardt P, Schremser EJ, Cooper GM. B-Raf inhibits programmed cell death downstream of cytochrome c release from mitochondria by activating the MEK/Erk pathway. Molecular and cellular biology. 1999;19(8):5308-15. Epub 1999/07/20.

[132] Wan PT, Garnett MJ, Roe SM, Lee S, Niculescu-Duvaz D, Good VM, et al. Mechanism of activation of the RAF-ERK signaling pathway by oncogenic mutations of B-RAF. Cell. 2004;116(6):855-67. Epub 2004/03/24.

[133] Smalley KS. Understanding melanoma signaling networks as the basis for molecular targeted therapy. The Journal of investigative dermatology. 2010;130(1):28-37. Epub 2009/07/03.

[134] Pollock PM, Harper UL, Hansen KS, Yudt LM, Stark M, Robbins CM, et al. High frequency of BRAF mutations in nevi. Nature genetics. 2003;33(1):19-20. Epub 2002/11/26.

[135] Michaloglou C, Vredeveld LC, Soengas MS, Denoyelle C, Kuilman T, van der Horst CM, et al. BRAFE600-associated senescence-like cell cycle arrest of human naevi. Nature. 2005;436(7051):720-4. Epub 2005/08/05.

[136] Lage H, Christmann M, Kern MA, Dietel M, Pick M, Kaina B, et al. Expression of DNA repair proteins hMSH2, hMSH6, hMLH1, O6-methylguanine-DNA methyltransferase and N-methylpurine-DNA glycosylase in melanoma cells with acquired drug resistance. International journal of cancer Journal international du cancer. 1999;80(5):744-50. Epub 1999/02/27.

[137] Ma S, Egyhazi S, Ringborg U, Hansson J. Immunohistochemical analysis of DNA mismatch repair protein and O6-methylguanine-DNA methyltransferase in melanoma metastases in relation to clinical response to DTIC-based chemotherapy. Oncology reports. 2002;9(5):1015-9. Epub 2002/08/09.

[138] Ma S, Egyhazi S, Martenhed G, Ringborg U, Hansson J. Analysis of O(6)-methylguanine-DNA methyltransferase in melanoma tumours in patients treated with dacarbazine-based chemotherapy. Melanoma research. 2002;12(4):335-42. Epub 2002/08/10.

[139] Li W, Melton DW. Cisplatin regulates the MAPK kinase pathway to induce increased expression of DNA repair gene ERCC1 and increase melanoma chemoresistance. Oncogene. 2012;31(19):2412-22. Epub 2011/10/15.

[140] Chen KG, Valencia JC, Gillet JP, Hearing VJ, Gottesman MM. Involvement of ABC transporters in melanogenesis and the development of multidrug resistance of melanoma. Pigment cell & melanoma research. 2009;22(6):740-9. Epub 2009/09/04.

[141] Depeille P, Cuq P, Mary S, Passagne I, Evrard A, Cupissol D, et al. Glutathione S-transferase M1 and multidrug resistance protein 1 act in synergy to protect melanoma cells from vincristine effects. Molecular pharmacology. 2004;65(4):897-905. Epub 2004/03/27.

[142] Ortega A, Benlloch M, Ferrer P, Segarra R, Asensi M, Obrador E, Estrela JM. GSH depletion in B16 melanoma cells: MRP 1-channeled drug extrusion, Bcl-2 antisense therapy and inhibition of {gamma}-glutamyltranspeptidase. AACR Meeting Abstracts 2004 2004: 122.

[143] Frank NY, Margaryan A, Huang Y, Schatton T, Waaga-Gasser AM, Gasser M, et al. ABCB5-mediated doxorubicin transport and chemoresistance in human malignant melanoma. Cancer research. 2005;65(10):4320-33. Epub 2005/05/19.

[144] Elliott AM, Al-Hajj MA. ABCB8 mediates doxorubicin resistance in melanoma cells by protecting the mitochondrial genome. Molecular cancer research : MCR. 2009;7(1): 79-87. Epub 2009/01/17.

[145] Frank NY, Pendse SS, Lapchak PH, Margaryan A, Shlain D, Doeing C, et al. Regulation of progenitor cell fusion by ABCB5 P-glycoprotein, a novel human ATP-binding cassette transporter. The Journal of biological chemistry. 2003;278(47):47156-65. Epub 2003/09/10.

[146] Chen KG, Szakacs G, Annereau JP, Rouzaud F, Liang XJ, Valencia JC, et al. Principal expression of two mRNA isoforms (ABCB 5alpha and ABCB 5beta) of the ATP-binding cassette transporter gene ABCB 5 in melanoma cells and melanocytes. Pigment cell research / sponsored by the European Society for Pigment Cell Research and the International Pigment Cell Society. 2005;18(2):102-12. Epub 2005/03/12.

[147] Huang Y, Anderle P, Bussey KJ, Barbacioru C, Shankavaram U, Dai Z, et al. Membrane transporters and channels: role of the transportome in cancer chemosensitivity and chemoresistance. Cancer research. 2004;64(12):4294-301. Epub 2004/06/19.

[148] Szakacs G, Annereau JP, Lababidi S, Shankavaram U, Arciello A, Bussey KJ, et al. Predicting drug sensitivity and resistance: profiling ABC transporter genes in cancer cells. Cancer cell. 2004;6(2):129-37. Epub 2004/08/25.

[149] Schatton T, Murphy GF, Frank NY, Yamaura K, Waaga-Gasser AM, Gasser M, et al. Identification of cells initiating human melanomas. Nature. 2008;451(7176):345-9. Epub 2008/01/19.

[150] Keshet GI, Goldstein I, Itzhaki O, Cesarkas K, Shenhav L, Yakirevitch A, et al. MDR1 expression identifies human melanoma stem cells. Biochemical and biophysical research communications. 2008;368(4):930-6. Epub 2008/02/19.

[151] Halliwell B. Oxidative stress and cancer: have we moved forward? The Biochemical journal. 2007;401(1):1-11. Epub 2006/12/08.

[152] Rasheed MH, Beevi SS, Geetha A. Enhanced lipid peroxidation and nitric oxide products with deranged antioxidant status in patients with head and neck squamous cell carcinoma. Oral Oncol. 2007;43(4):333-8. Epub 2006/07/22.

[153] Kumar B, Koul S, Khandrika L, Meacham RB, Koul HK. Oxidative stress is inherent in prostate cancer cells and is required for aggressive phenotype. Cancer research. 2008;68(6):1777-85. Epub 2008/03/15.

[154] Martin KR, Barrett JC. Reactive oxygen species as double-edged swords in cellular processes: low-dose cell signaling versus high-dose toxicity. Hum Exp Toxicol. 2002;21(2):71-5. Epub 2002/07/10.

[155] McCord JM. Superoxide radical: controversies, contradictions, and paradoxes. Proc Soc Exp Biol Med. 1995;209(2):112-7. Epub 1995/06/01.

[156] Lau A, Villeneuve NF, Sun Z, Wong PK, Zhang DD. Dual roles of Nrf2 in cancer. Pharmacological research : the official journal of the Italian Pharmacological Society. 2008;58(5-6):262-70. Epub 2008/10/08.

[157] Yanagawa T, Ishikawa T, Ishii T, Tabuchi K, Iwasa S, Bannai S, et al. Peroxiredoxin I expression in human thyroid tumors. Cancer letters. 1999;145(1-2):127-32. Epub 1999/10/26.

[158] Lee KW, Lee HJ. Biphasic effects of dietary antioxidants on oxidative stress-mediated carcinogenesis. Mech Ageing Dev. 2006;127(5):424-31. Epub 2006/03/08.

[159] Fruehauf JP, Meyskens FL, Jr. Reactive oxygen species: a breath of life or death? Clinical cancer research : an official journal of the American Association for Cancer Research. 2007;13(3):789-94. Epub 2007/02/10.

[160] Valko M, Rhodes CJ, Moncol J, Izakovic M, Mazur M. Free radicals, metals and antioxidants in oxidative stress-induced cancer. Chemico-biological interactions. 2006;160(1):1-40. Epub 2006/01/25.

[161] Campos AC, Molognoni F, Melo FH, Galdieri LC, Carneiro CR, D'Almeida V, et al. Oxidative stress modulates DNA methylation during melanocyte anchorage blockade associated with malignant transformation. Neoplasia. 2007;9(12):1111-21. Epub 2007/12/18.

[162] Donkena KV, Young CY, Tindall DJ. Oxidative stress and DNA methylation in prostate cancer. Obstet Gynecol Int. 2010;2010:302051. Epub 2010/07/31.

[163] Ziech D, Franco R, Pappa A, Malamou-Mitsi V, Georgakila S, Georgakilas AG, et al. The role of epigenetics in environmental and occupational carcinogenesis. Chemico-biological interactions. 2010;188(2):340-9. Epub 2010/07/06.

[164] Weitzman SA, Turk PW, Milkowski DH, Kozlowski K. Free radical adducts induce alterations in DNA cytosine methylation. Proceedings of the National Academy of Sciences of the United States of America. 1994;91(4):1261-4. Epub 1994/02/15.

[165] Turk PW, Laayoun A, Smith SS, Weitzman SA. DNA adduct 8-hydroxyl-2'-deoxyguanosine (8-hydroxyguanine) affects function of human DNA methyltransferase. Carcinogenesis. 1995;16(5):1253-5. Epub 1995/05/01.

[166] Turk PW, Weitzman SA. Free radical DNA adduct 8-OH-deoxyguanosine affects activity of Hpa II and Msp I restriction endonucleases. Free radical research. 1995;23(3): 255-8. Epub 1995/09/01.

[167] Christman JK, Sheikhnejad G, Marasco CJ, Sufrin JR. 5-Methyl-2'-deoxycytidine in single-stranded DNA can act in cis to signal de novo DNA methylation. Proceedings of the National Academy of Sciences of the United States of America. 1995;92(16): 7347-51. Epub 1995/08/01.

[168] Franco R, Schoneveld O, Georgakilas AG, Panayiotidis MI. Oxidative stress, DNA methylation and carcinogenesis. Cancer letters. 2008;266(1):6-11. Epub 2008/03/29.

[169] Sander CS, Hamm F, Elsner P, Thiele JJ. Oxidative stress in malignant melanoma and non-melanoma skin cancer. The British journal of dermatology. 2003;148(5):913-22. Epub 2003/06/06.

[170] Gidanian S, Mentelle M, Meyskens FL, Jr., Farmer PJ. Melanosomal damage in normal human melanocytes induced by UVB and metal uptake--a basis for the pro-oxidant state of melanoma. Photochemistry and photobiology. 2008;84(3):556-64. Epub 2008/03/12.

[171] Meyskens FL, Jr., McNulty SE, Buckmeier JA, Tohidian NB, Spillane TJ, Kahlon RS, et al. Aberrant redox regulation in human metastatic melanoma cells compared to normal melanocytes. Free radical biology & medicine. 2001;31(6):799-808. Epub 2001/09/15.

[172] Meyskens FL, Jr., Farmer P, Fruehauf JP. Redox regulation in human melanocytes and melanoma. Pigment cell research / sponsored by the European Society for Pigment Cell Research and the International Pigment Cell Society. 2001;14(3):148-54. Epub 2001/07/04.

[173] Meyskens FL, Jr., Berwick M. UV or not UV: metals are the answer. Cancer epidemiology, biomarkers & prevention : a publication of the American Association for Cancer Research, cosponsored by the American Society of Preventive Oncology. 2008;17(2):268-70. Epub 2008/02/13.

[174] Cooke MS, Evans MD, Dizdaroglu M, Lunec J. Oxidative DNA damage: mechanisms, mutation, and disease. FASEB journal : official publication of the Federation of American Societies for Experimental Biology. 2003;17(10):1195-214. Epub 2003/07/02.

[175] Pavel S, van Nieuwpoort F, van der Meulen H, Out C, Pizinger K, Cetkovska P, et al. Disturbed melanin synthesis and chronic oxidative stress in dysplastic naevi. Eur J Cancer. 2004;40(9):1423-30. Epub 2004/06/05.

[176] Smit NP, van Nieuwpoort FA, Marrot L, Out C, Poorthuis B, van Pelt H, et al. Increased melanogenesis is a risk factor for oxidative DNA damage--study on cultured melanocytes and atypical nevus cells. Photochemistry and photobiology. 2008;84(3): 550-5. Epub 2008/04/26.

[177] Leikam C, Hufnagel A, Schartl M, Meierjohann S. Oncogene activation in melanocytes links reactive oxygen to multinucleated phenotype and senescence. Oncogene. 2008;27(56):7070-82. Epub 2008/09/23.

[178] Gaudiano G, Koch TH. Redox chemistry of anthracycline antitumor drugs and use of captodative radicals as tools for its elucidation and control. Chemical research in toxicology. 1991;4(1):2-16. Epub 1991/01/01.

[179] Sengupta SK, Kelly C, Sehgal RK. "Reverse" and "symmetrical" analogues of actino-mycin D: metabolic activation and in vitro and in vivo tumor growth inhibitory ac-tivities. Journal of medicinal chemistry. 1985;28(5):620-8. Epub 1985/05/01.

[180] Roller A, Weller M. Antioxidants specifically inhibit cisplatin cytotoxicity of human malignant glioma cells. Anticancer research. 1998;18(6A):4493-7. Epub 1999/01/19.

[181] Thrall BD, Raha GA, Springer DL, Meadows GG. Differential sensitivities of murine melanocytes and melanoma cells to buthionine sulfoximine and anticancer drugs. Pigment cell research / sponsored by the European Society for Pigment Cell Research and the International Pigment Cell Society. 1991;4(5-6):234-9. Epub 1991/12/01.

[182] Iacobini M, Menichelli A, Palumbo G, Multari G, Werner B, Del Principe D. Involve-ment of oxygen radicals in cytarabine-induced apoptosis in human polymorphonu-clear cells. Biochemical pharmacology. 2001;61(8):1033-40. Epub 2001/04/05.

[183] Sakhi AK, Russnes KM, Thoresen M, Bastani NE, Karlsen A, Smeland S, et al. Pre-radiotherapy plasma carotenoids and markers of oxidative stress are associated with survival in head and neck squamous cell carcinoma patients: a prospective study. BMC Cancer. 2009;9:458. Epub 2009/12/23.

[184] Sabitha KE, Shyamaladevi CS. Oxidant and antioxidant activity changes in patients with oral cancer and treated with radiotherapy. Oral Oncol. 1999;35(3):273-7. Epub 2000/01/06.

[185] Kasapovic J, Pejic S, Stojiljkovic V, Todorovic A, Radosevic-Jelic L, Saicic ZS, et al. Antioxidant status and lipid peroxidation in the blood of breast cancer patients of different ages after chemotherapy with 5-fluorouracil, doxorubicin and cyclophos-phamide. Clin Biochem. 2010;43(16-17):1287-93. Epub 2010/08/18.

[186] Gupta A, Bhatt ML, Misra MK. Assessment of free radical-mediated damage in head and neck squamous cell carcinoma patients and after treatment with radiotherapy. Indian J Biochem Biophys. 2010;47(2):96-9. Epub 2010/06/05.

[187] Kim SK, Yang JW, Kim MR, Roh SH, Kim HG, Lee KY, et al. Increased expression of Nrf2/ARE-dependent anti-oxidant proteins in tamoxifen-resistant breast cancer cells. Free radical biology & medicine. 2008;45(4):537-46. Epub 2008/06/10.

[188] Osburn WO, Kensler TW. Nrf2 signaling: an adaptive response pathway for protec-tion against environmental toxic insults. Mutat Res. 2008;659(1-2):31-9. Epub 2008/01/01.

[189] Kim YJ, Ahn JY, Liang P, Ip C, Zhang Y, Park YM. Human prx1 gene is a target of Nrf2 and is up-regulated by hypoxia/reoxygenation: implication to tumor biology. Cancer research. 2007;67(2):546-54. Epub 2007/01/20.

[190] Maher JM, Dieter MZ, Aleksunes LM, Slitt AL, Guo G, Tanaka Y, et al. Oxidative and electrophilic stress induces multidrug resistance-associated protein transporters via the nuclear factor-E2-related factor-2 transcriptional pathway. Hepatology. 2007;46(5):1597-610. Epub 2007/08/03.

[191] Chan JY, Kwong M. Impaired expression of glutathione synthetic enzyme genes in
       mice with targeted deletion of the Nrf2 basic-leucine zipper protein. Biochimica et bi-
       ophysica acta. 2000;1517(1):19-26. Epub 2000/12/19.

[192] Xu Z, Chen L, Leung L, Yen TS, Lee C, Chan JY. Liver-specific inactivation of the
       Nrf1 gene in adult mouse leads to nonalcoholic steatohepatitis and hepatic neoplasia.
       Proceedings of the National Academy of Sciences of the United States of America.
       2005;102(11):4120-5. Epub 2005/03/02.

[193] Chen L, Kwong M, Lu R, Ginzinger D, Lee C, Leung L, et al. Nrf1 is critical for redox
       balance and survival of liver cells during development. Molecular and cellular biolo-
       gy. 2003;23(13):4673-86. Epub 2003/06/17.

[194] Ohtsuji M, Katsuoka F, Kobayashi A, Aburatani H, Hayes JD, Yamamoto M. Nrf1
       and Nrf2 play distinct roles in activation of antioxidant response element-dependent
       genes. The Journal of biological chemistry. 2008;283(48):33554-62. Epub 2008/10/02.

[195] Khandrika L, Kumar B, Koul S, Maroni P, Koul HK. Oxidative stress in prostate can-
       cer. Cancer letters. 2009;282(2):125-36. Epub 2009/02/03.

[196] Frohlich DA, McCabe MT, Arnold RS, Day ML. The role of Nrf2 in increased reactive
       oxygen species and DNA damage in prostate tumorigenesis. Oncogene. 2008;27(31):
       4353-62. Epub 2008/04/01.

[197] Kaspar JW, Niture SK, Jaiswal AK. Nrf2:INrf2 (Keap1) signaling in oxidative stress.
       Free radical biology & medicine. 2009;47(9):1304-9. Epub 2009/08/12.

[198] Wang XJ, Sun Z, Villeneuve NF, Zhang S, Zhao F, Li Y, et al. Nrf2 enhances resist-
       ance of cancer cells to chemotherapeutic drugs, the dark side of Nrf2. Carcinogenesis.
       2008;29(6):1235-43. Epub 2008/04/17.

[199] Padmanabhan B, Tong KI, Ohta T, Nakamura Y, Scharlock M, Ohtsuji M, et al. Struc-
       tural basis for defects of Keap1 activity provoked by its point mutations in lung can-
       cer. Molecular cell. 2006;21(5):689-700. Epub 2006/03/02.

[200] Singh A, Misra V, Thimmulappa RK, Lee H, Ames S, Hoque MO, et al. Dysfunctional
       KEAP1-NRF2 interaction in non-small-cell lung cancer. PLoS medicine.
       2006;3(10):e420. Epub 2006/10/06.

[201] Ohta T, Iijima K, Miyamoto M, Nakahara I, Tanaka H, Ohtsuji M, et al. Loss of Keap1
       function activates Nrf2 and provides advantages for lung cancer cell growth. Cancer
       research. 2008;68(5):1303-9. Epub 2008/03/05.

[202] Nioi P, Nguyen T. A mutation of Keap1 found in breast cancer impairs its ability to
       repress Nrf2 activity. Biochemical and biophysical research communications.
       2007;362(4):816-21. Epub 2007/09/08.

[203] Shibata T, Kokubu A, Gotoh M, Ojima H, Ohta T, Yamamoto M, et al. Genetic altera-
       tion of Keap1 confers constitutive Nrf2 activation and resistance to chemotherapy in
       gallbladder cancer. Gastroenterology. 2008;135(4):1358-68, 68 e1-4. Epub 2008/08/12.

[204] Matundan HH, Dellinger RW, Jr. FLM. Nrf2 Mediates Chemoresistance in Melanoma. Free Radical Biology and Medicine. 1 November 2011.;51:S126.

[205] Takatori T, Ogura M, Tsuruo T. Purification and characterization of NF-R2 that regulates the expression of the human multidrug resistance (MDR1) gene. Jpn J Cancer Res. 1993;84(3):298-303. Epub 1993/03/01.

[206] Hayashi A, Suzuki H, Itoh K, Yamamoto M, Sugiyama Y. Transcription factor Nrf2 is required for the constitutive and inducible expression of multidrug resistance-associated protein 1 in mouse embryo fibroblasts. Biochemical and biophysical research communications. 2003;310(3):824-9. Epub 2003/10/11.

[207] You A, Nam CW, Wakabayashi N, Yamamoto M, Kensler TW, Kwak MK. Transcription factor Nrf2 maintains the basal expression of Mdm2: An implication of the regulation of p53 signaling by Nrf2. Archives of biochemistry and biophysics. 2011;507(2): 356-64. Epub 2011/01/08.

[208] Hayes JD, Ashford ML. Nrf2 orchestrates fuel partitioning for cell proliferation. Cell metabolism. 2012;16(2):139-41. Epub 2012/08/14.

[209] So HS, Kim HJ, Lee JH, Lee JH, Park SY, Park C, et al. Flunarizine induces Nrf2-mediated transcriptional activation of heme oxygenase-1 in protection of auditory cells from cisplatin. Cell death and differentiation. 2006;13(10):1763-75. Epub 2006/02/18.

[210] Beyer TA, Xu W, Teupser D, auf dem Keller U, Bugnon P, Hildt E, et al. Impaired liver regeneration in Nrf2 knockout mice: role of ROS-mediated insulin/IGF-1 resistance. The EMBO journal. 2008;27(1):212-23. Epub 2007/12/07.

[211] Mitsuishi Y, Taguchi K, Kawatani Y, Shibata T, Nukiwa T, Aburatani H, et al. Nrf2 redirects glucose and glutamine into anabolic pathways in metabolic reprogramming. Cancer cell. 2012;22(1):66-79. Epub 2012/07/14.

[212] Sun Z, Huang Z, Zhang DD. Phosphorylation of Nrf2 at multiple sites by MAP kinases has a limited contribution in modulating the Nrf2-dependent antioxidant response. PloS one. 2009;4(8):e6588. Epub 2009/08/12.

[213] Niture SK, Jaiswal AK. INrf2 (Keap1) targets Bcl-2 degradation and controls cellular apoptosis. Cell death and differentiation. 2011;18(3):439-51. Epub 2010/09/25.

[214] Niture SK, Jaiswal AK. Nrf2 protein up-regulates antiapoptotic protein Bcl-2 and prevents cellular apoptosis. The Journal of biological chemistry. 2012;287(13):9873-86. Epub 2012/01/26.

Chapter 8

Sentinel Lymph Node Biopsy for Melanoma and Surgical Approach to Lymph Node Metastasis

Yasuhiro Nakamura and Fujio Otsuka

Additional information is available at the end of the chapter

1. Introduction

The surgical approach to cutaneous melanoma patients with clinically uninvolved regional lymph nodes has been controversial. Although most patients with melanoma have no clinically palpable nodal disease at the time of presentation, some patients whose primary tumor increases in thickness, has ulceration, and shows a high mitotic rate histologically harbor clinically undetectable regional lymph node metastasis[1].

While some authors have advocated wide excision of the primary tumor with elective lymph node dissection (ELND), others had recommended excision of the primary site alone and therapeutic lymph node dissection (TLND) only when clinical nodal disease is present. ELND is based on the concept that metastasis arises by passage of the tumor from the primary to the regional lymph nodes and distant sites, in which case early LND will prevent this metastatic progression. In contrast, TLND, which is a "watch and wait" approach, suggests that regional lymph node metastases are markers for disease progression and that hematogenous distant metastases could occur without lymph node metastasis. Four randomized prospective studies comparing ELND with TLND were reported[2-5]. The earlier 2 studies conducted in the 1970s demonstrated no overall survival advantage for ELND[2, 3]. Accordingly, ELND was once contested and largely abandoned. Thereafter, the latter 2 studies conducted in the 1990s suggested the tendency, albeit statistically insignificant, that patients with early regional metastases may benefit from ELND[4, 5]. However, in most melanoma patients with no clinical nodal disease, microscopic nodal disease is absent at presentation. These patients cannot benefit from ELND; if ELND were to be performed, they would suffer from the cost, time, and morbidity of an unnecessary operation.

With respect to this controversy surrounding ELND, the technique of lymphatic mapping and sentinel lymph node biopsy (SLNB) was introduced as a minimally invasive method for detection of microscopic regional lymph node metastases in the early 1990s[6]. Lymphatic mapping is based on the concept that the lymphatic drainage from the skin to the regional lymph node basins runs in an orderly, stepwise fashion. These lymphatic drainage patterns would be the same as the dissemination of melanoma through the lymphatic system and therefore predict the routes of metastatic spread of melanoma cells to the regional lymph nodes (Fig. 1). Morton et al. first reported the details of the SLN technique using intradermal blue dye injection around the primary site and reported that the SLN identification rate was 82% among 237 patients[6], which was considered a high identification rate at that time. In the early 1990s, several authors evaluated this concept by performing synchronous ELND at the time of SLNB[7-9]. A "false-negative" SLN was defined as microscopic metastasis in a non-SLN despite the SLN showing no metastasis. These studies indicated that 5.8% of patients had a false-negative SLN. In addition, Gershenwald et al. reported that only 4.1% (10/243) of patients with a histologically negative SLN developed a nodal recurrence in the previously mapped basin during a follow-up period of over 3 years[10]. This low false-negative rate supported the SLN concept described above.

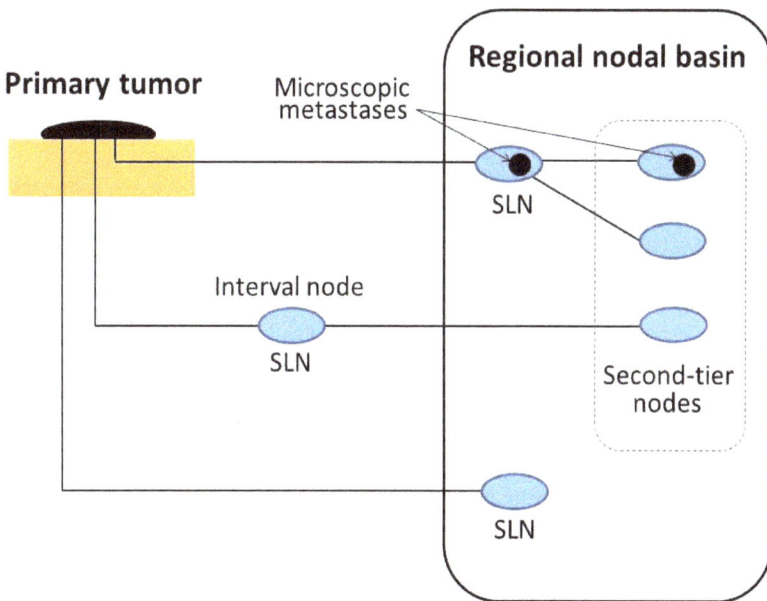

Figure 1. Lymphatic drainage from a primary tumor to sentinel lymph nodes. A sentinel node is sometimes located between the primary tumor and the regional nodal basins, in which case it is called an interval (unusual, in-transit, ectopic) node. If the SLN has microscopic nodal metastasis, some of the second-tier nodes may also have metastasis.

2. Technical advances in SLNB

Although the initial SLN identification rate using blue dye injections alone was approximately 82%[6], the advent of lymphoscintigraphy and the intraoperative hand-held gamma probe drastically improved the SLN identification rate. Studies comparing blue dye injection alone with combined techniques using blue dye, lymphoscintigraphy, and an intraoperative hand-held gamma probe showed a significant increase in SLN identification of up to 99% with the combined techniques[11, 12], which has come to be recognized as the standard technique of SLNB (Fig. 2). This combined technique also enables the surgeon to identify the interval (unusual, in-transit, ectopic) nodes located outside the named regional nodal basins (Fig. 3)[13-17]. The rate of interval SLN identification is reported to be approximately 5% to 10%, and the rate of microscopic metastasis in the interval nodes is approximately the same as that in the SLN in the regional nodal basins[14].

However, SLNB in the head and neck has particular problems because the lymphatic drainage in the head and neck is much more complex than those in the axillary and inguinal regions. Furthermore, the cervical and parotid lymph nodes are smaller and located in sites that are not easily accessible, for example in the parotid gland, through which the facial nerve passes [18, 19]. In addition, it is sometimes difficult to detect the lymphatic drainage and SLN with lymphoscintigraphy because the SLN is often close to the highly radioactive site where the tracer was injected, the so-called shine-through phenomenon[18, 19]. In addition, in some cases the naked eye cannot confirm that an SLN has been dyed blue even after injection of the blue dye because of the short staining period for blue dye in cervical SLNs resulting from the rapid and complex cervical lymphatic flow[19]. In our experience too, over half of the SLNs did not show any blue staining. Furthermore, some authors reported a high false-negative rate of up to 44%, which leads to increased morbidity[20-22]. This high rate may be caused by partially obstructed lymphatic vessels that do not allow for smooth flow of nanocolloids with a size of 6 to 12 nm[23]. Although several authors have reported a high identification rate in SLNB for head and neck melanoma[24-26], the identification rate of SLNs for the standard technique in the cervical region is generally less than that in the inguinal or axillary regions. In the MSLT-I trial reported by Morton et al., the SLN identification rate in the cervical region (84.5%) was clearly lower than that in the inguinal (99.3%) or axillary regions (96.6%)[18].

Several studies on the SLNB technique using indocyanine green (ICG) injection in skin cancer patients have demonstrated high SLN detection and identification rates, although these studies involved mainly axillary and inguinal SLNBs and only a small number of cervical SLNBs[23, 27-29]. ICG is a diagnostic reagent used in various examinations such as examination for cardiac output or hepatic function and retinal angiography. It has a size of only 2.1 nm, binds with albumin, and generates a peak wavelength of 840 nm near-infrared fluorescence when excited with 765-nm light[30]. Using a near-infrared camera intraoperatively, it is possible to observe the ICG as a subcutaneous lymphatic flow as well as SLNs in the fluorescence images after intradermal injection of ICG around the primary tumor. (Fig. 4) In our experience, the mean and median numbers of SLNs per basin were higher in the ICG group than in the standard-technique group. The small size of ICG allows a smooth flow along the lymphatic vessels. It may lead to detection of SLNs not detectable by lymphoscintigraphy (Fig. 4C, D) owing to poor flow of the radioactive tracer and may reduce the false-negative rate. Indeed, Stoffels et al. reported that 2 of 11 additional SLNs that were only identified by the ICG technique showed microscopic metastasis[23].

In addition, the recently introduced hybrid single-photon emission computed tomography with computed tomography (SPECT/CT) can visualize the exact anatomic location of the SLN and second-tier nodes, which would be of great help in identifying the SLN, especially those in the head and neck region[31, 32], as well as the interval nodes.

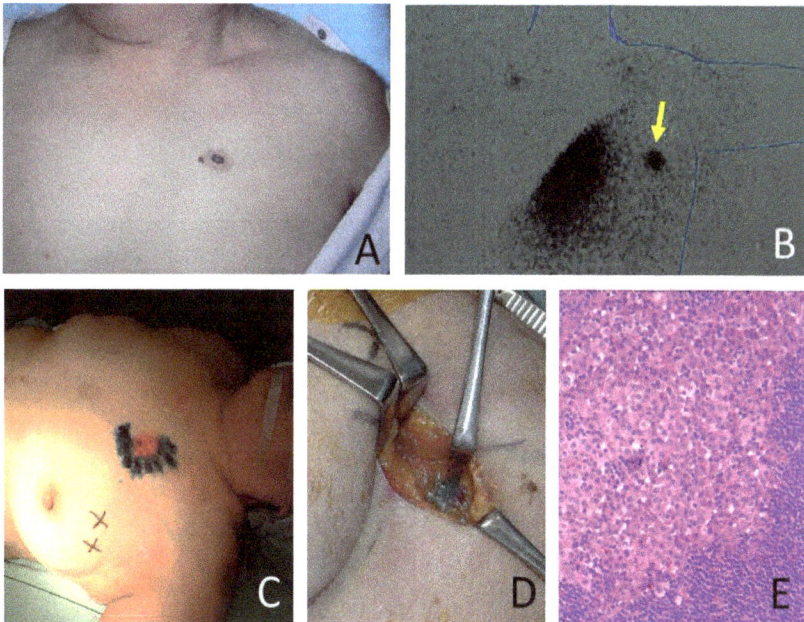

Figure 2. The technique of lymphatic mapping and sentinel lymph node biopsy (SLNB). (A) Primary melanoma on the left chest. (B) Lymphoscintigraphy shows accumulation of 99Tc-tin colloid which was intradermally injected around the primary tumor in the left axilla (arrow). (C) Intradermal injection of 2% isosulfan blue injection around the primary site. (D) The exploration of the location of SLN using a hand-held gamma-probe and identification of a blue-stained SLN. (E) Histopathologic detection of microscopic nodal metastasis.

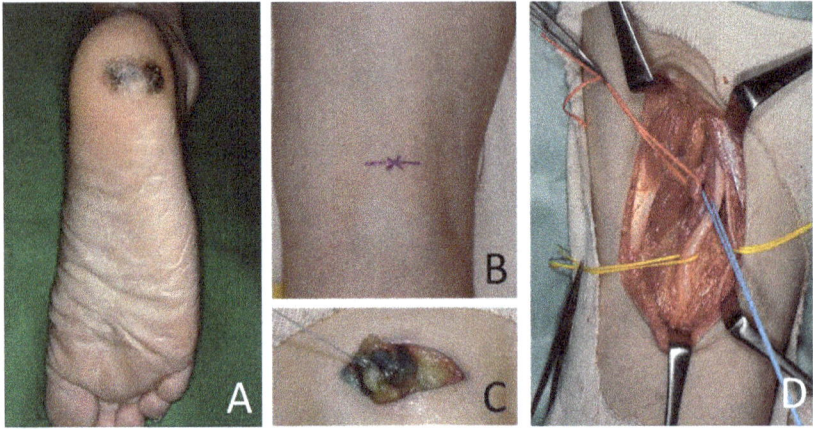

Figure 3. Detection of interval SLN. (A) Primary melanoma on the right heel. (B) Lymphoscintigraphy revealed accumulation in the right popliteal fossa. (C) Radioactive and blue-stained popliteal node, which had microscopic metastasis. (D) Popliteal lymph node dissection was performed.

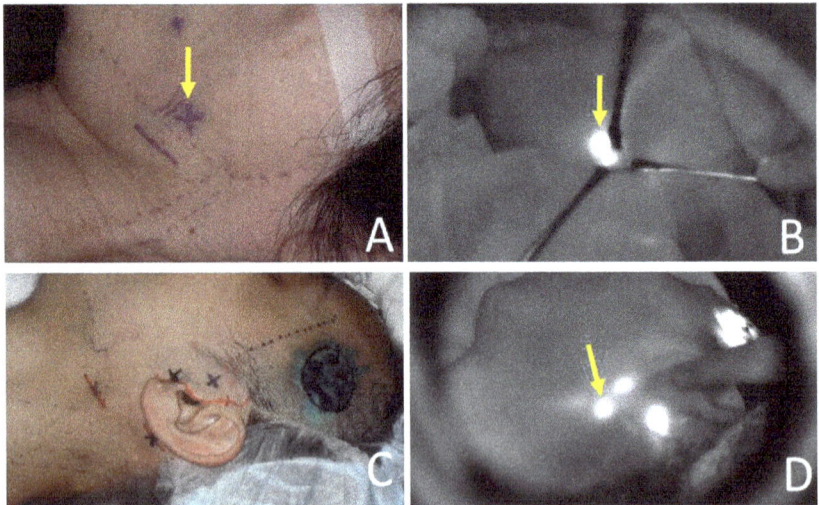

Figure 4. SLNB using ICG. (A) SLNB for melanoma of the nose. The X mark on the left mandible indicates accumulation of radioisotope (arrow). (B) A fluorescent submandibular SLN is visible through the incision using the near-infrared camera (arrow). (C) SLNB for melanoma of the left temporal region. The X marks indicate accumulation of radioisotope. (D) An additional fluorescent SLN (arrow), which was not detected by lymphoscintigraphy, is observed through the overlying skin.

3. Does SLNB-guided early lymph node dissection improve survival rate?

Whether patients who undergo complete lymph node dissection (CLND) after confirmation of a positive SLN have a better prognosis than patients who undergo TLND after occurrence of clinical nodal disease is controversial. The results of retrospective studies that compared survival after CLND for a positive SLN with survival after TLND for clinical nodal disease remain controversial. Several retrospective studies, including a multicentric study and a matched control study, demonstrated a significant survival benefit for patients who underwent CLND for a positive SLN[33, 34]. In addition, a survival benefit was also demonstrated for patients whose primary tumor thickness was between 1 mm and 4 mm and who underwent CLND for a positive SLN[35]. In contrast, other retrospective studies demonstrated no significant difference in overall survival between patients who underwent CLND for a positive SLN and those who underwent TLND for clinical nodal disease[36, 37].

The third interim analysis of the Multicenter Selective Lymphadenectomy Trial 1 (MLST-1), the only randomized control trial with available results, failed to demonstrate a 5-year survival advantage for the SLNB group when compared with the observation group and only a disease-free survival benefit for the SLNB group[38]. In a subgroup analysis, patients who underwent CLND for a positive SLN showed an improvement in 5-year survival of about 20% when compared with patients who underwent TLND after nodal observation and subsequently occurring clinical nodal disease (72.3% vs 52.4%; P=.004). The nodal recurrence was lower in patients who had a negative SLN (4.0%) than in those who had a positive SLN but were observed without early CLND (15.6%). From these results, the authors concluded that microscopic metastasis would develop within the lymph nodes and that early LND may lead to accurate staging and survival improvement.

However, whether SLNB and/or CLND would be a therapeutic procedure remains unclear, and several authors have questioned this conclusion from the results of the MLST-1. First, they claim that it was inappropriate to conclude that early CLND would improve survival because this result was based on a postrandomization subgroup analysis[39]. Second, they question whether all microscopic metastases will develop into clinical nodal disease. That is, some microscopic metastases may show indolent behavior and not develop into clinical nodal disease for a long time. In that case, comparison of the nodal recurrence rate between the 2 arms described above is an inappropriate analysis[37]. As a result, all that is currently clear is that SLNB can provide staging information that predicts prognosis and may impact clinical management.

4. Complete lymph node dissection

4.1. The role of complete lymph node dissection

The therapeutic value of CLND and appropriate selection of patients for CLND remain questionable. The role of CLND in patients with positive SLNs is also a clinically important question because only 10% to 25% of patients with positive SLNs will have additional micro-scopic metastasis in non-SLNs[40-42], which means that approximately 80% of patients with positive SLNs may be spared CLND. Several authors categorized the SLN as several varia-bles and tried to find a reliable indicator of non-SLN status[43, 44]. However, it remains un-clear what size of microscopic metastasis of the SLN or which histopathologic location of metastasis in the SLN, such as subcapsular, parenchymal, multifocal, and extensive, would be a reliable indicator of non-SLN status[44].

The choice of the extent of CLND is ultimately decided by the individual surgeon. Few spe-cific recommendations are available in the published guidelines, with the common descrip-tion being "a thorough dissection" and reports of low levels of evidence supporting the appropriate surgical extent of CLND of the cervical, axillary, and inguinal regions[45-47].

5. Neck dissection

5.1. Extent of dissection and regional recurrence rate

The purpose of neck dissection is to control regional disease; it has little impact on overall sur-vival. However, the extent of neck dissection is still controversial and various extents of neck dissection have been advocated by several authors. Radical neck dissection (RND) including removal of level I-V (Fig. 5A) and nonlymphatic tissue such as the sternocleidomastoid muscle, the internal jugular vein, and the spinal accessary nerve has been the gold standard for neck dissection for melanoma[48]. Despite extensive areas of dissection, O'Brien et al. reported that regional control with RND was unsatisfactory, with regional recurrence of 28% in patients with all nodal disease and of 34% in patients with clinical nodal disease[48].

Generally, RND is associated with significant morbidity. Therefore, some authors have con-sidered modified RND (MRND) or functional neck dissection including preservation of any or all of the sternocleidomastoid muscle, the internal jugular vein, and the spinal accessory nerve[49, 50]. In studies of patients with clinical nodal disease, several authors demonstrat-ed that regional recurrence rates were 14-32% after RND, 0% after MRND, and 23% to 29% after selective neck dissection (SND), which is not statistically significant among the groups[51-53]. Byers also reported a 16% recurrence rate after MRND[54]. From these stud-ies, MRND has been advocated even in the setting of clinical nodal disease.

In addition, as an even more selective approach, the lymphatic drainage patterns of head and neck melanoma have been described by O'Brien et al. based on a consecutive series of over 270 neck dissections and parotidectomies (Fig. 5B)[52]. As described above, although several authors reported relatively high regional recurrence rates of 23% to 29% after SND, these studies include clinical N2-N3 (multiple involved nodes) disease, which will have a higher risk of recurrence than N1 disease[51, 52]. In a study of 37 consecutive patients with clinically N1 neck disease reported by White et al., 6 patients underwent RND, 24, MRND, and 7, SND. None of the 3 groups had any cases of local recurrence during a mean follow-up of 46 months[55], indicating that SND may be an alternative to RND or MRND for the clinically N1 neck in melanoma[55].

Furthermore, the appropriate extent of dissection is also unclear in patients with positive SLNs. Pu et al. reported 23 consecutive patients with positive SLNs who underwent MRND or superficial parotidectomy. Of those patients, 21 (91.3%) had no additional positive non-SLNs and only 2 (8.7 %) had 1 additional positive non-SLN[56]. No patient developed a regional local recurrence during a mean follow-up period of 23.7 months. The low prevalence of additional positive non-SLNs in MRND specimens suggests that when microscopic SLN metastasis exists, nodal disease is confined to the SLN alone in most patients [56] and SND may be selected.

As for parotid gland nodes, patients with clinically palpable parotid nodes have a 28% to 58% risk of microscopic metastasis in the cervical nodes[57-59]. Although neck dissection should be included when clinical parotid disease is present, the need to treat the parotid nodes when clinical nodal disease of the neck is present is controversial. In such cases, many surgeons selectively perform superficial parotidectomy combined with a neck dissection based on O'Brien's lymphatic map (Fig. 5B) or the protocol of the individual institute[60].

However, the lymphatic drainage in the head and neck is generally complex and 8% to 43% of patients have unexpected drainage patterns in the occipital, postauricular, and contralateral nodes (Fig. 5A).[26, 61-64] Therefore, SND should be tailored to the individual patient according to the location of the SLN and second-tier nodes.

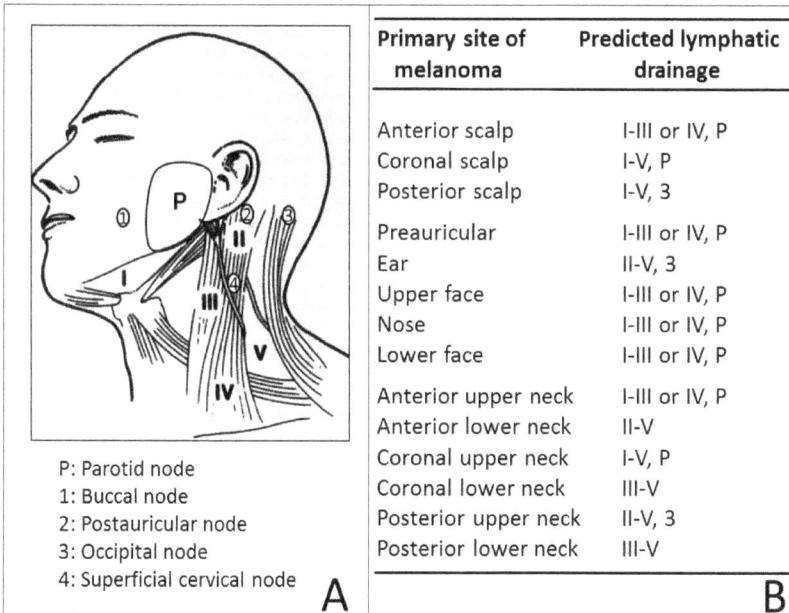

Primary site of melanoma	Predicted lymphatic drainage
Anterior scalp	I-III or IV, P
Coronal scalp	I-V, P
Posterior scalp	I-V, 3
Preauricular	I-III or IV, P
Ear	II-V, 3
Upper face	I-III or IV, P
Nose	I-III or IV, P
Lower face	I-III or IV, P
Anterior upper neck	I-III or IV, P
Anterior lower neck	II-V
Coronal upper neck	I-V, P
Coronal lower neck	III-V
Posterior upper neck	II-V, 3
Posterior lower neck	III-V

P: Parotid node
1: Buccal node
2: Postauricular node
3: Occipital node
4: Superficial cervical node

A   B

Figure 5. A)Lymphatic anatomy of the head and neck showing the 5 major lymph node levels and superficial nodes (B) Predicted lymphatic drainage and extent of neck dissection recommended by O'Brien et al.

5.2. Complication rate and technical variables

Significant complications associated with radical neck dissection may include injury to the facial and spinal accessory nerves, chylous fistula, and skin flap necrosis[65]. Although it is generally accepted that the rate of morbidity is reduced by MRND and further reduced by SND, detailed complication rates in the treatment of melanoma have not been reported. According to the literature, neck dissection and parotidectomy is usually safe when appropriately planned preoperatively and when performed by well-experienced surgeons.

Technical variables mainly include skin incisions. Commonly used incisions are single Y, T, or double Y-type incisions, which provide optimal exposure of the entire neck. However, the edge of the flap sometimes has a poor blood supply and breakdown can result in the exposure of the major vessels. The three-point suture line gives a high incidence of postoperative scar contracture[66, 67]. The Mcfee incision was designed to eliminate the three-point exposure line, giving a good cosmetic result. However, the exposure is difficult, particularly in a short fat neck, and excessive traction of the skin flaps can result in damaging of the skin edges[67]. Large, single incisions such as the curtain flap, apron flap, U-flap, and Hockey stick incision offer a good blood supply and most of the scar lies within the relaxed skin tension lines of the neck[68]. Each incision should be selected appropriately according to the extent of the neck dissection.

6. Axillary lymph node dissection

6.1. Extent of dissection and regional recurrence

Axillary LND for patients with melanoma is performed for local control and staging[69]; the therapeutic value is still unclear. The axillary nodes are divided into level I, II, and III nodes. Level I nodes are lateral to the lateral edge of the pectoralis minor muscle. Level II nodes are between the medial and lateral edges of the pectoralis minor muscle. Level III nodes are medial to the medial edge of the pectorarlis minor muscle, in the apex of the axilla. The generally recommended extent of dissection is from level I to III nodes because of the various drainage patterns in the second-tier nodes as well as the potentially increased risk of recurrence with a lesser dissection[70, 71]. Several authors recommended a more extensive dissection including the supraaxillary fat pad because approximately 14% of patients will have metastatic nodes in this area[69, 72]. In contrast, several authors have questioned whether a level III dissection is necessary in all melanoma patients with a positive SLN and advocated that level III dissection should be included only when suspicious nodes are present in this level [73-75]. Namm et al. also advocated that level I and II dissection should be performed for positive-SLN patients because of the low regional recurrence rate and low postoperative morbidity and concluded that level III dissection is not necessary for regional control in patients with microscopic metastasis[76].

As for the regional recurrence rate, unfortunately, most studies grouped together all of the dissected levels. Several authors reported a 10% to 19% regional recurrence rate during about a 30-month median follow-up[77-79]; however, in all 3 of those studies, the extent of dissection was not documented. Veenstra et al. reported a 4% regional recurrence rate and documented which levels were included when axillary LND was performed; however, they did not tease out the axillary recurrence rate specifically[80]. In the case of level I and II dissection for patients with a positive SLN, a low recurrence rate of 4% during a median follow-up of approximately 39-month was reported[76].

6.2. Complication rate and technical variables

Wrightson et al. reported a 19.9% complication rate among 262 patients undergoing axillary LND, most of which was thought to be level I-III dissection, for a positive SLN[81]. Several authors reported a complication rate of 14% to 21% for wound infection and of 19% to 36% for lymphocele when performing level I–III dissections[82, 83]. In contrast, Numm et al. reported that postoperative complications occurred in 11% of patients, with infectious complications in 8% when performing level I and II dissection. However, comparative studies of level I-II dissection with and level I-III dissection have not been published. Although the definition of lymphedema varies among studies, a long-term lymphedema rate was reported to be 1% to 12%[72, 75, 81].

Evidence of an optimal surgical technique for axillary LND has not been shown. As technical modifications, 2 incisions are mainly used. One is a transverse incision from the lateral edge of the pectoralis major muscle to the border of the latissimus dorsi muscle, and the other is an extended incision following the contour of the pectoralis major into the axillary apex and then down the medial arm[72, 84]. However, these incision variables would not affect the complication rate. Lawton et al. advocated preservation of the pectoralis major, the interpectoral, and the latissimus dorsi fascia during axillary LND to try to reduce lymphedema[84]. Over 110 elective and therapeutic fascia-preserving axillary LNDs developed a 5% incidence of long-term lymphedema, which is the same as or slightly lower than the incidence rates reported by the studies [72, 75, 81] described above. Optimal surgical exposure for level III dissection sometimes requires transection of the pectoralis minor muscle, and several authors suggested routine en bloc dissection of the pectoralis minor for TLND[16, 72, 75]. The long thoracic and thoracodorsal nerves are routinely preserved, although the intercostobrachial nerves are often sacrificed in TLND[73, 75]. As a result, no modifications clearly improve the complication rate, and only the extent of dissection impacts the complication rate.

7. Ilioinguinnal lymph node dissection

7.1. Extent of dissection and regional recurrence rate

The dissection areas subject to most controversy are inguinal LND alone or ilioinguinal LND (inguinal LND + iliac/obturator (pelvic) LND). When iliac or obturator node involvement is suspected clinically or radiologically, additional pelvic LND is generally recommended[74, 85-87]. For patients with clinically palpable nodal disease in the ingui-nal region alone, additional pelvic LND has not been widely accepted because of the lack of overall survival advantage[88, 89]. However, some authors advocated ilioinguinal LND because the rate of pelvic lymph node involvement in patients with palpable ingui-nal disease is 27% to 52%[87-92]. In a study of predictive factors for pelvic nodal status, Strobbe et al. reported that the Cloquet node has a limited sensitivity of 65% to predict involvement of the pelvic nodes and that the negative predictive value is 78%. In pa-tients with clinical inguinal nodal disease, a tumor-positive Cloquet node had a 69% risk (positive predictive value) of additional positive nodes[91]. They also showed that the number of positive nodes in the inguinal region is not a reliable predictive factor for the pelvic nodal status, with a sensitivity of 41% and a negative predictive value of 78%[91].

Furthermore, the extent of dissection is more controversial in positive inguinal SLN patients. Van der Ploeg et al. reported that there is no lymphatic drainage to the inferior lateral zone, which is just lateral to the femoral artery and inferior to the level of saphenofemoral junction in the inguinal area, in patients with a positive SLN and advocated that this area need not be included in LND for such patients[93]. Pelvic nodes also seem unlikely to be involved when an inguinal SLN shows only microscopic metastasis[94, 95]. Several authors reported that 9% to 17 % of patients with a positive inguinal SLN also have positive pelvic nodes when ilioinguinal LND is performed[96-98]. In addition, a study evaluating lymphatic flow using lymphoscintigraphy and/or SPECT/CT demonstrated that over 50% of patients with a posi-tive SLN showed second-tier nodal drainage to the pelvic nodes[93]. This study suggests that a selective pelvic LND based on the location of the second-tier nodes may be appropri-ate in positive SLN patients[93, 99].

As for the regional recurrence rate, published recurrence rates after inguinal or ilioinguinal LND for patients with clinical nodal disease is 0% to 33.6% (inguinal LND: 11.7%-13%; ilioinguinal LND: 0%-17.9%)[74, 85-89]. Sterne et al. reported that patients with palpable no-dal disease who underwent inguinal LND alone had a regional recurrence rate of 12.5% (2 of 16 patients), whereas for those who underwent ilioinguinal LND, it was 0% (0 of 25 patients) [85]. Pearlman et al. reported a modification of inguinal LND that does not violate the femo-ral sheath. However, a 16% rate of regional recurrence was reported[100].

7.2. Complication rate and technical variables

In the field of urology, classical inguinal LND has traditionally been associated with an 80% to 100% risk of surgical morbidity[101]. In the treatment of melanoma, several authors re-ported that 20% to 77% of patients who underwent inguinal LND had postoperative mor-bidity such as skin necrosis and wound dehiscence (7%-55%), wound infection (5%-15%), lymphocele/seroma (2%-46%), and lymphedema (5%-64%).[102] Although concerns have been raised about the potential for increased morbidity in patients undergoing an additional pelvic LND[87, 103], the addition of pelvic LND to inguinal LND did not significantly in-crease the risk for postoperative wound complication[87, 101, 104, 105]. However, lymphe-dema was more common after inguinal LND alone in some studies, although 1 study specifically evaluating the incidence of lymphedema found no difference between the 2 procedures[87, 106, 107]. The lack of consensus about the complications of additional pelvic LND may suggest that when clinically indicated, concern about increased morbidity should not be a reason to avoid ilioinguinal LND, although patients may suffer from the operating time and cost.

The commonly described technical variables of ilioinguinal LND include different type of skin incision, thick skin flap, preservation of the large saphenous vein, transposition of the sartorius muscle over the femoral vessels, continuity dissection with division of the inguinal ligament, and trimming of the skin edges at the time of closure[108].

Several skin incisions are used: a Lazy-S incision from just medial to the anterior superior iliac spine to the inferior margin of the femoral triangle, paired oblique incisions (Fig. 6A), or an oblique/transverse incision above the inguinal crease with a longitudinal incision below and a skin bridge between[73, 84, 100]. Lazy-S incision provides optimal exposure and less subcutaneous lymphatic disruption[108]. In contrast, paired oblique incisions or an oblique/transverse incision can avoid an incision in the inguinal crease to reduce skin necrosis and wound dehiscence[84]. Recently, however, Spillane et al. reported minimal-access 3- to 6-cm-long paired incisions above and below the inguinal ligament, which showed no significant difference in wound and lymphedema complications[109]. A thick skin flap elevated at the level of the Scarpa fascia may improve skin necrosis and wound dehiscence rates; however, a 26% to 34% rate of skin necrosis and wound infection was reported[84, 100]. The preservation of the saphenous vein and the sartorius transposition flap for vessel coverage were designed to improve lymphedema rates, with no incidence of lymphedema[100]. When performing ilioinguinal LND, technical variables include a continuity dissection by dividing the inguinal ligament or an abdominal wall incision above and parallel to the inguinal ligament (Fig. 6B) to expose the retroperitoneal space[73, 84, 86]. Although advantages of inguinal ligament division include optimal exposure and possible continuity dissection, the main disadvantage is possible long-term abdominal wall weakness that may lead to abdominal incisional hernia. As another modification, Lawton et al. advocated fascia-preserving ilioinguinal LND, which is similar to the modified axillary dissection described above in the section on axillary LND, and the long-term lymphedema rate was 14%. Video-assisted endoscopic inguinal LND is currently investigated as a minimally invasive and less morbid approach but is not widely used[110, 111].

Despite such modifications, a comparative study reported by Sabel et al. demonstrated no significant difference in wound and lymphedema complications between modified inguinal LND (incision avoiding the inguinal crease, saphenous vein preservation, or sartorius transposition) and conventional inguinal LND[107]. However, although insignificant, saphenous vein preservation decreased the lymphedema rate from 30% to 13% and the wound complication rate from 20% to 7%. An incision avoiding the inguinal crease also decreased the wound complication rate from 21% to 9%, which is also statistically insignificant. Thus, these modifications seem to offer promise in decreasing morbidity.

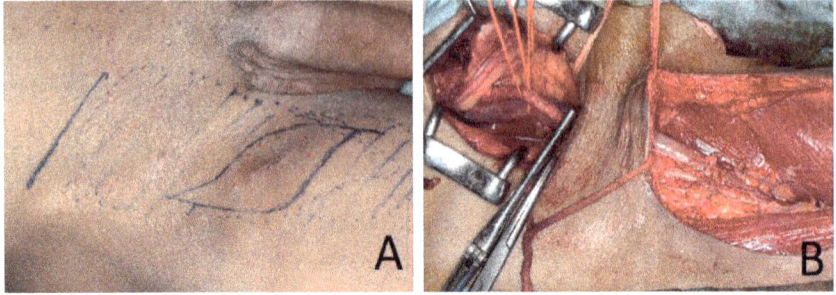

Figure 6. Ilioinguinal LND using paired incisions. (A) Incision lines. The incision below the inguinal crease is fusiform to include the skin overlying the metastatic node. (B) Operating field after dissection. The abdominal wall was incised parallel to the inguinal ligament, which was preserved under the bipedicle flap.

As another procedure in an attempt to decrease lymphocele, Nakamura et al. reported a simple method using intraoperative injection of isosulfan blue during inguinal LND without modifications to identify leakage from an injured lymphatic vessels for the prevention of lymphocele (Fig. 7)[112]. There was no incidence of lymphocele in the isosulfan blue injection group and the lymphatic drainage output from the inguinal region was clearly less, leading to early removal of the suction catheter.

Despite many technical variables, it is difficult to evaluate each technique because of the different study designs, variable definitions of complications, and different patient populations. Multicenter, randomized prospective trials with a standardized definition of complications are required in the future.

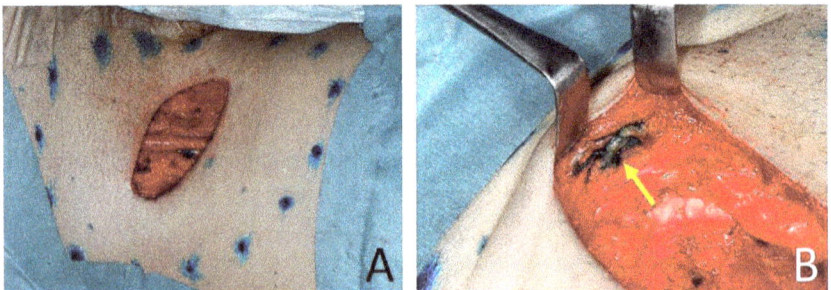

Figure 7. Intraoperative injection of blue dye during inguinal LND for detection of injured lymphatic vessels. (A) Intracutaneous injection of isosulfan blue around the right inguinal region just after inguinal LND. (B) Blue-staining lymphatic leak (arrow) in the surgical field, which was ligated.

8. Adjuvant radiation therapy

Regional recurrence occurs in 20% to 50% of patients after TLND. High-risk factors associated with regional recurrence include a cervical lymph node basin, large lymph nodes, multiple positive lymph nodes, and extracapsular extension[113]. Patients with such risk factors are appropriate candidates for adjuvant radiation therapy, and several nonrandomized studies have demonstrated that adjuvant radiation therapy after CLND for patients with regional nodal disease can reduce the risk of regional recurrence to between 5% and 20% [114-118]. In a prospective phase II study by the Trans Tasman Radiation Oncology Group (TROG Study 96.06) of adjuvant radiation therapy after CLND for patients with regional nodal disease, the regional control rate was 91%[118].

Although adjuvant radiation therapy can be effective in achieving regional control after TLND, it increases chronic lymphedema, particularly in the inguinal region, which is the major morbidity associated with TLND[119].

9. Conclusions

The surgical approach to regional lymph node metastasis of cutaneous melanoma is challenging. SLNB allows accurate staging of nodal status and prediction of prognosis. A positive SLN should be treated with CLND for regional control. However, the impact on SLNB on overall survival remains unclear, and the appropriate surgical extent of CLND in the cervical, axillary, and inguinal regions is also debated. More research is required to provide evidence-based guidelines for surgeons about the extent of LND and to investigate the factors that may lead to a more patient-tailored approach.

Acknowledgements

We thank Ms F. Miyamasu, associate professor of the Medical English Communications Center, University of Tsukuba, for expert English revision.

This work was partly supported by the National Cancer Center Research and Development Fund (23-A-22), and the Japanese Association of Dermatologic Surgery.

Author details

Yasuhiro Nakamura* and Fujio Otsuka

*Address all correspondence to: ynakamurta3@yahoo.co.jp

Department of Dermatology, Faculty of Medicine, University of Tsukuba, Tsukuba, Japan

References

[1] Balch CM, Soong SJ, Gershenwald JE et al. Prognostic factors analysis of 17,600 melanoma patients: validation of the American Joint Committee on Cancer melanoma staging system. J Clin Oncol 2001; 19: 3622-34.

[2] Sim FH, Taylor WF, Pritchard DJ, Soule EH. Lymphadenectomy in the management of stage I malignant melanoma: a prospective randomized study. Mayo Clin Proc 1986; 61: 697-705.

[3] Veronesi U, Adamus J, Bandiera DC et al. Inefficacy of immediate node dissection in stage 1 melanoma of the limbs. N Engl J Med 1977; 297: 627-30.

[4] Cascinelli N, Morabito A, Santinami M, MacKie RM, Belli F. Immediate or delayed dissection of regional nodes in patients with melanoma of the trunk: a randomised trial. WHO Melanoma Programme. Lancet 1998; 351: 793-6.

[5] Balch CM, Soong S, Ross MI et al. Long-term results of a multi-institutional randomized trial comparing prognostic factors and surgical results for intermediate thickness melanomas (1.0 to 4.0 mm). Intergroup Melanoma Surgical Trial. Ann Surg Oncol 2000; 7: 87-97.

[6] Morton DL, Wen DR, Wong JH et al. Technical details of intraoperative lymphatic mapping for early stage melanoma. Arch Surg 1992; 127: 392-9.

[7] Ross MI, Reintgen D, Balch CM. Selective lymphadenectomy: emerging role for lymphatic mapping and sentinel node biopsy in the management of early stage melanoma. Semin Surg Oncol 1993; 9: 219-23.

[8] Reintgen D, Cruse CW, Wells K et al. The orderly progression of melanoma nodal metastases. Ann Surg 1994; 220: 759-67.

[9] Thompson JF, McCarthy WH, Bosch CM et al. Sentinel lymph node status as an indicator of the presence of metastatic melanoma in regional lymph nodes. Melanoma Res 1995; 5: 255-60.

[10] Gershenwald JE, Colome MI, Lee JE et al. Patterns of recurrence following a negative sentinel lymph node biopsy in 243 patients with stage I or II melanoma. J Clin Oncol 1998; 16: 2253-60.

[11] Kapteijn BA, Nieweg OE, Liem I et al. Localizing the sentinel node in cutaneous melanoma: gamma probe detection versus blue dye. Ann Surg Oncol 1997; 4: 156-60.

[12] Gershenwald JE, Tseng CH, Thompson W et al. Improved sentinel lymph node localization in patients with primary melanoma with the use of radiolabeled colloid. Surgery 1998; 124: 203-10.

[13] Uren RF, Howman-Giles R, Thompson JF et al. Lymphoscintigraphy to identify sentinel lymph nodes in patients with melanoma. Melanoma Res 1994; 4: 395-9.

[14] Sumner WE, 3rd, Ross MI, Mansfield PF et al. Implications of lymphatic drainage to unusual sentinel lymph node sites in patients with primary cutaneous melanoma. Cancer 2002; 95: 354-60.

[15] Thompson JF, Uren RF, Shaw HM et al. Location of sentinel lymph nodes in patients with cutaneous melanoma: new insights into lymphatic anatomy. J Am Coll Surg 1999; 189: 195-204.

[16] Uren RF, Howman-Giles R, Thompson JF et al. Interval nodes: the forgotten sentinel nodes in patients with melanoma. Arch Surg 2000; 135: 1168-72.

[17] Uren RF, Thompson JF, Howman-Giles R. Sentinel nodes. Interval nodes, lymphatic lakes, and accurate sentinel node identification. Clin Nucl Med 2000; 25: 234-6.

[18] Morton DL, Cochran AJ, Thompson JF et al. Sentinel node biopsy for early-stage melanoma: accuracy and morbidity in MSLT-I, an international multicenter trial. Ann Surg 2005; 242: 302-11; discussion 11-3.

[19] Hayashi T, Furukawa H, Oyama A et al. Sentinel lymph node biopsy using real-time fluorescence navigation with indocyanine green in cutaneous head and neck/lip mucosa melanomas. Head Neck 2012; 34: 758-61.

[20] Thomas JM. Sentinel lymph node biopsy in malignant melanoma. BMJ 2008; 336: 902-3.

[21] Veenstra HJ, Wouters MW, Kroon BB, Olmos RA, Nieweg OE. Less false-negative sentinel node procedures in melanoma patients with experience and proper collaboration. J Surg Oncol 2011; 104: 454-7.

[22] Thomas JM. Caution with sentinel node biopsy in cutaneous melanoma. Br J Surg 2006; 93: 129-30.

[23] Stoffels I, von der Stuck H, Boy C et al. Indocyanine green fluorescence-guided sentinel lymph node biopsy in dermato-oncology. J Dtsch Dermatol Ges 2012; 10: 51-7.

[24] Wagner JD, Park HM, Coleman JJ, 3rd, Love C, Hayes JT. Cervical sentinel lymph node biopsy for melanomas of the head and neck and upper thorax. Arch Otolaryngol Head Neck Surg 2000; 126: 313-21.

[25] Chao C, Wong SL, Edwards MJ et al. Sentinel lymph node biopsy for head and neck melanomas. Ann Surg Oncol 2003; 10: 21-6.

[26] Fincher TR, O'Brien JC, McCarty TM et al. Patterns of drainage and recurrence following sentinel lymph node biopsy for cutaneous melanoma of the head and neck. Arch Otolaryngol Head Neck Surg 2004; 130: 844-8.

[27] Namikawa K, Yamazaki N. Sentinel lymph node biopsy guided by indocyanine green fluorescence for cutaneous melanoma. Eur J Dermatol 2011; 21: 184-90.

[28] Fujisawa Y, Nakamura Y, Kawachi Y, Otsuka F. A custom-made, low-cost intraoperative fluorescence navigation system with indocyanine green for sentinel lymph node biopsy in skin cancer. Dermatology 2011; 222: 261-8.

[29] Polom K, Murawa D, Rho YS, Spychala A, Murawa P. Skin melanoma sentinel lymph node biopsy using real-time fluorescence navigation with indocyanine green and indocyanine green with human serum albumin. Br J Dermatol 2012; 166: 682-3.

[30] Benson RC, Kues HA. Fluorescence properties of indocyanine green as related to angiography. Phys Med Biol 1978; 23: 159-63.

[31] Uren RF. SPECT/CT Lymphoscintigraphy to locate the sentinel lymph node in patients with melanoma. Ann Surg Oncol 2009; 16: 1459-60.

[32] Vermeeren L, van der Ploeg IM, Olmos RA et al. SPECT/CT for preoperative sentinel node localization. J Surg Oncol 2010; 101: 184-90.

[33] Morton DL, Hoon DS, Cochran AJ et al. Lymphatic mapping and sentinel lymphadenectomy for early-stage melanoma: therapeutic utility and implications of nodal microanatomy and molecular staging for improving the accuracy of detection of nodal micrometastases. Ann Surg 2003; 238: 538-49; discussion 49-50.

[34] Kretschmer L, Hilgers R, Mohrle M et al. Patients with lymphatic metastasis of cutaneous malignant melanoma benefit from sentinel lymphonodectomy and early excision of their nodal disease. Eur J Cancer 2004; 40: 212-8.

[35] Nowecki ZI, Rutkowski P, Michej W. The survival benefit to patients with positive sentinel node melanoma after completion lymph node dissection may be limited to the subgroup with a primary lesion Breslow thickness greater than 1.0 and less than or equal to 4 mm (pT2-pT3). Ann Surg Oncol 2008; 15: 2223-34.

[36] Pasquali S, Mocellin S. The anticancer face of interferon alpha (IFN-alpha): from biology to clinical results, with a focus on melanoma. Curr Med Chem 2010; 17: 3327-36.

[37] van Akkooi AC, Bouwhuis MG, de Wilt JH, Kliffen M, Schmitz PI, Eggermont AM. Multivariable analysis comparing outcome after sentinel node biopsy or therapeutic lymph node dissection in patients with melanoma. Br J Surg 2007; 94: 1293-9.

[38] Morton DL, Thompson JF, Cochran AJ et al. Sentinel-node biopsy or nodal observation in melanoma. N Engl J Med 2006; 355: 1307-17.

[39] Ross MI, Gershenwald JE. How should we view the results of the Multicenter Selective Lymphadenectomy Trial-1 (MSLT-1)? Ann Surg Oncol 2008; 15: 670-3.

[40] Govindarajan A, Ghazarian DM, McCready DR, Leong WL. Histological features of melanoma sentinel lymph node metastases associated with status of the completion lymphadenectomy and rate of subsequent relapse. Ann Surg Oncol 2007; 14: 906-12.

[41] Gershenwald JE, Andtbacka RH, Prieto VG et al. Microscopic tumor burden in sentinel lymph nodes predicts synchronous nonsentinel lymph node involvement in patients with melanoma. J Clin Oncol 2008; 26: 4296-303.

[42] Vuylsteke RJ, Borgstein PJ, van Leeuwen PA et al. Sentinel lymph node tumor load: an independent predictor of additional lymph node involvement and survival in melanoma. Ann Surg Oncol 2005; 12: 440-8.

[43] Francischetto T, Spector N, Neto Rezende JF et al. Influence of sentinel lymph node tumor burden on survival in melanoma. Ann Surg Oncol 2010; 17: 1152-8.

[44] van der Ploeg AP, van Akkooi AC, Schmitz PI, Koljenovic S, Verhoef C, Eggermont AM. EORTC Melanoma Group sentinel node protocol identifies high rate of submicrometastases according to Rotterdam Criteria. Eur J Cancer 2010; 46: 2414-21.

[45] Marsden JR, Newton-Bishop JA, Burrows L et al. Revised U.K. guidelines for the management of cutaneous melanoma 2010. Br J Dermatol 2010; 163: 238-56.

[46] Garbe C, Peris K, Hauschild A et al. Diagnosis and treatment of melanoma: European consensus-based interdisciplinary guideline. Eur J Cancer 2010; 46: 270-83.

[47] Gershenwald JE, Ross MI. Sentinel-lymph-node biopsy for cutaneous melanoma. N Engl J Med 2011; 364: 1738-45.

[48] O'Brien CJ, Gianoutsos MP, Morgan MJ. Neck dissection for cutaneous malignant melanoma. World J Surg 1992; 16: 222-6.

[49] Calearo CV, Teatini G. Functional neck dissection. Anatomical grounds, surgical technique, clinical observations. Ann Otol Rhinol Laryngol 1983; 92: 215-22.

[50] O'Brien CJ, Coates AS, Petersen-Schaefer K et al. Experience with 998 cutaneous melanomas of the head and neck over 30 years. Am J Surg 1991; 162: 310-4.

[51] Turkula LD, Woods JE. Limited or selective nodal dissection for malignant melanoma of the head and neck. Am J Surg 1984; 148: 446-8.

[52] O'Brien CJ, Petersen-Schaefer K, Ruark D, Coates AS, Menzie SJ, Harrison RI. Radical, modified, and selective neck dissection for cutaneous malignant melanoma. Head Neck 1995; 17: 232-41.

[53] Jonk A, Strobbe LJ, Kroon BB et al. Cervical lymph-node metastasis from cutaneous melanoma of the head and neck: a search for prognostic factors. Eur J Surg Oncol 1998; 24: 298-302.

[54] Byers RM. The role of modified neck dissection in the treatment of cutaneous melanoma of the head and neck. Arch Surg 1986; 121: 1338-41.

[55] White N, Yap LH, Srivastava S. Lymphadenectomy for melanoma in the clinically N1 neck: radical, modified radical, or selective? J Craniofac Surg 2009; 20: 385-8.

[56] Pu LL, Wells KE, Cruse CW, Shons AR, Reintgen DS. Prevalence of additional positive lymph nodes in complete lymphadenectomy specimens after positive sentinel lymphadenectomy findings for early-stage melanoma of the head and neck. Plast Reconstr Surg 2003; 112: 43-9.

[57] O'Brien CJ, McNeil EB, McMahon JD, Pathak I, Lauer CS. Incidence of cervical node involvement in metastatic cutaneous malignancy involving the parotid gland. Head Neck 2001; 23: 744-8.

[58] Caldwell CB, Spiro RH. The role of parotidectomy in the treatment of cutaneous head and neck melanoma. Am J Surg 1988; 156: 318-22.

[59] Barr LC, Skene AI, Fish S, Thomas JM. Superficial parotidectomy in the treatment of cutaneous melanoma of the head and neck. Br J Surg 1994; 81: 64-5.

[60] Klop WM, Veenstra HJ, Vermeeren L, Nieweg OE, Balm AJ, Lohuis PJ. Assessment of lymphatic drainage patterns and implications for the extent of neck dissection in head and neck melanoma patients. J Surg Oncol 2011; 103: 756-60.

[61] O'Brien CJ, Uren RF, Thompson JF et al. Prediction of potential metastatic sites in cutaneous head and neck melanoma using lymphoscintigraphy. Am J Surg 1995; 170: 461-6.

[62] Pathak I, O'Brien CJ, Petersen-Schaeffer K et al. Do nodal metastases from cutaneous melanoma of the head and neck follow a clinically predictable pattern? Head Neck 2001; 23: 785-90.

[63] Lin D, Franc BL, Kashani-Sabet M, Singer MI. Lymphatic drainage patterns of head and neck cutaneous melanoma observed on lymphoscintigraphy and sentinel lymph node biopsy. Head Neck 2006; 28: 249-55.

[64] Reynolds HM, Smith NP, Uren RF, Thompson JF, Dunbar PR. Three-dimensional visualization of skin lymphatic drainage patterns of the head and neck. Head Neck 2009; 31: 1316-25.

[65] Leong SP. Role of selective sentinel lymph node dissection in head and neck melanoma. J Surg Oncol 2011; 104: 361-8.

[66] Attie JN. A single transverse incision for radical neck dissection. Surgery 1957; 41: 498-502.

[67] Macfee WF. Transverse incisions for neck dissection. Ann Surg 1960; 151: 279-84.

[68] Dancey AL, Srivastava S. Experience with the modified hockey stick incision for block dissection of neck. J Plast Reconstr Aesthet Surg 2006; 59: 1276-9.

[69] Balch CM. Axillary lymph node dissection: differences in goals and techniques when treating melanoma and breast cancer. Surgery 1990; 108: 118-9.

[70] Garbe C, Hauschild A, Volkenandt M et al. Evidence-based and interdisciplinary consensus-based German guidelines: systemic medical treatment of melanoma in the adjuvant and palliative setting. Melanoma Res 2008; 18: 152-60.

[71] Essner R. Surgical treatment of malignant melanoma. Surg Clin North Am 2003; 83: 109-56.

[72] Karakousis CP, Hena MA, Emrich LJ, Driscoll DL. Axillary node dissection in malignant melanoma: results and complications. Surgery 1990; 108: 10-7.

[73] Karakousis CP. Therapeutic node dissections in malignant melanoma. Ann Surg Oncol 1998; 5: 473-82.

[74] Meyer T, Merkel S, Gohl J, Hohenberger W. Lymph node dissection for clinically evident lymph node metastases of malignant melanoma. Eur J Surg Oncol 2002; 28: 424-30.

[75] Serpell JW, Carne PW, Bailey M. Radical lymph node dissection for melanoma. ANZ J Surg 2003; 73: 294-9.

[76] Namm JP, Chang AE, Cimmino VM, Rees RS, Johnson TM, Sabel MS. Is a level III dissection necessary for a positive sentinel lymph node in melanoma? J Surg Oncol 2012; 105: 225-8.

[77] Gershenwald JE, Berman RS, Porter G, Mansfield PF, Lee JE, Ross MI. Regional nodal basin control is not compromised by previous sentinel lymph node biopsy in patients with melanoma. Ann Surg Oncol 2000; 7: 226-31.

[78] Clary BM, Brady MS, Lewis JJ, Coit DG. Sentinel lymph node biopsy in the management of patients with primary cutaneous melanoma: review of a large single-institutional experience with an emphasis on recurrence. Ann Surg 2001; 233: 250-8.

[79] Leiter U, Buettner PG, Bohnenberger K et al. Sentinel lymph node dissection in primary melanoma reduces subsequent regional lymph node metastasis as well as distant metastasis after nodal involvement. Ann Surg Oncol 2010; 17: 129-37.

[80] Veenstra HJ, van der Ploeg IM, Wouters MW, Kroon BB, Nieweg OE. Reevaluation of the locoregional recurrence rate in melanoma patients with a positive sentinel node compared to patients with palpable nodal involvement. Ann Surg Oncol 2010; 17: 521-6.

[81] Wrightson WR, Wong SL, Edwards MJ et al. Complications associated with sentinel lymph node biopsy for melanoma. Ann Surg Oncol 2003; 10: 676-80.

[82] Kretschmer L, Thoms KM, Peeters S, Haenssle H, Bertsch HP, Emmert S. Postoperative morbidity of lymph node excision for cutaneous melanoma-sentinel lymphonodectomy versus complete regional lymph node dissection. Melanoma Res 2008; 18: 16-21.

[83] de Vries M, Vonkeman WG, van Ginkel RJ, Hoekstra HJ. Morbidity after axillary sentinel lymph node biopsy in patients with cutaneous melanoma. Eur J Surg Oncol 2005; 31: 778-83.

[84] Lawton G, Rasque H, Ariyan S. Preservation of muscle fascia to decrease lymphedema after complete axillary and ilioinguinofemoral lymphadenectomy for melanoma. J Am Coll Surg 2002; 195: 339-51.

[85] Sterne GD, Murray DS, Grimley RP. Ilioinguinal block dissection for malignant mela-
      noma. Br J Surg 1995; 82: 1057-9.

[86] Strobbe LJ, Jonk A, Hart AA, Nieweg OE, Kroon BB. Positive iliac and obturator no-
      des in melanoma: survival and prognostic factors. Ann Surg Oncol 1999; 6: 255-62.

[87] Hughes TM, A'Hern RP, Thomas JM. Prognosis and surgical management of patients
      with palpable inguinal lymph node metastases from melanoma. Br J Surg 2000; 87:
      892-901.

[88] Mann GB, Coit DG. Does the extent of operation influence the prognosis in patients
      with melanoma metastatic to inguinal nodes? Ann Surg Oncol 1999; 6: 263-71.

[89] Kretschmer L, Neumann C, Preusser KP, Marsch WC. Superficial inguinal and radi-
      cal ilioinguinal lymph node dissection in patients with palpable melanoma metasta-
      ses to the groin--an analysis of survival and local recurrence. Acta Oncol 2001; 40:
      72-8.

[90] Shen P, Conforti AM, Essner R, Cochran AJ, Turner RR, Morton DL. Is the node of
      Cloquet the sentinel node for the iliac/obturator node group? Cancer J 2000; 6: 93-7.

[91] Strobbe LJ, Jonk A, Hart AA et al. The value of Cloquet's node in predicting melano-
      ma nodal metastases in the pelvic lymph node basin. Ann Surg Oncol 2001; 8: 209-14.

[92] Allan CP, Hayes AJ, Thomas JM. Ilioinguinal lymph node dissection for palpable
      metastatic melanoma to the groin. ANZ J Surg 2008; 78: 982-6.

[93] van der Ploeg IM, Kroon BB, Valdes Olmos RA, Nieweg OE. Evaluation of lymphatic
      drainage patterns to the groin and implications for the extent of groin dissection in
      melanoma patients. Ann Surg Oncol 2009; 16: 2994-9.

[94] Jansen L, Nieweg OE, Peterse JL, Hoefnagel CA, Olmos RA, Kroon BB. Reliability of
      sentinel lymph node biopsy for staging melanoma. Br J Surg 2000; 87: 484-9.

[95] Estourgie SH, Nieweg OE, Valdes Olmos RA, Hoefnagel CA, Kroon BB. Review and
      evaluation of sentinel node procedures in 250 melanoma patients with a median fol-
      low-up of 6 years. Ann Surg Oncol 2003; 10: 681-8.

[96] Santinami M, Carbone A, Crippa F et al. Radical dissection after positive groin senti-
      nel biopsy in melanoma patients: rate of further positive nodes. Melanoma Res 2009;
      19: 112-8.

[97] Spillane AJ, Haydu L, McMillan W, Stretch JR, Thompson JF. Quality assurance pa-
      rameters and predictors of outcome for ilioinguinal and inguinal dissection in a con-
      temporary melanoma patient population. Ann Surg Oncol 2011; 18: 2521-8.

[98] Chu CK, Delman KA, Carlson GW, Hestley AC, Murray DR. Inguinopelvic lympha-
      denectomy following positive inguinal sentinel lymph node biopsy in melanoma:
      true frequency of synchronous pelvic metastases. Ann Surg Oncol 2011; 18: 3309-15.

[99]   van der Ploeg IM, Valdes Olmos RA, Kroon BB, Nieweg OE. Tumor-positive sentinel node biopsy of the groin in clinically node-negative melanoma patients: superficial or superficial and deep lymph node dissection? Ann Surg Oncol 2008; 15: 1485-91.

[100] Pearlman NW, Robinson WA, Dreiling LK, McIntyre RC, Jr., Gonzales R. Modified ilioinguinal node dissection for metastatic melanoma. Am J Surg 1995; 170: 647-9; discussion 9-50.

[101] Spiess PE, Hernandez MS, Pettaway CA. Contemporary inguinal lymph node dissection: minimizing complications. World J Urol 2009; 27: 205-12.

[102] Chang SB, Askew RL, Xing Y et al. Prospective assessment of postoperative complications and associated costs following inguinal lymph node dissection (ILND) in melanoma patients. Ann Surg Oncol 2010; 17: 2764-72.

[103] Hughes TM, Thomas JM. Combined inguinal and pelvic lymph node dissection for stage III melanoma. Br J Surg 1999; 86: 1493-8.

[104] Ravi R. Morbidity following groin dissection for penile carcinoma. Br J Urol 1993; 72: 941-5.

[105] Karakousis CP, Driscoll DL. Groin dissection in malignant melanoma. Br J Surg 1994; 81: 1771-4.

[106] Beitsch P, Balch C. Operative morbidity and risk factor assessment in melanoma patients undergoing inguinal lymph node dissection. Am J Surg 1992; 164: 462-5; discussion 5-6.

[107] Sabel MS, Griffith KA, Arora A et al. Inguinal node dissection for melanoma in the era of sentinel lymph node biopsy. Surgery 2007; 141: 728-35.

[108] Karakousis CP. Therapeutic node dissections in malignant melanoma. Semin Surg Oncol 1998; 14: 291-301.

[109] Spillane AJ, Tucker M, Pasquali S. A pilot study reporting outcomes for melanoma patients of a minimal access ilio-inguinal dissection technique based on two incisions. Ann Surg Oncol 2011; 18: 970-6.

[110] Delman KA, Kooby DA, Rizzo M, Ogan K, Master V. Initial experience with videoscopic inguinal lymphadenectomy. Ann Surg Oncol 2011; 18: 977-82.

[111] Ising IM, Bembenek A, Gutzmer R, Kockerling F, Moesta KT. Enhanced postoperative lymphatic staging of malignant melanoma by endoscopically assisted iliacoinguinal dissection. Langenbecks Arch Surg 2012; 397: 429-36.

[112] Nakamura Y, Fujisawa Y, Maruyama H, Furuta J, Kawachi Y, Otsuka F. Intraoperative mapping with isosulfan blue of lymphatic leakage during inguinal lymph node dissection (ILND) for skin cancer for the prevention of postoperative lymphocele. J Surg Oncol 2011; 104: 657-60.

[113] Lee RJ, Gibbs JF, Proulx GM, Kollmorgen DR, Jia C, Kraybill WG. Nodal basin recur-
       rence following lymph node dissection for melanoma: implications for adjuvant radi-
       otherapy. Int J Radiat Oncol Biol Phys 2000; 46: 467-74.

[114] Ballo MT, Strom EA, Zagars GK et al. Adjuvant irradiation for axillary metastases
       from malignant melanoma. Int J Radiat Oncol Biol Phys 2002; 52: 964-72.

[115] Ballo MT, Bonnen MD, Garden AS et al. Adjuvant irradiation for cervical lymph
       node metastases from melanoma. Cancer 2003; 97: 1789-96.

[116] Ballo MT, Zagars GK, Gershenwald JE et al. A critical assessment of adjuvant radio-
       therapy for inguinal lymph node metastases from melanoma. Ann Surg Oncol 2004;
       11: 1079-84.

[117] Ballo MT, Ross MI, Cormier JN et al. Combined-modality therapy for patients with
       regional nodal metastases from melanoma. Int J Radiat Oncol Biol Phys 2006; 64:
       106-13.

[118] Burmeister BH, Mark Smithers B, Burmeister E et al. A prospective phase II study of
       adjuvant postoperative radiation therapy following nodal surgery in malignant mel-
       anoma-Trans Tasman Radiation Oncology Group (TROG) Study 96.06. Radiother
       Oncol 2006; 81: 136-42.

[119] Agrawal S, Kane JM, 3rd, Guadagnolo BA, Kraybill WG, Ballo MT. The benefits of
       adjuvant radiation therapy after therapeutic lymphadenectomy for clinically ad-
       vanced, high-risk, lymph node-metastatic melanoma. Cancer 2009; 115: 5836-44.

Chapter 9

Management of Acral Lentiginous Melanoma

Yoshitaka Kai and Sakuhei Fujiwara

Additional information is available at the end of the chapter

1. Introduction

Cutaneous malignant melanoma is the most common cause of mortality from skin cancers in Caucasian populations. The incidence rates of malignant melanoma show considerable variation worldwide. Annual incidence rates per 100,000 people vary between about 40 in Australia and New Zealand to about 20 in the United States [1,2]. In contrast, a significantly lower incidence rate has been reported in Asian populations with rates of 0.65 to 1/100,000 [3-5]. In addition, the most common sites of melanoma occurrence in Asians are the extremities at a rate of about 50% of all cases [6,7], compared to only 2-3% in Caucasian populations [8].

In 1976, RJ Reed first described the fourth variant of melanoma as "pigmented lesions on the extremities, particularly on palmoplantar regions, that are characterized by a lentiginous (radial) growth phase evolving over months or years to a dermal (vertical) invasive stage" [9]. He named this anatomical subgroup of melanoma as "plantar lentiginous melanoma (PLM) ", which had a characteristic lentiginous, radial component of melanocytic proliferation and mentioned for the first time that this subgroup was the most common in Blacks and the very poor prognosis group [10].

In 1986, malignant melanoma was classified into four subtypes by Clark et al. according to histological features; nodular melanoma (NM), superficial spreading melanoma (SSM), lentigo maligna melanoma (LMM) and acral lentiginous melanoma (ALM) [11]. In the United States, the incidence rates of SSM, NM, LMM and ALM are approximately 70%, 15%, 13% and 2-3% respectively [12,13]. Although, ALM is the most common expression of malignant melanoma in Asian and Black populations, the rate of ALM is 41% in Japan [14], 65% in Korea [15] and 62% in the American Blacks [16].

The prognosis of each subtype differs due to delayed diagnosis rather than an actual differences in the biological nature of tumour and the prognosis of ALM is generally poorer than other subtypes [17]. The lesion, especially on soles and nail beds, is likely to be overlooked by patients. Moreover, Metzger et al. found that ALM had a high likelihood of being clinically mis-diagnosed as a benign melanocytic lesion, which leads to a delay in the initiation of treatment [18]. However, this report was made in the pre-dermoscopic era and now it has become much easier with dermoscopy to distinguish the early stage of ALM from a benign lesion.

Human extremities, especially palms and soles, are not exposed to ultraviolet light and there is no evidence of overexposure to UV light as a risk factor of ALM [19]. In contrast, UV light plays an important role in the pathogenesis of LMM.

In 2005, Bastian et al. proposed new classification of melanoma according to genetic altera-tions at different sites. They classified melanoma into four distinct groups, each of which has a different degree of exposure to UV light: chronic sun-damaged melanoma (CSD) which nearly corresponds to LMM, non-CSD melanoma which also corresponds to SSM, acral mel-anoma (AM) which also corresponds to ALM, and mucosal melanoma [20]. They found that 81% of non-CSD melanoma had mutations in BRAF or N-RAS and the other groups had no mutations in either gene. Otherwise, melanoma with wild-type BRAF or N-RAS frequently had an increase in the number of copies of the genes for cyclin-dependent kinase 4 (CDK4) and cyclin D1 (CCND1). Furthermore, a recent study showed that AM and mucosal melano-ma had frequent mutation or amplification of the KIT gene [21]. Although these findings have led to molecular targeted therapy today, this new therapeutic approach has just begun and therefore we will only touch upon these new directions.

Today, there are some difficulties and controversies in the treatment of ALM caused by the anatomical and biological specificity of ALM. The standardized treatment of ALM is not easy to establish due to the unique characteristics. This chapter includes our experiences and a review of the literature focusing on the surgical treatment of ALM, and in particular, dis-cusses the controversies surrounding the treatment of ALM.

Clinical presentation and dermoscopic findings of ALM

ALM occurs more frequently on lower extremities than on upper extremities. In our insti-tute, 41 cases of all 61 ALM cases occurred on lower extremities. The soles of the feet are the most frequent sites of ALM, where 56% of ALM on lower extremities occurred. In contrast, most frequent sites on upper extremities are fingernails, where 45% of ALM on upper ex-tremities appeared.

Clinically, ALMs begin with pale brown macules, enlarge slowly and form irregularly pig-mented, asymmetric macular lesions with notching at the periphery over the years. After that, nodules appear on the pigmented lesion and form ulceration. In the past ALM was considered to occur from benign malanocytic lesions, however, de novo synthesis in major cases of ALM has been confirmed by dermoscopic findings (see below). Due to the very slow progress, it tends to be overlooked and even when the tumour becomes larger, it is easily underestimated.

Histologically, "(1) the radial growth phase consists of lentiginous dysplastic melanocytes, extending along the basal cell layer, with extension of single atypical melanocytes up into the thickened epidermis; (2) the vertical growth phase usually consists of a progressive central plaque-like thickening of malignant cells in the papillary dermis, with (3) extension of the spindle cells into the deeper levels, accompanied by prominent dysplasia; (4) there is epidermal hyperplasia with elongation of the rete ridges and acanthosis and central ulceration; and (5) host immune response is active, with areas of tumor regression" [22].

	Location	Case Number (%)
	Thigh	1 (1.6)
	Lower leg	6 (9.8)
	Dorsum of foot	1 (1.6)
Lower extremities	Sole	23 (37.7)
	Toe	8 (13.1)
	Toenail	2 (3.3)
	Total	41
	Upper arm	0 (0)
	Forearm	1 (1.6)
	Dorsum of Hand	1 (1.6)
Upper extremities	Palm	4 (6.6)
	Finger	4 (6.6)
	Fingernail	9 (14.8)
	Total	19
Unknown		1 (1.6)
Total		61 (100)

Table 1. Primary sites of cutaneous melanoma experienced in our institute from 2004 to 2011

Dermoscopic observations help the diagnosis in the early stage of ALM. In 66 cases of volar skin melanomas, irregular diffuse pigmentation (60%) with variable shades from tan to black without parallel disposition of pigment (figure 1a) and the parallel ridge pattern (53%) with pigmentation along the ridges (figure 1b) were the two most prevalent patterns [23]. According to Saida et al., the sensitivity and specificity of the parallel ridge pattern in diagnosing all melanoma on volar skins were 86% and 99% respectively and those of irregular diffuse pigmentation were 85% and 97% respectively. Only in diagnosing melanoma in situ on volar skin, the sensitivity of parallel ridge pattern (86%) was significantly higher than that of irregular diffuse pigmentation (69%) [24]. A parallel furrow pattern with pigmentation along the furrows (figure 1c) and a lattice-like pattern with longitudinal and transversal thicker lines surrounding the eccrine pores (figure 1d) are more common in melanocytic nevi. The sensitivity and specificity of a parallel furrow pattern or lattice-like pattern in diagnosing melanocytic nevi were 67% and 93% respectively [24].

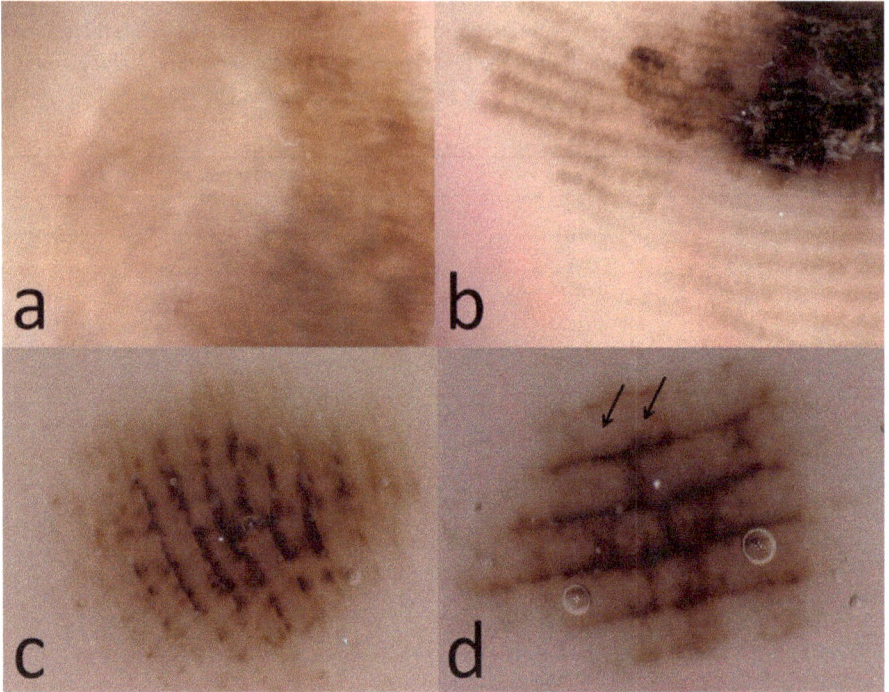

Figure 1. Dermoscopy of early stage ALM (a,b) and melanocytic nevi (c,d). (a) Irregular diffuse pigmentation, (b) parallel ridge pattern, (c) parallel furrow pattern, (d) lattice-like pattern with longitudinal and transversal thicker lines surrounding the eccrine pores (arrows).

Ulceration on nodules following pigmented macules reveals a polymorphous vascular pattern with a combination of milky-red areas (95%) which are larger areas of fuzzy or unfocused milky-red colour corresponding to an elevated part of the lesion, linear irregular vessels (49%), dotted vessels (43%) and hairpin vessels (41%) [25].

2. Subungual melanoma

The incidence of subungual melanoma also has a racial difference. It is more frequent in Asian and Blacks than in Caucasians. Its frequency has been reported to be approximately 2-4% in all cutaneous melanomas in Caucasians and 10% in Japanese [26]. Of the 108 subungual melanomas in Japan, the cases involving fingers and toes were 76% and 24% respectively. On both fingers and toes, the thumb and the great toe were the most common sites [26]. Among the subungual melanoma, the occurrence rate of ALM on the fingernail is higher than on toenails. According to the literature, of 64 cases of subungual melanoma, 55% cases occurred on the thumbnail, 27% on the nail of the great toe, 2-4% on the nail of the index, middle and ring finger, 1.6% on the nail of the second toe [27].

It is known that subungual melanoma has a very poor prognosis among all subtypes of cutaneous melanomas. The reason for this is because the majority of subungual melanomas are already been quite deep when diagnosed [28]. Delayed diagnosis of subungual melanoma is common because it is very difficult to distinguish the early stage of subungual melanoma from longitudinal melanonychia. According to Cohen et al., 38 of 43 patients (88%) had delayed diagnosis and the median delay time was 24 months (range 4 to 132) [29].

Subungual melanomas begin with fine pigmented striata which could not be clinically distinguished from benign longitudinal melanonychia at an early stage and grow wider with colour variegation and the presence of nail plate fissuring or splitting eventually forming a triangular shape which has a broader proximal lesion rather than a distal lesion, blurred lateral borders and Hutchinson's sign - indicating the peripheral pigmentation beyond the nail apparatus [30].

Baran et al. mentioned the clinical clues to the diagnosis of subungual melanoma in detail. Hutchinson's sign is the most important sign of subungual melanoma. Other clues are when longitudinal melanonychia (a) begins in a single digit of a person over six decades or more, (b) develops abruptly in a previous normal nail plate, (c) becomes suddenly darker or wider, (d) occurs in either the thumb, index finger or giant toe, (e) is accompanied by nail destruction or disappearance, (f) has colour variegation, (g) has a wide band and so on [31].

In addition to these clinical clues, dermoscopy provides useful information for the diagnosis of subungual melanoma. The prominent dermoscopic features of subungual melanoma are brown pigmentation of the background with longitudinal brown to black lines which are irregular in their colouration, spacing, thickness and parallelism [32]. This irregularity was significantly associated with melanoma when compared with all other benign diseases. The micro-Hutchinson's sign is the suspicious dermoscopic feature, which consists of the irregular lines in the cuticle area and can be observed only on dermoscopy [32,33].

Since the early stage of subungual melanoma has minimal histopathological change, it may be difficult to distinguish subungual melanoma from benign lesion with only histopathological findings. Thus, both clinical features, including present history and histopathological findings, are necessary for diagnosis.

We propose a diagnostic algorithm for the early stage of subungual melanoma (figure 2). When a case falls under any of the clinical features mentioned above (a-g), dermoscopic examination is recommended. If Hutchinson's sign and colour change in overall nail to dark black are present, excisional biopsy is recommended. When those characteristic appearances are absent, but a nail streak has irregularity, biopsy is also recommended. On the contrary, when nail streaks are monotonous pale brown, subungual melanoma is not suspicious. Even if a streak is dark brown or black, no irregularity of lines on dermoscopy allows careful follow-up without biopsies. If the streak increases in width or has colour variegation during a period of follow-up, the necessity of excision or biopsy should be discussed according to further dermoscopic examination.

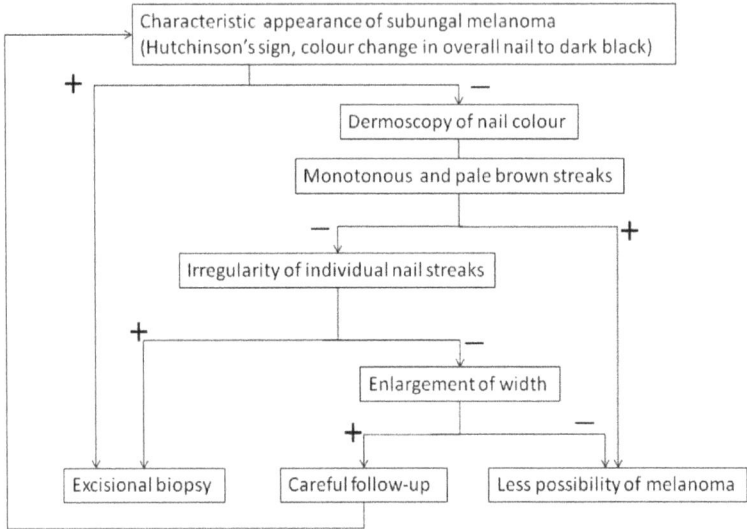

Figure 2. Diagnostic algorithm for early stage subungual melanoma.

Since nail biopsies cause cosmetic problems, biopsy methods should be selected as follows. If streaks are more likely to be melanoma, complete excisional biopsies are desirable. If it is less likely, punch biopsies around the origin of the longitudinal melanonychia (which is frequently located on the nail matrix) can be chosen. When excisional biopsies are performed, we should keep in mind that an insufficient margin at the proximal side of the nail may cause incision in between the lesional nail matrix without including the whole lesion. Ultrasound echography provides useful information on the location of the nail matrix [34], so that a sufficient margin can be ensured. Furthermore, it is desirable that extent of the excisional biopsy includes the periosteum of the distal phalanx. Since the distance between the nail matrix and bone is extremely close at the proximal side, excisional biopsies excluding periosteum may incise the nail matrix and leave some lesion on the body. Excisional biopsies including the periosteum causes very little disadvantage compared with those excluding the periosteum and afterwards good granulation tissue will be formed on the bone when the artificial dermis is used. If it is histopathologically diagnosed as subungual melanoma, a local wide excision is selected, excluding the case when a sufficient margin is ensured at the previous excisional biopsy.

Excisional biopsies in a good manner allow us to determine correct tumour thickness, which provides important information on the choice of SLNB, local wide excision and chemotherapy. However, biopsy specimens easily break down if the biopsy procedure for histological examination is not performed well, which may cause incorrect choices for treatment.

If nail destruction is present under diagnosis of subungual melanoma, amputation of the distal phalanx will be applied on the assumption that the lesion invades the periosteum or bone. However, not all cases of nail destruction are accompanied with invasion. Some cases of nail destruction may be melanomas in situ. Since the distance between nail bed and bone is wider at the distal side than at the proximal side, the possibility of avoiding amputation is higher when the nail destruction is modest and located at the distal side of the nail.

Moehrle et al. proposed 'functional' surgery for subungual melanoma, by which the amputation of the distal phalanx could be avoided and the more digital function could be preserved [35]. The tumour was surgically removed with measurable excision margins and a partial resection of the distal part of the distal phalanx was performed with a Luer instrument. After the resection, three-dimensional histology was performed as described in the literature [36]. Two of 31 patients had local recurrence after this operation. This method did not lead to shorter survival when compared to amputation, thus, it is worth considering.

3. Wide local excision

According to a review of the literature on the margins of radical excision for melanomas thinner than 2mm, the French Cooperative Group Trial [37] and the Scandinavian Melanoma Group Study [38] compared 2cm with 5cm margins and the World Health Organization (WHO) Melanoma Program Trial 10 [39] compared 1cm with 3cm margins. All three trials demonstrated no benefits for wider margins.

Although a 5mm margin for melanoma in situ is frequently recommended in some national guidelines, Kunishige et al. demonstrated that 86% of 1120 melanomas in situ were successfully excised with a 6mm margin and 98.9% with a 9mm margin. They concluded that a 6mm margin for melanomas in situ was inadequate and a 9mm margin was necessary [40].

A 1cm margin of excision has been proposed for melanomas less than 1mm thick and a wider margin for more than 1mm thick [41,42]. Although many national guidelines recommend that a 1 cm margin is appropriate for 1-2mm thick invasive melanoma, this is less clear because there has been very little data indicating that a 1cm margin for 1-2mm thick melanoma is safer than 2cm margin [43]. For more than 2mm thick melanomas, a 2cm margin is considered to be sufficient in almost all cases. Depth of excision has been recommended to be at least the level of muscle fascia and deeper excision under it has not been shown to improve outcome [43-45].

For melanomas on the extremities, especially on fingers, amputation impairs the function. Thus, even if finger amputation is necessary, it is desirable that the defect is smaller so that functional impairment can be minimal. Detailed histopathological examination of resected specimens may allow surgeons to excise a smaller part of the fingers. We show the pathological specimen as illustrated on Figure 3. Because the resected margins are usually intricately curved, the specimen is divided into several parts so that a marginal side of each part becomes planar and paraffin sections can be made so that the whole surface of the marginal side can be examined. This technique provides highly accurate detection of continuous lesions with a small possibility of missing skip lesions. If the margin is negative, additional excision is not necessary and that provides preservation of more digital functions.

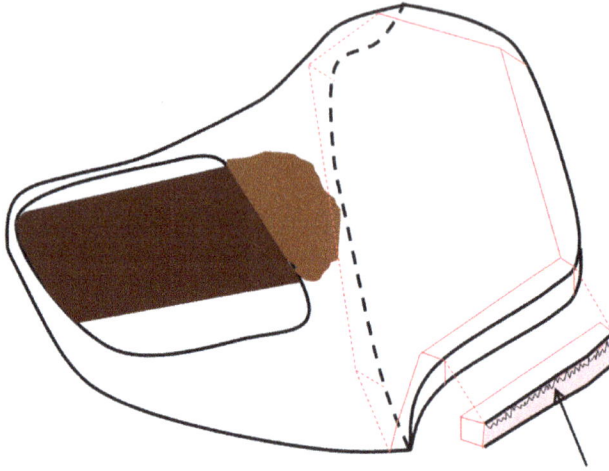

Figure 3. How to make pathological specimen of an amputated finger tip was illustrated. In order to examine the tumor cells at the marginal side accurately and continuously, curved rim of the excised margin was cut as linear as possible, and the outside of the margin is examined. (arrow)

4. Sentinel lymph node biopsy

Sentinel lymph node biopsy (SLNB) has become the standard procedure used to determine whether a tumour has metastasized to lymph nodes and more accurate staging of the melanoma. It is a less invasive technique than lymph node dissection allowing patients with node negative (N0) melanoma to avoid unnecessary lymph node dissection. In the case of SLN positive melanoma, additional surgery of lymph node dissection is necessary.

The false-negative rate in SLN mapping for melanoma has been reported to be very low with a rate of 0 to 2 % [46-49]. The multicenter selective lymphadenectomy trial-1 (MSLT-1) demonstrated immediate lymph node dissection following microscopic positive node at SLNB could bring about better prognosis than the lymph node dissection after clinical nodal observation [50].

For more correct mapping of SLNs, a combination of blue dye and radioisotope ^{99m}Tc labelled phytate is generally used. SLNs are identified by the presence of blue stained lymph vessels and lymph nodes, and the radioactivity measured by gamma probe. Furthermore, distinction between SLNs and secondary non-SLNs is achieved by using pre-operative dynamic cutaneous lymphoscintigraphy [51].

Although most melanomas drain to conventional regional nodes, unexpected drainage outside of these basins is observed in some cases. Pre-operative lymphscintigraphy and a hand-held gamma probe are required for detection of these interval SLNs. According to a single-institution study in Japan, SLNs were identified in 253 nodal basins from 117 patients and interval SLNs were found in six patients. They recognized 41 (17%) SLN metastases in 246 conventional nodal basins and one (14%) in seven interval SLNs [52].

5. Sentinel lymph node biopsy on upper extremities

Tumours on upper extremities almost always drain to the axillary region. The axillary region is divided into three parts based on the pectoralis minor. Level 1, 2 and 3 are located lateral, deep and medial to the pectoralis minor respectively. Outside this conventional region, SLNs are recognized in the cubital region and other areas. Figure 4 is the local sites of SLNs in our experience of 10 cases.

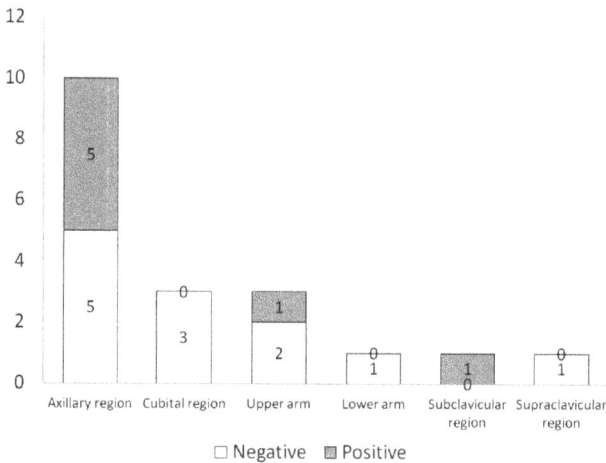

Figure 4. The sites of SLNs in primary melanomas on upper extremities.

SLNs were identified in all 10 cases (100%) for the axillary region, three cases (30%) for the cubital region, three cases (30%) for the upper arm, one case (10%) for the forearm, one case (10%) for the subclavicular region (level 3) and one case (10%) for the supraclavicular region. In all 10 cases, SLNs were present in anatomic level 1 of the axillary region. Although it has been considered that there is very little chance of finding SLNs in level 3, one case with SLN in level 3 was present in our data.

SLNs between the primary lesion and the axillary region are regarded as interval nodes on the upper extremities. Manganomi et al. reported that the interval SLN identification rate on upper extremities was 0.4% (two out of 480 cases) [53] and Kelly et al. reported 3.8% (16 out of 423 cases) [54]. Cubital region is the most common site of interval SLN on upper extremities. In our 3 cases of interval SLNs identified in cubital region, those were present on cubital fossa and on ulnar side of cubital region. We have experienced five cases of other interval region rather than cubital region.

Tumours on upper extremities rarely drain to the subclavicular region (level 3) rather than to level 1 or 2. Our case with SLNs on the subclavicular region had positive with non-positive SLNs in level 11 and no SLNs in level 2 (Figure 5).

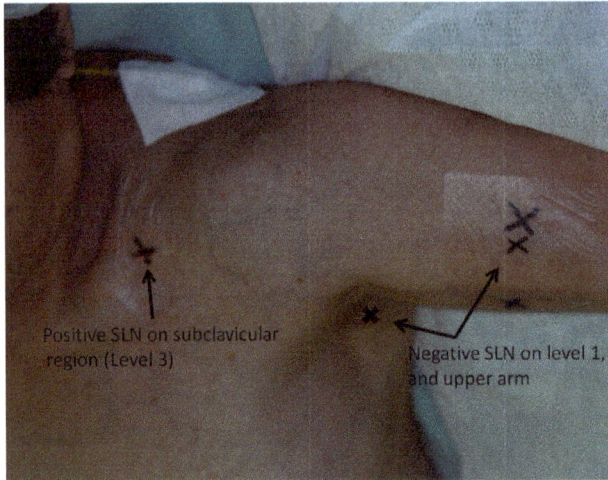

Figure 5. The case with positive SLN in level 3 and non-positive SLNs in level 1 and the upper arm. This metastatic pattern is extremely rare.

There may be cases where it is uncertain whether or not SLNB should be applied when tumour thickness is unknown. Some literature demonstrated that the patients with primary lesions on their extremities have a lower risk of misidentification of SLNs, even after wide local excision, than patients with axial primary lesions [55-59]. Tumors on central trunk may drain to both bilateral, or both axillary and inguinal regions. By contrast, tumours on extremities tend to drain more simply to the expected region. Although it is preferable that wide local excision and SLNB are performed at the same time, SLNB after wide local excision is less disruptive to lymphatic drainage in the case of primary lesions on the extremities than on axial sites.

6. Sentinel lymph node biopsy on lower extremities

In almost all cases, tumours on lower extremities drain to the inguinal region. Figure 6 demonstrates lymphatic drainage for 23 cases with tumours on lower extremities in our institute. Of all 23 cases, the lymph node identification rate was 23 cases (100%) for the inguinal region, five cases (21%) for the popliteal region and 10 cases (43%) for the pelvic region (nine cases for external iliac lymph nodes and one case for the obturator region). Three of the 23 cases with SLN on the inguinal region had positive nodes and there were no positive nodes on the popliteal and pelvic region.

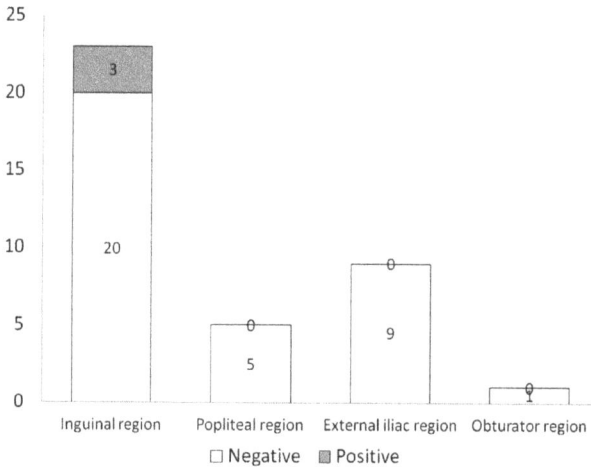

Figure 6. The sites of SLNs in primary melanomas on lower extremities.

One of the problems with SLNB of lower extremities is the presence of pelvic SLNs. Kaoutzanis et al. showed 11 of 82 cases with tumour on lower extremities had SLNs on the pelvic region and underwent SLNB [60]. They also showed that 19 of 82 cases (24%) had positive SLNs and all the positive SLNs were located in the inguinal region. No positive SLNs were present in the pelvic region as our cases.

Even in SLNB, removing the lymph nodes in the external iliac and obturator region is a relatively invasive technique. It is still controversial whether or not SLNs in the pelvic region should be harvested because SLNs in the pelvic region may be considered as secondary or third lymphatic basin, even when radioisotope is accumulated in pelvic lymph nodes.

Even now there is no consensus on the clinical definition of an SLN [61]. The SLN has been described as the hottest node, the blue node, first node visualized on lymphoscintigraphy and a node with radioactivity greater than twice or three times background radioactivity [61-63]. McMaster et al. recommended that all blue nodes and all nodes that measure 10% or higher of the 'ex vivo' radioactive count of hottest SLNs should be removed in order to decrease false-negative cases [64]. In our institute, SLN is defined as the node which showed higher than one tenth of the radioactivity of the hottest node. Because radioactivity depends on the distance from the surface of skin to the nodes, the measured radioactivity of the pelvic lymph nodes from the surface of skin is much less than superficial lymph nodes and tends to be underestimated [65]. Therefore, Bagaria et al. provided an answer that the background radioactivity of the regional nodal basin was measured before incision and all blue nodes and all hot nodes that have radioactivity greater than the background were harvested [61]. According to Soteldo et al., the rate of the cases that had metastasized lymph nodes in the pelvic region after SLNB that had indicated non-positive SLNs in the inguinal region was 2.4% [65]. This indicated that there might be cases with positive lymph nodes in the pelvic region with non-positive lymph nodes in the inguinal region. This rate should not be underestimated and gives a reason for removing SLNs in the pelvic region.

On the other hand, there have been no published results of positive pelvic lymph nodes with negative inguinal SLNs for melanoma located below the knee. Pelvic lymph nodes for melanoma located below the knee were considered as secondary lymphatic basin because they were not stained blue and the radioactivity of the pelvic lymph nodes was significantly less than that of the inguinal nodes removed from the same patients [66]. By contrast, the pelvic lymph nodes for melanoma located on the trunk and thigh are possibly SLNs. In the case of melanoma below the knee in which there is a risk or difficulty in removing the pelvic lymph nodes, for example the case of pelvic adhesion after surgery in the pelvis, SLNB could be clinically avoided in terms of the cost-benefit relationship.

There are two approaches to removing the pelvic lymph nodes. One is the technique with incision above the inguinal ligament and the other is the technique with median incision in the lower abdomen. Each technique has an advantage. With median incision, it is easier to approach a deep site in the pelvic region such as the obturator area or the external iliac region near to the common iliac region. By contrast, it is easier and less invasive to approach the external iliac region near to the inguinal ligament with an incision above the inguinal ligament.

7. Lymph node dissection

Lymph node dissection is the primary management for regional lymph node metastasis. It is applied in cases of clinical metastasis, positive SLNs after SLNB and histological lymphatic invasion for a resected or biopsied primary lesion. Surgical technique, extent of dissection, morbidity and complication vary widely in the published literature. Although lymph node dissection has been a standard treatment and the technique has not drastically changed for many years, even now there is much controversy surrounding lymph node dissection. Some of the controversies will be mentioned in the following section.

8. Axillary lymph node dissection

Since the tumours on upper extremities drain to the axillary region, axillary dissection is necessary and performed by way of cure or local control of the metastatic melanoma in the upper extremities. On the area of axillary dissection, it is controversial whether a level 3 dissection should be included. Namm et al. reported that the local recurrence rate of axillary dissection including level 1 and 2was 5 % (14 cases out of 270 cases) [67]. Guggenheim et al. also reported a rate of 4.5% after axillary dissection which mainly included level 1 and 2 [68]. On the other hand, according to Kretschmer et al., the local recurrence rate was 9.5% (six out of 63 cases) after dissection including level 1,2 and 3. There is no direct evidence that dissection including level 3 is superior to dissection without level 3 [69].

The complication rate of dissection for level 1and 2 is less severe than that of dissection for level 1,2 and 3. The rates of infection and seroma after the former operation were 8% and 2% respectively, whereas those for the latter operation were 20% and 18% [67,70].

There are very few reported cases in which positive SLNs in level 3 were harvested except for our case. In addition, the lymph node ratio (LNR: the ratio of involved lymph nodes to total retrieved nodes in lymph node dissection) provides prognostic information [71-73]. There is very little possibility that positive lymph nodes are harvested only in level 3 without positive SLNs in level 1 or 2. Although there is data not on upper extremities but on lower extremities, a larger number of cases involved lymph nodes in the inguinal region with a higher rate of pelvic lymph node metastases [74]. This indicates that the number of superficial involved lymph nodes is related to the possibility of metastasis in the deep region. It has been reported that the size of SLN metastases predicts other nodal disease and survival in malignant melanoma [75,76]. Due to these findings, axillary dissection including level 3 is not always necessary when there are one or two micrometastatic lymph nodes in level 1, but it is necessary when a case falls under any of the following conditions:

- There is a relatively large clinically involved lymph node in level 1 or 2.

- There are many metastatic lymph nodes in level 1 or 2.

- There is negative SLNs in level 3 with positive lymph nodes in level 1 or 2.

- There are positive SLNs in level 3.

- There are involved lymph nodes in level 3 evaluated with radiological examination such as computed tomography (CT).

9. Inguinal and pelvic lymph node dissection

There is also controversy surrounding inguinal and pelvic lymph node dissection. The most controversial question is whether routine dissection with the primary tumour on lower extremities includes only a superficial inguinal lymph node dissection (SLND) or includes additional iliac and obturator lymph node dissection (deep pelvic/inguinal lymph node dissection : DLND) [77]. Like the axillary dissection, decision on the area to be dissected is difficult from the viewpoint of local control, overall survival and complications.

Hughes et al. reported that in cases of palpable inguinal lymph node metastases, pelvic lymph node recurrence occurred in one of 72 patients who had DLND and seven of 60 patients who had SLND (p=0.01) [74]. In this study, patients with one positive superficial node and those with more than one positive superficial node were 17% and 51% of 72 patients with DLND respectively. The number of positive superficial lymph nodes and the presence of extracapsular spread were significant prognostic factors for overall survival [77].

In addition, the patients who had DLND with the presence of pelvic lymph node metastases had significantly poorer five year survival than the patients without the pelvic lymph node metastases. However, there was no difference in postoperative morbidity between SLND and DLND [74]. Van der Ploeg et al. also reported that survival and local control did not differ for patients with palpable inguinal metastases treated by DLND or SLND and pelvic lymph node metastases was a significant prognostic factor [78]. In their series of 169 patients with palpable nodes in the inguinal region, five year estimated overall survival rates were 33% for DLND and 29% for SLND.

However, there is no evidence on how the recurrence affects quality of life when DLND is not performed and how the recurrence occurs in the pelvic region for melanomas on lower extremities. It is likely that enlargement of a tumour in pelvic region causes lymphedema, congestion of lower extremities, ileus and so on. Although these symptoms may be due to DLND, also it is possible that DLND increases patients' quality of life during the remaining life time by decreasing the risk of recurrence in the pelvic region. However, there is no evidence indicating this.

Cloquet's node is an indicator of pelvic lymph node metastases. According to Shen et al.'s study, positive pelvic lymph nodes were identified in the DLND specimen from 20 of 30 (67%) patients with a positive Cloquet's node and negative pelvic lymph nodes were identified from 27 of 35 (77%) patients with a negative Cloquet's node (p=0.0019) [79].

Pre-operative computed tomography (CT) is also a good tool to use in predicting the metastasis. Out of 44 patients with negative pelvic lymph nodes evaluated with pre-operative CT, 40 patients had in fact histologically negative pelvic lymph nodes (negative predictive value = 90.9%). On the other hand, the positive predictive value of pre-operative CT for pelvic metastases, was 59% [78].

A recent study shows pre-operative lymphoscintigraphy can be used to guide the extent of inguinal lymph node dissection [66]. Chu et al. reported on 42 cases of DLND with positive inguinal SLNs. The frequency of synchronous pelvic disease was five of 42 (11.9%) [80]. All five cases with pelvic disease had primary melanomas on extremities. Upon review on the lymphoscintigraphic findings, pelvic drainage was present in four of five cases with pelvic disease (80%) and in 18 of the 32 cases (56%) without pelvic disease, though neither was statistically significant. This strategy is based on the idea that when lymphoscintigraphy shows secondary nodes to be located in the next drainage basin, this basin should be included as the dissecting area [66]. More data is necessary to prove that treatment based on the idea improves the mortality and local control.

For now, there is no guideline on choosing between SLND and DLND. However, many findings provide useful information and surgeons should actively select DLND when a case falls under any of the following conditions:

- There is a palpable inguinal metastasis.
- There is more than one superficial lymph node metastasis.
- CT indicates metastatic pelvic lymph nodes.
- There is a Cloquet's lymph node metastasis.
- Lymphoschintigraphy indicates SLNs in the pelvic region with a superficial lymph node metastasis.

10. Molecular targeted therapy

Recent discoveries in cell signalling have provided greater understanding of the biology that underlines melanoma and these advances are being exploited to provide targeted drugs and new therapeutic approaches [81]. In some cases of ALM and mucosal melanoma, the mutations of KIT, a transmenbrane receptor tyrosine kinase, are reported and these mutations lead to marked expression of KIT in tumour cells. These cases have marked a tendency to respond to imatinib mesylate which inhibits tyrosine kinase. Although case reports are accumulating [82,83], more data, including long-term control and prognostic data, will be necessary to confirm the effect of this agent.

11. Conclusion

Controversies remain regarding the surgical treatment of ALM as described above, thus, international guidelines are yet to be established.

It is not still known whether the thickness of the nail tumour is the same as that on other sites because the distance between the nail bed and bone is very narrow and a mild degree of invasion can reach the bone easily. Considering the poor prognosis of cases with subungual melanoma, the tumour thickness of the subungual melanoma needs to be evaluated. Because biopsies of the nail bed may cause cosmetic and occasionally functional problems, surgeons may hesitate to do biopsies and lose a vital chance of early diagnosis. Suspicious lesions should be actively biopsied with fully informed consent. When taking a wait-and-see approach, careful observation is necessary so as not to overlook any minor change of dermoscopic findings.

On the excision margins around the primary lesion, 2cm is regarded as sufficient for invasive melanomas. Although some guidelines suggest a 0.5 cm margin for melanomas in situ, some data indicated that resection with 0.5 cm margin caused significant high rates of local recurrence. As mentioned here according to the report, a 1cm surgical margin is a better answer for melanomas in situ, except for tumours on cosmetic or functional sites such as the face or fingers. When an excision margin is less than 1cm, more careful histological examination and follow-up are necessary.

Although SLNB is the standard technique for the management of malignant melanoma, the definition of SLN itself has not been established. This creates differences in the extent of SLNB between each institute. SLNs in patients with melanomas on upper extremities are very rarely located in level 3. There are very few cases with positive SLNs only in level 3 without positive SLNs in level 1or 2, thus, the lymph nodes in level 3 can be regarded as secondary nodes for melanomas on upper extremities in almost all cases. Surgeons should also pay additional attention to SLNs in other sites such as supraclavicular, the cubital region and interval nodes.

There is controversy around the management of lymph nodes in the pelvic region. According to the literature, there were patients without positive SLNs in the inguinal region, who had metastatic lymph nodes in the pelvic region during follow-up. Thus, at the moment, it is better not to regard all pelvic lymph nodes as secondary nodes and not to exclude all pelvic lymph nodes from SLNs. There are no reported cases with primary melanomas below the knee in which only positive pelvic lymph nodes are present without positive inguinal lymph nodes. Thus, surgeons should decide whether to harvest pelvic lymph nodes taking into consideration the sites of primary lesion, Brethlow thickness and the possibility of complication on a case by case basis.

Whether or not dissection in cases with primary lesions on upper extremities should include the extent of level 3 is controversial. When a case falls under any of the lists described above, the dissection including level 3 should be actively performed. However, not all cases with positive lymph nodes in level 1 or 2 need to undergo dissection including level 3.

Similarly, it is difficult to choose between SLND and DLND in the case of primary melanomas on lower extremities. The cases which are likely to have metastatic lymph nodes in the pelvic region were mentioned above. It is better that the indication of DLND is determined by referring to the list.

Author details

Yoshitaka Kai and Sakuhei Fujiwara*

*Address all correspondence to: fujiwara@oita-u.ac.jp

Department of Dermatology, Faculty of Medicine, Oita University, Oita, Japan

References

[1] Sneyd M, Cox B. The control of melanoma in New Zealand. New Zealand Medical Journal 2006;119 U2169.

[2] Parkin DM, Bray F, Ferlay J, Pisani P. Global cancer statistics, 2002. CA: A Cancer Journal for Clinicians 2005; 55(2) 74-108

[3] Ishihara K, Saida T, Otsuka F, Yamazaki N; Prognosis and Statistical Investigation Committee of the Japanese Skin Cancer Society. Statistical profiles of malignant melanoma and other skin cancers in Japan: 2007 update. International Journal of Clinical Oncology 2008; 13(1) 33-41.

[4] Makredes M, Hui SK, Kimball AB. Melanoma in Hong Kong between 1983 and 2002: a decreasing trend in incidence observed in a complex socio-political and economic setting. Melanoma Research 2010; 20(5) 427-430.

[5] Chang JW. Cutaneous melanoma: Taiwan experience and literature review. Chang Gung Medical Journal 2010; 33(6) 602-612.

[6] Luk NM, Ho CL, Choi CL, Wong KH, Yu KH, Yeung WK. Clinicopathological features and prognostic factors of cutaneous melanoma among Hong Kong Chinese. Clinical and Experimental Dermatology 2004;29(6) 600-604.

[7] Chen YJ, Wu CY, Chen JT, Shen JL, Chen CC, Wang HC. Clinicopathologic analysis of malignant melanoma in Taiwan. Journal of American Academy of Dermatology 1999;41(6) 945-949.

[8] Bradford PT, Goldstein AM, McMaster ML, Tucker MA. Acral lentiginous melanoma. Incidence and survival patterns in the United States 1986-2005. Archives of Dermatology 2009;145(4) 427-434.

[9] Reed, RJ. New Concepts in Surgical Pathology of the Skin. New York: John Wiley & Sons; 1976.

[10] Reed RJ, Ichinose H, Krementz ET. Plantar lentiginous melanoma: a distinctive variant of human cutaneous malignant melanoma. American Journal of Surgical Pathology 1977;1(2) 131-143.

[11] Clark, W. H., Jr., Elder, D. E. & Van Horn, M. The biologic forms of malignant melanoma. Human Pathology 1986; 17(5) 443-450.

[12] Surveillance, Epidemiology and End Results (SEER) Program. National Cancer Institute, DCCPS,Surveillance Research Program, Cancer Statistics Branch. 2008 SEER*Stat Database. (www.seer.cancer.gov).

[13] Markovic SN, Erickson LA, Rao RD, et al. Malignant Melanoma in the 21st Century, Part 1:Epidemiology, Risk Factors, Screening, Prevention, and Diagnosis. Mayo Clinic Proceedings 2007;82(3) 364-380.

[14] Ishihara, K., Saida, T., Otsuka, F. & Yamazaki, N. Statistical profiles of malignant melanoma and other skin cancers in Japan. International Journal of Clinical Oncology 2007; 13(1) 33-41.

[15] Mi Ryung Roh, Jihyun Kim, and Kee Yang Chung. Treatment and Outcomes of Melanoma in Acral Location in Korean Patients. Yonsei Medical Journal 2010;51(4) 562-568.

[16] Krementz ET, Sutherland CM, Carter RD, Ryan RF. Malignant melanoma in the American Black. Annals of Surgery 1976; 183(5) 533-542.

[17] Paek SC, Sober AJ, Tsao H, Mihm MC Jr, Johnson TM. Cutaneous melanoma. In: Wolff K, Goldsmith LA, Katz SI, Gilchrest BA, Paller AS, Leffell DJ.(ed.) Fitzpatrick's dermatology in general medicine. 7th ed. New York: McGraw-Hill; 2008. p1134-1157.

[18] Metzger S, Ellwanger U, Stroebel W, Schiebel U, Rassner G, Fierlbeck G. Extent and consequences of physician delay in the diagnosis of acral melanoma. Melanoma Research 1998;8(2) 181-186.

[19] Phan A, Touzet S, Dalle S, Ronger-Savlé S, Balme B, Thomas L. Acral lentiginous melanoma: a clinicoprognostic study of 126 cases. British Journal of Dermatology 2006; 155(3) 561-569.

[20] Curtin JA, Fridlyand J, Kageshita T, Patel HN, Busam KJ, Kutzner H, Cho KH, Aiba S, Bröcker EB, LeBoit PE, Pinkel D, Bastian BC. Distinct sets of genetic alterations in melanoma. New England Journal of Medicine 2005; 353(20) 2135-2147.

[21] Curtin JA, Busam K, Pinkel D, Bastian BC. Somatic activation of KIT in distinct subtypes of melanoma. Journal of Clinical Oncology 2006; 24(26) 4340-4346.

[22] Krementz ET, Feed RJ, Coleman WP 3rd, Sutherland CM, Carter RD, Campbell M. Acral lentiginous melanoma. A clinicopathologic entity.Annals of Surgery 1982; 195(5) 632-645.

[23] Phan A, Dalle S, Touzet S, Ronger-Savlé S, Balme B, Thomas L.British Journal of Dermatology 2010; 162(4) 765-771.

[24] Saida T, Miyazaki A, Oguchi S, Ishihara Y, Yamazaki Y, Murase S, Yoshikawa S, Tsuchida T, Kawabata Y, Tamaki K. Archives of Dermatology 2004; 140(10) 1233-1238.

[25] Moloney FJ, Menzies SW. Key points in the dermoscopic diagnosis of hypomelanotic melanoma and nodular melanoma. Journal of Dermatology 2011; 38(1) 10-15.

[26] Miura S, Jimbow K. Clinical characteristics of subungual melanomas in Japan: case report and a questionnaire survey of 108 cases. Journal of Dermatology 1985; 12(5) 393-402.

[27] Seui M, Takematsu H, Hosokawa M, Obata M, Tomita Y, Kato T, Takahashi M, Mihm MC Jr. Acral melanoma in Japan. Journal of Investigative Dermatology 1983; 80(1 Suppl):56s-60s

[28] Patterson RH, Helwig EB. Subungual malignant melanoma: a clinical-pathologic study. Cancer 1980; 46(9) 2074-2087.

[29] Cohen T, Busam KJ, Patel A, Brady MS. Subungual melanoma: management considerations. American Journal of Surgery 2008; 195(2) 244-248.

[30] Di Chiacchio N, Hirata SH, Enokihara MY, Michalany NS, Fabbrocini G, Tosti A. Dermatologists' accuracy in early diagnosis of melanoma of the nail matrix. Archives of Dermatology 2010; 146(4) 382-387.

[31] Baran R, Kechijian P. Longitudinal melanonychia (melanonychia striata): diagnosis and management. Journal of the American Academy of Dermatology 1989; 21(6) 1165-1175.

[32] Ronger S, Touzet S, Ligeron C, Balme B, Viallard AM, Barrut D, Colin C, Thomas L. Dermoscopic examination of nail pigmentation. Archives of Dermatology 2002; 138(10) 1327-1333.

[33] Koga H, Saida T, Uhara H. Key point in dermoscopic differentiation between early nail apparatus melanoma and benign longitudinal melanonychia. Journal of Dermatology 2011; 38(1) 45-52.

[34] Jemec GB, Serup J. Ultrasound structure of the human nail plate. Archives of Dermatology 1989; 125(5) 643-646.

[35] Moehrle M, Metzger S, Schippert W, Garbe C, Rassner G, Breuninger H. "Functional" surgery in subungual melanoma. Dermatologic Surgery 2003; 29(4) 366-374.

[36] Breuninger H, Schlagenhauff B, Stroebel W, Schaumburg-Lever G, Rassner G. Patterns of local horizontal spread of melanomas: consequences for surgery and histopathologic investigation. American Journal of Surgical Pathology 1999; 23(12) 1493-1498.

[37] Khayat D, Rixe O, Martin G, Soubrane C, Banzet M, Bazex JA, Lauret P, Vérola O, Auclerc G, Harper P, Banzet P; French Group of Research on Malignant Melanoma. Surgical margins in cutaneous melanoma (2 cm versus 5 cm for lesions measuring less than 2.1-mm thick). Cancer 2003; 97(8) 1941-1946.

[38] Cohn-Cedermark G, Rutqvist LE, Andersson R, Breivald M, Ingvar C, Johansson H, Jönsson PE, Krysander L, Lindholm C, Ringborg U. Long term results of a randomized study by the Swedish Melanoma Study Group on 2-cm versus 5-cm resection margins for patients with cutaneous melanoma with a tumor thickness of 0.8-2.0 mm. Cancer 2000; 89(7) 1495-1501.

[39] Veronesi U, Cascinelli N, Adamus J, Balch C, Bandiera D, Barchuk A, Bufalino R, Craig P, De Marsillac J, Durand JC, et al. Thin stage I primary cutaneous malignant melanoma. Comparison of excision with margins of 1 or 3 cm. New England Journal of Medicine 1988; 318(18) 1159-1162.

[40] Kunishige JH, Brodland DG, Zitelli JA. Surgical margins for melanoma in situ. Journal of the American Academy of Dermatology 2012; 66(3) 438-444.

[41] Karakousis CP. Surgical treatment of malignant melanoma. Surgical Clinics of North America 1996; 76(6) 1299-1312.

[42] Ng AK, Jones WO, Shaw JH. Analysis of local recurrence and optimizing excision margins for cutaneous melanoma. British Journal of Surgery 2001; 88(1) 137-142.

[43] Testori A, Rutkowski P, Marsden J, Bastholt L, Chiarion-Sileni V, Hauschild A, Eggermont AM. Surgery and radiotherapy in the treatment of cutaneous melanoma. Annals of Oncology 2009; Suppl 6:vi22-29.

[44] Kenady DE, Brown BW, McBride CM. Excision of underlying fascia with a primary malignant melanoma: effect on recurrence and survival rates. Surgery 1982; 92(4) 615-618.

[45] Holmström H. Surgical management of primary melanoma. Seminars in Surgical Oncology 1992; 8(6) 366-369.

[46] Morton DL, Wen DR, Wong JH, Economou JS, Cagle LA, Storm FK, Foshag LJ, Cochran AJ. Technical details of intraoperative lymphatic mapping for early stage melanoma. Archives of Surgery 1992; 127(4) 392-399.

[47] Ross MI, Reintgen D, Balch CM. Selective lymphadenectomy: emerging role for lymphatic mapping and sentinel node biopsy in the management of early stage melanoma. Seminars in Surgical Oncology 1993; 219-223.

[48] Reintgen D, Cruse CW, Wells K, Berman C, Fenske N, Glass F, Schroer K, Heller R, Ross M, Lyman G, et al. The orderly progression of melanoma nodal metastases. Annals of Surgery 1994; 220(6) 759-767.

[49] Thompson JF, McCarthy WH, Bosch CM, O'Brien CJ, Quinn MJ, Paramaesvaran S, Crotty K, McCarthy SW, Uren RF, Howman-Giles R. Sentinel lymph node status as an indicator of the presence of metastatic melanoma in regional lymph nodes.Melanoma Research 1995; 5(4) 255-260.

[50] Morton DL, Thompson JF, Cochran AJ, Mozzillo N, Elashoff R, Essner R, Nieweg OE, Roses DF, Hoekstra HJ, Karakousis CP, Reintgen DS, Coventry BJ, Glass EC, Wang HJ; MSLT Group. Sentinel-node biopsy or nodal observation in melanoma. New England Journal of Medicine 2006; 355(13) 1307-1317.

[51] Morton DL, Cochran AJ, Thompson JF, Elashoff R, Essner R, Glass EC, Mozzillo N, Nieweg OE, Roses DF, Hoekstra HJ, Karakousis CP, Reintgen DS, Coventry BJ, Wang HJ; Multicenter Selective Lymphadenectomy Trial Group. Sentinel node biopsy for early-stage melanoma: accuracy and morbidity in MSLT-I, an international multicenter trial. Annals of Surgery 2005; 242(3) 302-313.

[52] Matsumoto T, Shibata S, Yasue S, Sakakibara A, Yokota K, Sawada M, Kono M, Kato K, Shimoyama Y, Tomita Y. Interval sentinel lymph nodes in patients with cutaneous melanoma: a single-institution study in Japan. Journal of Dermatology 2010; 37(7) 629-634.

[53] Manganoni AM, Farfaglia R, Sereni E, Farisoglio C, Pizzocaro C, Marocolo D, Gavazzoni F, Pavoni L, Calzavara-Pinton P. Interval sentinel lymph nodes: an unusual lo-

calization in patients with cutaneous melanoma. Dermatology Research and Practice 2011; Epub 2011 May 4.

[54] McMasters KM, Chao C, Wong SL, Wrightson WR, Ross MI, Reintgen DS, Noyes RD, Cerrito PB, Edwards MJ; Sunbelt Melanoma Trial Group. Interval sentinel lymph nodes in melanoma. Archives of Surgery 2002; 137(5) 543-9.

[55] Gannon CJ, Rousseau DL Jr, Ross MI, Johnson MM, Lee JE, Mansfield PF, Cormier JN, Prieto VG, Gershenwald JE. Accuracy of lymphatic mapping and sentinel lymph node biopsy after previous wide local excision in patients with primary melanoma. Cancer 2006;107(11) 2647-2652.

[56] Leong SP, Thelmo MC, Kim RP, Gokhale R, Rhee JY, Achtem TA, Morita E, Allen RE Jr, Kashani-Sabet M, Sagebiel RW. Delayed harvesting of sentinel lymph nodes after previous wide local excision of extremity melanoma. Annals of Surgical Oncology 2003; 10(2) 196-200.

[57] Uren RF, Howman-Giles RB, Shaw HM, Thompson JF, McCarthy WH. Lymphoscintigraphy in high-risk melanoma of the trunk: predicting draining node groups, defining lymphatic channels and locating the sentinel node. Journal of Nuclear Medicine 1993; 34(9) 1435-1440.

[58] Sumner WE 3rd, Ross MI, Mansfield PF, Lee JE, Prieto VG, Schacherer CW, Gershenwald JE. Implications of lymphatic drainage to unusual sentinel lymph node sites in patients with primary cutaneous melanoma. Cancer 2002; 95(2) 354-360.

[59] Porter GA, Ross MI, Berman RS, Lee JE, Mansfield PF, Gershenwald JE. Significance of multiple nodal basin drainage in truncal melanoma patients undergoing sentinel lymph node biopsy. Annals of Surgical Oncology 2000; 7(4) 256-261.

[60] Kosmidis C, Efthimiadis C, Anthimidis G, Grigoriou M, Vasiliadou K, Ioannidou G, Makedou F, Baka S. Acral lentiginous melanoma: a case control study and guidelines update. Case Reports in Medicine 2011; Epub 2011 Apr 6.

[61] Bagaria SP, Faries MB, Morton DL. Sentinel node biopsy in melanoma: technical considerations of the procedure as performed at the John Wayne Cancer Institute. Journal of Surgical Oncology 2010; 101(8) 669-676.

[62] Nieweg OE, Tanis PJ, Kroon BB. The definition of a sentinel node. Annals of Surgical Oncology 2001; 8(6) 538-541.

[63] Morton DL, Bostick PJ. Will the true sentinel node please stand?. Annals of Surgical Oncology 1999; 6(1) 12-14.

[64] McMasters KM, Reintgen DS, Ross MI, Wong SL, Gershenwald JE, Krag DN, Noyes RD, Viar V, Cerrito PB, Edwards MJ. Sentinel lymph node biopsy for melanoma: how many radioactive nodes should be removed?. Annals of Surgical Oncology 2001; 8(3) 192-197.

[65] Soteldo J, Ratto EL, Gandini S, Trifirò G, Mazzarol G, Tosti G, Rastrelli M, Verrecchia F, Baldini F, Testori A. Pelvic sentinel lymph node biopsy in melanoma patients: is it worthwhile?. Melanoma Research 2010; 20(2) 133-137.

[66] Kaoutzanis C, Barabás A, Allan R, Hussain M, Powell B. When should pelvic sentinel lymph nodes be harvested in patients with malignant melanoma?. Journal of Plastic, Reconstructive & Aesthetic Surgery 2012; 65(1) 85-90.

[67] Namm JP, Chang AE, Cimmino VM, Rees RS, Johnson TM, Sabel MS. Is a level III dissection necessary for a positive sentinel lymph node in melanoma?. Journal of Surgical Oncology 2012; 105(3) 225-228.

[68] Guggenheim MM, Hug U, Jung FJ, Rousson V, Aust MC, Calcagni M, Künzi W, Giovanoli P. Morbidity and recurrence after completion lymph node dissection following sentinel lymph node biopsy in cutaneous malignant melanoma. Annals of Surgery 2008; 247(4) 687-693.

[69] Kretschmer L, Preusser KP. Standardized axillary lymphadenectomy improves local control but not survival in patients with palpable lymph node metastases of cutaneous malignant melanoma. Langenbeck's Archives of surgery 2001; 386(6) 418-425.

[70] Kretschmer L, Thoms KM, Peeters S, Haenssle H, Bertsch HP, Emmert S. Postoperative morbidity of lymph node excision for cutaneous melanoma-sentinel lymphonodectomy versus complete regional lymph node dissection. Melanoma Research 2008; 18(1) 16-21.

[71] Xing Y, Badgwell BD, Ross MI, Gershenwald JE, Lee JE, Mansfield PF, Lucci A, Cormier JN. Lymph node ratio predicts disease-specific survival in melanoma patients. Cancer 2009; 115(11) 2505-2513.

[72] Spillane AJ, Cheung BL, Winstanley J, Thompson JF. Lymph node ratio provides prognostic information in addition to american joint committee on cancer N stage in patients with melanoma, even if quality of surgery is standardized. Annals of Surgery 2011; 253(1) 109-115.

[73] Spillane AJ, Winstanley J, Thompson JF. Lymph node ratio in melanoma: A marker of variation in surgical quality?. Cancer 2009; 115(11) 2384-2387.

[74] Hughes TM, A'Hern RP, Thomas JM. Prognosis and surgical management of patients with palpable inguinal lymph node metastases from melanoma. British Journal of Surgery 2000; 87(7) 892-901.

[75] Pearlman NW, McCarter MD, Frank M, Hurtubis C, Merkow RP, Franklin WA, Gonzalez R, Lewis K, Roaten JB, Robinson WA. Size of sentinel node metastases predicts other nodal disease and survival in malignant melanoma. Americal Journal of Surgery 2006; 192(6) 878-881.

[76] Carlson GW, Murray DR, Lyles RH, Staley CA, Hestley A, Cohen C. The amount of metastatic melanoma in a sentinel lymph node: does it have prognostic significance?. Annals of Surgical Oncology 2003; 10(5) 575-581.

[77] Mack LA, McKinnon JG. Controversies in the management of metastatic melanoma to regional lymphatic basins. Journal of Surgical Oncology 2004; 86(4) 189-199.

[78] van der Ploeg AP, van Akkooi AC, Schmitz PI, van Geel AN, de Wilt JH, Eggermont AM, Verhoef C. Therapeutic surgical management of palpable melanoma groin metastases: superficial or combined superficial and deep groin lymph node dissection. Annals of Surgical Oncology 2011; 18(12) 3300-3308.

[79] Shen P, Conforti AM, Essner R, Cochran AJ, Turner RR, Morton DL. Is the node of Cloquet the sentinel node for the iliac/obturator node group?. Cancer Journal 2000; 6(2) 93-97.

[80] Chu CK, Delman KA, Carlson GW, Hestley AC, Murray DR. Inguinopelvic lymphadenectomy following positive inguinal sentinel lymph node biopsy in melanoma: true frequency of synchronous pelvic metastases. Annals of Surgical Oncology 2011; 18(12) 3309-3315.

[81] Gray-Schopfer V, Wellbrock C, Marais R. Melanoma biology and new targeted therapy. Nature 2007; 445(7130) 851-857.

[82] [82]Yamaguchi M, Harada K, Ando N, Kawamura T, Shibagaki N, Shimada S. Marked response to imatinib mesylate in metastatic acral lentiginous melanoma on the thumb. Clinical and Experimental Dermatology 2011; 36(2) 174-177.

[83] Itoh M, Goto A, Wakasugi H, Yoshida Y, Matsunaga Y, Fujii K, Suzuki K, Yonezawa K, Abe T, Arimura Y, Shinomura Y. Anorectal melanoma with a KIT-activating mutation, which is a target for tyrosine kinase inhibitor. International Journal of Clinical Oncology 2011; 16(4) 428-434.

Chapter 10

Cutaneous Melanoma – Surgical Treatment

Mario Santinami, Roberto Patuzzo,
Roberta Ruggeri, Gianpiero Castelli,
Andrea Maurichi, Giulia Baffa and Carlotta Tinti

Additional information is available at the end of the chapter

1. Introduction

1.1. Excision margins for primary tumor

Although surgical excision of the primary melanoma is internationally accepted as the treatment of choice, several questions concerning the follow-up schedule are still debated controversially. Incision biopsies should be avoided, except in selected cases (wide lesions or critical anatomic locations). Excision biopsy is preferred to give the dermatopathologist an optimal specimen and to allow evaluation of the excision margins for residual tumor. Since the beginning of the last century, the recommendation has been to excise a primary melanoma with safety margins. In 1907 Handley [1] analyzed the pattern of satellite metastases in melanoma and recommended excision of the primary tumor with a margin of 1 inch (2.54 cm) from the edge of the tumor. In the 1970s and 1980s, safety margins of 5 cm, independent of tumor thickness, were the surgical standard.[2] The World Health Organization Melanoma Group performed the first surgical trial to compare lower safety margins of 1 and 3 cm in primary melanomas with less than 2 mm of tumor thickness.[3] The group found no differences in survival and only slightly increased local recurrence rates in the patients with narrower excision margins. These results led to the recommendation of 1-cm margins in patients with primary melanomas with less than 1 mm tumor thickness. Later comparisons of 5- and 2-cm safety margins in thick primary melanomas revealed no significant advantages for the 5-cm margins.[4] A recent trial, however, comparing 1- and 3-cm safety margins in thick primary melanoma with 2 mm and more tumor thickness showed an increased rate of local recurrence in those with the small safety margins and a simultaneous trend towards decreased survival rates. These findings indicate that the safety margin cannot be reduced to zero in melanoma.[5] Different national guidelines now give uniform recommendations for the excision of primary melanoma.[6-9]

2. Sentinel lymph node biopsy and lymph node dissection

Metastasis to regional nodes is the most important prognostic factor in patients with early-stage melanoma and has been shown to occur in approximately 20% of patients with intermediate-thickness tumors.[10,11] As such, it is critically important to identify those patients for whom the expected benefits of resecting regional lymph nodes outweigh the risks of surgical morbidity. The technique of lymphatic mapping and sentinel lymph node (SLN) biopsy for melanoma has emerged during the last 2 decades as a minimally invasive approach to evaluate regional lymph node basins in patients with intermediate- and high-risk primary cutaneous melanoma. Goals of SLN biopsy include accurate nodal staging, identification of patients with clinically occult, microscopic lymph node disease who may benefit from further treatment, regional nodal control, and a possible survival benefit.[12,13] Moreover, this approach may also identify a subset of patients for whom further treatment is not indicated, sparing them from unnecessary surgical procedures or systemic therapies.[12,13] In this review, we examine the evolution of SLN biopsy as a technique, the preoperative assessment and operative strategy, the pathologic evaluation of the SLN, the current practice guidelines, the prognostic significance of SLN biopsy findings, and the potential complications of the procedure and address some of the current areas of controversies in the field. Sentinel lymph node (SLN) biopsy is commonly used in melanoma and has been endorsed by the American Joint Committee on Cancer (AJCC) as a valuable staging procedure for patients with melanoma who are at risk of clinically occult nodal metastases. This highly accurate and low-morbidity staging procedure should be used to guide treatment decisions (ie, completion lymph node dissection [CLND] and adjuvant therapy) as well as entry into clinical trials.[14] To develop and formalize guideline recommendations for the use of SLN biopsy in oncology practice, the American Society of Clinical Oncology (ASCO) and Society of Surgical Oncology (SSO) convened a joint Expert Panel in order to better define what are the indications for SLN biopsy as well as what is the role of CLND. SLN biopsy is recommended for patients with intermediate-thickness cutaneous melanomas (Breslow thickness, 1 to 4 mm) of any anatomic site. Routine use of SLN biopsy in this population provides accurate staging. Although there are few studies focusing specifically on patients with thick melanomas (T4; Breslow thickness, > 4 mm), use of SLN biopsy in this population may be recommended for staging purposes and to facilitate regional disease control. There is insufficient evidence to support routine SLN biopsy for patients with thin melanomas (T1; Breslow thickness, < 1 mm), although it may be considered in selected patients with high-risk features when the benefits of pathologic staging may outweigh the potential risks of the procedure. Such risk factors may include ulceration or mitotic rate $\geq 1/mm^2$, especially in the subgroup of patients with melanomas 0.75 to 0.99 mm in Breslow thickness. After a positive SLN biopsy, 97.5% of patients underwent CLND, and 20.1% were found to have additional positive lymph nodes. Overall, the recurrence rate in the same nodal basin after a positive

SLN biopsy was 7.5%, despite CLND in nearly all patients.[15] Overall, the SLN biopsy procedure is well tolerated and associated with low complication rates.[16] Although clinical
variables such as older age have been variably reported as lower risk factors,[17-19] there
are no specific variables that can reliably identify patients with intermediate-thickness melanomas at low risk for metastases. The definition of intermediate-thickness melanoma varied
by study. Nevertheless, it is clinically consistent with contemporary staging systems to define intermediate-thickness melanomas as those measuring 1 to 4 mm.[20] Clinical judgment
must be used when considering SLN biopsy in patients with comorbid medical conditions.
The individual risks and benefits of the procedure should be weighed against the operative
and anesthetic risks as well as potential competing causes of mortality. Complications after
SLN biopsy are uncommon. The overall complication rate reported in the Multicenter Selective Lymphadenectomy Trial I (MSLT I) was 10.1% after SLN biopsy compared with 32.7%
after CLND.[21] The most common complications after SLN removal documented in MSLT I
included seroma (5.5%), infection (4.6%), and wound separation (1.2%). The Sunbelt Melanoma Trial similarly showed a low overall rate of complications from SLN biopsy (4.6%)
compared with CLND (23.2%).[16,17] Most complications were noted to be short-term issues that resolved over time with wound care and selective use of antibiotics. Accurate identification of patients with node-negative (stage I or II) or node-positive (stage III) disease
improves staging and may facilitate regional disease control and decision making for treatment with adjuvant therapy.[14,22] With substantive changes in the melanoma staging
guidelines in 2002, the AJCC staging system effectively linked disease stage and prognosis.
[23,24] At that time, the number of nodal metastases and whether nodal disease was occult
or clinically apparent (ie, how the N category was defined with regard to burden of disease)
were noted to be the most significant independent predictors of survival in patients with
stage III melanomas. With later iterations of the last AJCC staging system,[10] additional re-
finements were made in the N category based on the prognostic value of distinguishing micrometastases (as would be diagnosed after SLN biopsy) from macrometastases.[25,26] A
melanoma macrometastasis is detected by clinical examination (not by size criteria) and confirmed pathologically, whereas a melanoma micrometastasis is a clinically occult nodal
metastasis that is detected by a pathologist on microscopic examination of lymph nodes,
with or without immunohistochemistry, and is not limited by any minimum or maximum
size threshold. Recognizing the value of examining SLNs to detect low volumes of metastatic disease (aggregates of only a few cells), the current staging system[10,27] incorporates the
use of immunohistochemistry and eliminates any minimum size threshold for defining nodal metastases. Molecular diagnostics, such as reverse transcriptase-polymerase chain reaction, have unproven prognostic significance, and these results are not used to define positive
nodes. As a result, more refined definitions of the N category are now used for classification.
Distinct differences in classifications have validated prognostic significance. For example, 5-
year survival ranges from 70% for patients with one SLN positive with micrometastatic disease to 39% for patients with > four involved nodes or with nodes that are extensively
involved (eg, matted nodes).[1] Although SLN biopsy has been widely accepted for the pathologic staging of patients with intermediate-thickness melanomas, somewhat more controversy exists regarding the value of this procedure for patients with thick primary tumors

(T4; Breslow thickness, > 4 mm). Conventional wisdom asserts that patients with thick melanomas have a high risk of systemic disease at the time of diagnosis and that no survival benefit can be derived from removal of regional lymph nodes. However, among patients without distant disease, it can be argued that those with thick melanomas have indications for SLN biopsy similar to those of patients with intermediate-thickness melanomas and derive the same benefits from SLN biopsy as a pathologic staging procedure. One of the main advantages of SLN biopsy in patients with thick melanomas is better regional disease control, which is especially important in a population with > 30% chance of lymph node involvement.[25,28] Evidence from multiple retrospective studies has demonstrated that SLN biopsy provides important staging and prognostic information for patients with thick melanomas. Seven of eight published studies-each evaluating SLN biopsy in > 100 patients with T4 melanomas-have shown that SLN biopsy is a significant predictor of overall survival. [11,25,26,28-33] The one study that did not show a significant difference in overall survival demonstrated a significant difference in disease-free survival.[29] A majority (70%) of melanomas diagnosed are thin melanomas (T1; Breslow thickness, < 1 mm).[34] In general, the routine use of SLN biopsy in patients with thin melanomas has not been advocated, because the overall risk of nodal involvement is estimated to be only approximately 5.1%,[35] although there are reports of positive SLNs in up to 20% of patients in subsets with thin melanomas (especially those that are 0.75 to 0.99 mm in thickness with ulceration and/or mitotic rate ≥ 1/mm^2).[27] An individualized approach to SLN biopsy for patients with thin melanomas has been advocated in many treatment centers based on risk factors that have been shown to be associated with SLN metastasis. Further investigation is also needed to better identify the subgroups of patients with thin melanomas with a greater risk of nodal metastasis. CLND is recommended for all patients with a positive SLN biopsy. CLND achieves regional disease control, although whether CLND after a positive SLN biopsy improves survival is the subject of the ongoing Multicenter Selective Lymphadenectomy Trial II (MSLT II). Currently, CLND is the standard recommendation for patients with tumor-positive SLNs. The goals of CLND are to improve survival rates, maximize regional disease control, and minimize operative morbidity. Whether CLND improves survival is the subject of the ongoing prospective randomized MSLT II study.[36] The main objective of MSLT II is to determine if there is a therapeutic benefit to removing any non-SLNs in patients who have already had their tumor-positive SLN removed. In MSLT I, patients with demonstrated nodal metastases had a survival advantage with early intervention compared with those who had a delayed lymphadenectomy when they presented with clinically evident nodal metastases.[5] Hence, although two goals of CLND are regional disease control and cure, there is currently insufficient evidence to determine whether omission of CLND is safe. In the two large prospective randomized trials (ie, the Sunbelt Melanoma Trial and MSLT I), the rate of positive non-SLNs among patients who underwent CLND for a tumor-positive SLN was 16%.[17,37] In a retrospective multi-institutional study by Wong et al,[38] which included 134 highly selected patients with positive SLNs who did not undergo CLND, regional nodal metastasis was a component of first recurrence in 15% of these patients. Therefore, it is reasonable to conclude from these data that the risk of developing regional nodal metastasis as a first site of recurrence, if no CLND is performed, is at least 15% to 20%.[39,40] In MSLT I, the rate of regional nodal recurrence after CLND was 4.2%[5]; in the Sunbelt Melanoma Trial, it was 4.9% (unpublished data). These rates are much lower than the 15% rate of regional nodal recurrence as a site of first metastasis and the 41% overall regional nodal recurrence rate when CLND was not performed, reported in the study by Wong et al.[37] Until final results of MSLT II are available, we will not be able to determine, with higher-level evidence, the impact of CLND on regional disease control. Until that time, the best available evidence suggests that CLND is effective at achieving regional disease control in the majority of patients with positive SLNs. MSLT I showed no benefit of CLND with regard to overall survival, likely because only a minority of patients (16%) had tumor-positive SLNs, and the majority of the patients in the study would not have been helped by removal of regional lymph nodes.[37] However, the 5-year survival rate for patients with tumor-positive SLNs who underwent CLND was 72.3% compared with 52.4% for patients who did not undergo SLN biopsy and developed palpable nodal disease (hazard ratio, 0.51; 95% CI, 0.32 to 0.81; P =.004). CLND should be performed until there is convincing evidence that it does not improve regional disease control or survival. CLND is associated with risks of long-term morbidity, especially lymphedema. However, morbidity with CLND may be considerably worse when it is delayed until there is clinically evident disease. The observed increases in morbidity for patients who have undergone therapeutic lymphadenectomy for palpable disease and the increased morbidity associated with radiation therapy support the continued use of CLND for patients with a positive SLN biopsy rather than delayed CLND for palpable disease. There is a need for future clinical trials to address many unresolved research questions related to the use of SLN biopsy in patients with melanoma. These include: determining precise criteria for selecting which patients should undergo SLN biopsy, determining whether early identification of metastases in the SLN truly improves survival or merely represents lead-time bias, identifying which criteria for individualized risks best inform appropriate risk stratification for patients at high risk for relapse and those for whom CLND and/or adjuvant therapy are suitable, and establishing the role of prognostic markers from the primary melanoma and SLN to help assign appropriate risk stratification. Results from MSLT II, in which patients were randomly assigned to CLND or observation, will help determine whether there is any benefit to CLND after a positive sentinel node in patients with melanoma. Answers to these questions will assist clinicians and patients with making decisions and ultimately help to identify patients who may avoid expensive and intrusive procedures in staging and follow-up.

3. Treatment of *in transit* metastases

In 5–8% of cases, melanoma patients will develop in-transit metastasis (IT-mets). Standard regional treatment options include surgical resection, isolated limb perfusion (ILP), isolated limb infusion (ILI) and Electrochemotherapy. As regional recurrence often precedes systemic disease, amputative surgery is in general no longer practiced, although old series of radical surgery have demonstrated that some patients with IT-mets confined to the limb can be cured.[42,43] Simple surgical resection may suffice for incidental and low numbers of IT-mets. In cases of rapid recurrences and multiple IT-mets, other techniques must provide an attractive treatment option that can improve local control markedly and thereby quality of life. ILP, developed by Creech et al., achieves a 20-fold higher concentration of chemotherapeutic drugs when compared with systemic therapy.[44,45] Melphalan-based ILP (M-ILP) has been the standard treatment and has been reported to achieve overall complete response (CR) rates in the range of about 50%.[46]In general large IT-mets showed a poor response and inhomogeneous uptake comparable with locally advanced soft tissue sarcomas (STS). The introduction of tumor necrosis factor-α (TNF) changed this situation dramatically. Large tumors now reacted very well to ILP.[47] This led to a successful multicenter trial in Europe and the approval of TNF-based ILP (TM-ILP) for unresectable extremity soft tissue sarcomas (STS).[48] Similar encouraging results were reported for the use of TNF in ILP for melanoma patients.[49] Preclinical and clinical studies suggested that a reduction of the dose of TNF to 1 mg for the arm and 2 mg for the leg might be as effective as the higher doses.[50-53]Isolated limb infusion (ILI) is a minimally invasive technique for delivering high-dose regional chemotherapy in locally advanced melanoma. It was first described by Thompson et al. in 1994 from the Sydney Melanoma Unit as a simplified alternative to ILP [54,55]. Percutaneous arterial and venous catheters are placed in the affected extremity by interventional radiologists and a tourniquet is placed proximal to the catheter tips to allow isolation of the limb from the systemic circulation. High-dose chemotherapy (e.g. melphalan and actinomycin-D) is infused into a hyperthermic, hypoxic limb via the arterial catheter and blood is withdrawn from the venous catheter to be re-infused into the arterial side. Therefore, it is a quicker, safer, and cheaper procedure with reported response rates comparable to ILP.[56,57] Although the primary indication for this technique is melanoma, it has been successfully applied to other tumors such as soft-tissue sarcomas,[58] Merkel cell tumor,[59] and cutaneous T-cell lymphoma.[60]

Electrochemotherapy (ECT) represents an effective therapeutic option for skin tumors that has received experimental and clinical support in recent years.[61-71] The European standard operating procedures for ECT emphasize the technical aspects of the procedure and have established this treatment in clinical practice.[72,73] In recent years, the effectiveness of ECT treatment has been confirmed in several small series of patients with melanoma.[71] At present, ECT is employed routinely with encouraging results not only for superficial tumor control but also to preserve quality of life.[70]Patients with regional or distant skin or subcutaneous metastases, with or without visceral disease, could undergo this technique. Eligibility criteria were the following: melanoma stage IIIC–IV (American Joint Committee on Cancer, 6th edition)[74] lesions no deeper than 3 cm suitable for electrode insertion; no anticancer treatments 4 weeks before and 8 weeks after ECT; age more than 18 years; and an Eastern Cooperative Oncology Group performance status equal to or less than 2. Exclusion criteria included: allergy to Bleomycin; pulmonary, cardiac or liver impairment; epilepsy; life expectancy less than 3 months; active infection; brain metastases; and cardiac pacemaker in patients with chest wall metastases. Bleomycin is administered intravenously (15 000 units/m^2 in a bolus administered over 60 s) and was followed, within 8 min after intravenous injection, by the application of brief electric pulses to each tumor nodule. Electric currents were delivered by means of a 2–3-cm long needle electrode according to lesion size.

The electrodes were connected to a pulse generator (Cliniporator™; Igea, Modena, Italy). This generator produces high voltages (up to 1000 V), but delivered as a compressed train of eight pulses at a frequency of 5000 Hz and 100 μs duration, and therefore well tolerated by the patient. The software controls and stores the applied voltage and the actual current delivered to each tumor. ECT could be repeated every 8–12 weeks according to local response, the appearance of new lesions and the patient's tolerance of the treatment.

4. Surgical approach for distant metastases

Conventional teaching maintains that resection is not indicated in patients with distant metastases, except for palliation. This dogma stems from the concept that patients with multiple metastases usually also have occult micrometastases and circulating tumor cells. However the results of surgical treatment of stage IV melanoma patients have improved considerably over the past two decades. Recent studies [75] provide further evidence of the beneficial role of surgery for distant metastases of melanoma. Our findings indicate a survival advantage for a surgical approach, even in patients with high-risk visceral metastases or multiple metastases that may require multiple operations for complete resection. At least 55 % of stage IV patients may be eligible to undergo surgery as part of their treatment plan and the surgeon should play an integral role in evaluation and treatment planning for all patients with stage IV recurrence of melanoma. One potential therapeutic advantage of resection is that it may delay disease progression by interrupting the metastatic cascade associated with hematogenous seeding of cells to other sites.[76]In addition, it immediately reduces tumor burden and thereby decreases tumor-induced immune suppression.[77] Finally, metastasectomy may enhance the patient's endogenous immune defences or response to adjuvant immunotherapy and thus maintain a complete clinical remission. Surgery for distant metastases has been improved by development of more advanced imaging techniques that can detect lesions as small as 5–10 mm.[78] These techniques can differentiate patients with multiple versus limited metastases, allowing surgeons to better judge the extent of disease and plan the operative procedure necessary for complete resection. In addition, modern advances in anaesthesia, surgical techniques and supportive care have reduced operative mortality from multiple metastasectomy with a corresponding reduction in morbidity and finally, shorter postsurgical hospitalizations have decreased the total costs of cancer surgery. Surgical therapy for stage IV disease remains controversial. The development of metastases is a complex process and the rationale for surgical resection of metastatic melanoma is multifactorial. First, reduction of tumor burden through surgical resection limits disease progression by interrupting the metastatic cascade associated with haematogenous seeding of cells to other sites. Unlike chemotherapy, surgery can easily eradicate tumor masses 2 cm or larger. Second, surgery may reverse tumor-induced immunosuppression, restoring immune function and inhibiting metastatic progression. Third, most patients tolerate surgical resection to a much greater extent than they can tolerate adverse effects of systemic therapy and recurrences after initial metastasectomy can also be treated through a secondary resection of metastases. Last, metastasectomy does not preclude systemic therapy;

however, if metastasectomy is delayed, increasing tumor burden may make disease unresectable. In addition the advent of newer and better systemic therapies makes the role of surgical resection more relevant today than ever before. Timing of surgery versus systemic treatment is another important end point. The development of new and effective drugs in the systemic treatment of stage IV melanoma patients have been reported recently, with the BRAF inhibitor Vemurafinib and the monoclonal antibody Ipilimumab; other targeted drugs are being developed, and some are currently being tested in the clinical setting. Thus a therapeutic strategy combining new drugs with aggressive surgery in selected cases of melanoma metastatic disease could be designed in the following years.

Author details

Mario Santinami[1], Roberto Patuzzo[1], Roberta Ruggeri[1], Gianpiero Castelli[1], Andrea Maurichi[1], Giulia Baffa[1] and Carlotta Tinti[1]

1 Melanoma Sarcoma Unit Fondazione Istituto Tumori Milano, Italy

Dermatology Unit Ospedale Umberto I Siracusa, Italy

References

[1] W.S. Handley. The pathology of melanotic growths in relation to their operative treatment. Lancet, i: 927-996,1907

[2] R. Kaufmann. Surgical management of primary melanoma. Clin Exp Dermatol 25: 476–481, 2000

[3] U. Veronesi, N. Cascinelli, J. Adamus et al.Thin stage I primary cutaneous malignant melanoma. Comparison of excision with margins of 1 or 3 cm. N Engl J Med 318:1159–1162,1988.

[4] U. Ringborg, R. Andersson, J. Eldh et al. Resection margins of 2 versus 5 cm for cutaneous malignant melanoma with a tumor thickness of 0.8 to 2.0 mm: randomized study by the Swedish Melanoma Study Group. Cancer 77:1809–1814,1996.

[5] J.M. Thomas, J. Newton-Bishop, R. A'Hern et al.Excision margins in high-risk malignant melanoma N Engl J Med 350:757–766, 2004.

[6] R. Dummer, R. Panizzon, P.H. Bloch, et al.Updated Swiss guidelines for the treatment and follow-up of cutaneous melanoma.Dermatology 210: 39–44, 2005.

[7] R. Dummer, A. Hauschild, L. Jost. Cutaneous malignant melanoma: ESMO clinical recommendations for diagnosis, treatment and follow-up. Ann Oncol 19 (Suppl 2): ii86–ii88, 2008.

[8]   C. Garbe, A. Hauschild, M. Volkenandt et al.Evidence and interdisciplinary consen-
      sus-based German guidelines: surgical treatment and radiotherapy of melanoma.
      Melanoma Res, 18: 61–67, 2008.

[9]   R. Essner, J.H. Lee, L.A. Wanek, et al.Contemporary surgical treatment of advanced-
      stage melanoma. Arch Surg 139: 961–966, 2004.

[10] Balch CM, Gershenwald JE, Soong SJ, et al. Final version of 2009 AJCC melanoma
      staging and classification. J Clin Oncol 27:6199-6206, 2009.

[11] Balch CM, Gershenwald JE, Soong SJ. Multivariate analysis of prognostic factors
      among 2,313 patients with stage III melanoma: Comparison of nodal micrometasta-
      ses versus macrometastases. J Clin Oncol 28:2452–2459, 2010.

[12] Gershenwald JE, Ross MI. Sentinel-lymph-node biopsy for cutaneous melanoma. N
      Engl J Med 364: 1738–1745, 2011.

[13] Ross MI, Thompson JF, Gershenwald JE. Sentinel lymph node biopsy for melanoma: crit-
      ical assessment at its twentieth anniversary. Surg Oncol Clin North Am 20: 57–78, 2011.

[14] Balch CM, Morton DL, Gershenwald JE, et al.Sentinel node biopsy and standard of
      care for melanoma. J Am Acad Dermatol 60:872–875, 2009.

[15] Valsecchi ME, Silbermins D, de Rosa N, et al. Lymphatic mapping and sentinel
      lymph node biopsy in patients with melanoma: A meta-analysis. J Clin Oncol
      29:1479–1487,2011.

[16] Wrightson WR, Wong SL, Edwards MJ, et al. Complications associated with sentinel
      lymph node biopsy for melanoma. Ann Surg Oncol 10:676–680,2003.

[17] McMasters KM, Noyes RD, Reintgen DS, et al. Lessons learned from the Sunbelt Mel-
      anoma Trial. J Surg Oncol 86:212–223, 2004.

[18] Sondak VK, Taylor JM, Sabel MS, et al. Mitotic rate and younger age are predictors of
      sentinel lymph node positivity: Lessons learned from the generation of a probabilis-
      tic model. Ann Surg Oncol 11:247–258,2004.

[19] Sabel MS, Rice JD, Griffith KA, et al.Validation of statistical predictive models meant
      to select melanoma patients for sentinel lymph node biopsy. Ann Surg Oncol 19:287–
      293, 2012.

[20] Edge SB, Byrd DR, Compton CC, et al. AJCC Cancer Staging Manual, Springer, New
      York, NY,ed 7, 2010.

[21] Morton DL, Cochran AJ, Thompson JF, et al.Sentinel node biopsy for early-stage mel-
      anoma: Accuracy and morbidity in MSLT-I, an international multicenter trial. Ann
      Surg 242:302–311, discussion 311-313, 2005.

[22] Eggermont AM, Suciu S, Santinami M, et al. Adjuvant therapy with pegylated inter-
      feron alfa-2b versus observation alone in resected stage III melanoma: Final results of
      EORTC 18991, a randomised phase III trial. Lancet 372:117–126, 2008.

[23] Balch CM, Buzaid AC, Soong SJ, et al.Final version of the American Joint Committee on Cancer staging system for cutaneous melanoma. J Clin Oncol 19:3635–3648, 2001.

[24] Balch CM, Soong SJ, Gershenwald JE, et al. Prognostic factors analysis of 17,600 melanoma patients: Validation of the American Joint Committee on Cancer melanoma staging system. J Clin Oncol 19:3622–3634, 2001.

[25] Gershenwald JE, Mansfield PF, Lee JE, et al.Role for lymphatic mapping and sentinel lymph node biopsy in patients with thick (≥ 4 mm) primary melanoma. Ann Surg Oncol 7:160–165, 2000.

[26] Ferrone CR, Panageas KS, Busam K, et al.Multivariate prognostic model for patients with thick cutaneous melanoma: Importance of sentinel lymph node status. Ann Surg Oncol 9:637–645, 2002.

[27] Balch CM, Gershenwald JE, Soong SJ, et al. Update on the melanoma staging system: The importance of sentinel node staging and primary tumor mitotic rate. J Surg Oncol 104:379–385, 2011.

[28] Gajdos C, Griffith KA, Wong SL, et al.Is there a benefit to sentinel lymph node biopsy in patients with T4 melanoma? Cancer 115:5752–5760,2009.

[29] Essner R, Chung MH, Bleicher R, et al.Prognostic implications of thick (≥ 4 mm) melanoma in the era of intraoperative lymphatic mapping and sentinel lymphadenectomy. Ann Surg Oncol 9:754–761,2002.

[30] Carlson GW, Murray DR, Hestley A, et al.Sentinel lymph node mapping for thick (≥ 4 mm) melanoma: Should we be doing it? Ann Surg Oncol 10:408–415,2003.

[31] Thompson JF, Shaw HM.The prognosis of patients with thick primary melanomas: Is regional lymph node status relevant, and does removing positive regional nodes influence outcome? Ann Surg Oncol 9:719–722,2002.

[32] Gutzmer R, Satzger I, Thoms KM, et al.Sentinel lymph node status is the most important prognostic factor for thick (≥ 4 mm) melanomas. J Dtsch Dermatol Ges 6:198–203,2008.

[33] Scoggins CR, Bowen AL, Martin RC 2nd, et al.Prognostic information from sentinel lymph node biopsy in patients with thick melanoma. Arch Surg 145:622–627,2010.

[34] Criscione VD, Weinstock MA. Melanoma thickness trends in the United States 1988-2006. J Invest Dermatol 130:793–797,2010.

[35] Andtbacka RH, Gershenwald JE. Role of sentinel lymph node biopsy in patients with thin melanoma. J Natl Compr Canc Netw 7:308–317,2009.

[36] Amersi F, Morton DL.The role of sentinel lymph node biopsy in the management of melanoma. Adv Surg 41:241–256,2007.

[37] Morton DL, Thompson JF, Cochran AJ, et al.Sentinel-node biopsy or nodal observation in melanoma. N Engl J Med 355:1307–1317,2006

[38] Wong SL, Morton DL, Thompson JF, et al. Melanoma patients with positive sentinel nodes who did not undergo completion lymphadenectomy: A multi-institutional study. Ann Surg Oncol 13:809–816, 2006

[39] Kingham TP, Panageas KS, Ariyan CE, et al. Outcome of patients with a positive sentinel lymph node who do not undergo completion lymphadenectomy. Ann Surg Oncol 17:514–520, 2010

[40] Calabro A, Singletary SE, Balch CM. Patterns of relapse in 1,001 consecutive patients with melanoma nodal metastases. Arch Surg 124:1051–1055, 1989.

[41] Wong SL, Brady MS, Busam KJ, et al.Results of sentinel lymph node biopsy in patients with thin melanoma. Ann Surg Oncol 13:302–309,2006.

[42] Jaques DP, Coit DGet al. Major amputation for advanced malignant melanoma. Surg Gynecol Obstet 169:1–6,1989.

[43] Karakousis CP, Choe KJ, Holyoke ED. Biologic behavior and treatment of intransit metastasis of melanoma. Surg Gynecol Obstet 150:29–32,1980.

[44] Creech O, Jr., Krementz ET, Ryan RF, et al. Chemotherapy of cancer: regional perfusion utilizing an extracorporeal circuit. Ann Surg 148:616–32,1958.

[45] Benckhuijsen C, Kroon BB, van Geel AN, et al. Regional perfusion treatment with melphalan for melanoma in a limb: an evaluation of drug kinetics. Eur J Surg Oncol 14:157–63, 1988.

[46] Vrouenraets BC, Nieweg OE, Kroon BB. Thirty-five years of isolated limb perfusion for melanoma: indications and results. Br J Surg 83:1319–28,1996.

[47] Eggermont AM, Schraffordt Koops H, Lienard D, et al. Isolated limb perfusion with high-dose tumor necrosis factor-alpha in combination with interferon-gamma and melphalan for nonresectable extremity soft tissue sarcomas: a multicenter trial. J Clin Oncol 14:2653–65,1996

[48] Eggermont AM, Schraffordt Koops H, Klausner JM, et al. Isolated limb perfusion with tumor necrosis factor and melphalan for limb salvage in 186 patients with locally advanced soft tissue extremity sarcomas. The cumulative multicenter European experience. Ann Surg 224:756–64; discussion 764–5,1996

[49] Lejeune FJ, Lienard D, Leyvraz S, et al. Regional therapy of melanoma. Eur J Cancer 29A: 606–12, 1993.

[50] de Wilt JH, Manusama ER, van Tiel ST, et al. Prerequisites for effective isolated limb perfusion using tumour necrosis factor alpha and melphalan in rats. Br J Cancer 80:161–6, 1999

[51] Bonvalot S, Laplanche A, Lejeune F, et al. Limb salvage with isolated perfusion for soft tissue sarcoma: could less TNF-alpha be better? Ann Oncol 16:1061–8, 2005.

[52] Hill S, Fawcett WJ, Sheldon J, et al. Low-dose tumour necrosis factor alpha and melphalan in hyperthermic isolated limb perfusion. Br J Surg 80:995–7, 1993

[53] Rossi CR, Foletto M, Mocellin S, et al. Hyperthermic isolated limb perfusion with low-dose tumor necrosis factor-alpha and melphalan for bulky in-transit melanoma metastases. Ann Surg Oncol 11:173–7, 2004.

[54] J.F. Thompson, R.C. Waugh, C.W. Schacherer et al. Isolated limb infusion with melphalan for recurrent limb melanoma: a simple alternative to isolated limb perfusion. Reg Cancer Treat 7:188–192, 1994.

[55] J.F. Thompson, P.C. Kam, R.C. Waugh et al.Isolated limb infusion with cytotoxic agents: a simple alternative to isolated limb perfusion. Semin Surg Oncol 14: 238–247,1998.

[56] P. Lindnér, A. Doubrovsky, P.C.A. Kam et al.Prognostic factors after isolated limb infusion with cytotoxic agents for melanoma.Ann Surg Oncol, 9: 127–136, 2002.

[57] H.M. Kroon, M. Moncrieff, P.C.A. Kam et al.Outcomes following isolated limb infusion for melanoma. A 14-year experience.Ann Surg Oncol, 15: 3003–3013, 2008.

[58] M.S. Brady, K. Brown, A. Patel et al.A phase II trial of isolated limb infusion with melphalan and dactinomycin for regional melanoma and soft tissue sarcoma of the extremity.Ann Surg Oncol, 13: 1123–1129, 2006.

[59] A.S. Gupta, S. Heinzmann, E.A. Levine. Successful treatment of in transit metastases in Merkel's cell carcinoma with isolated hyperthermic limb perfusion. South Med J, 91: 289–292, 1998.

[60] E. Elhassadi, E. Egan, G. O'Sullivan et al. Isolated limb infusion with cytotoxic agent for treatment of localized refractory cutaneous T-cell lymphoma. Clin Lab Haematol, 4: 279–281, 2006.

[61] Belehradek M, Domenge C, Luboinski B, et al. Electrochemotherapy, a new antitumor treatment: first clinical phase I–II trial report. Cancer 72: 3694–3700, 1993.

[62] Mir LM, Orlowski S. Mechanisms of electrochemotherapy. Adv Drug Del Rev 35: 107–118,1999.

[63] Mir LM, Glass LF, Sersa G, et al. Effective treatment of cutaneous and subcutaneous malignant tumours by electrochemotherapy. Br J Cancer 77: 2336–2342,1998.

[64] Rols MP, Bachaud JM, Giraud P, et al. Electrochemotherapy of cutaneous metastases in malignant melanoma. Melanoma Res 10: 468–474,2000.

[65] Byrne MC, Thompson JF, Johnston H, et al. Treatment of metastatic melanoma using electroporation therapy with bleomycin (electrochemotherapy). Melanoma Res 15: 45–51,2005.

[66] Gaudy C, Richard MA, Folchetti G, et al. Randomized controlled study of electroche-motherapy in the local treatment of skin metastases of melanoma. J Cutan Med Surg 10: 115–121,2006.

[67] Larkin JO, Collins CG, Aarons S, et al. Electrochemotherapy: aspects of preclinical development and early clinical experience. Ann Surg 245: 469–479,2007.

[68] Serša G, Štabuc B, Čemažar M, et al. Electrochemotherapy with cisplatin: the system-ic antitumour effectiveness of cisplatin can be potentiated locally by the application of electric pulses in the treatment of malignant melanoma skin metastases. Melano-ma Res 10: 381–385,2000.

[69] Domenge C, Orlowski S, Luboinski B, et al. Antitumour electrochemotherapy: new advances in the clinical protocol. Cancer 77: 956–963,1996.

[70] Campana LG, Mocellin S, Basso M, et al. Bleomycin-based electrochemotherapy: clin-ical outcome from a single institution's experience with 52 patients. Ann Surg Oncol 6: 191–199,2009.

[71] Kis E, Oláh J, Ócsai H, et al. Electrochemotherapy of cutaneous metastases of mela-noma—a case series study and systematic review of the evidence. Dermatol Surg 37: 816–824,2011.

[72] Marty M, Serša G, Garbay JR, et al. Electrochemotherapy—an easy, highly effective and safe treatment of cutaneous and subcutaneous metastases: results of ESOPE study. EJC Suppl 4: 3–13,2006.

[73] Mir LM, Gehl J, Sersa G, et al. Standard operating procedures of the electrochemo-therapy: instructions for the use of bleomycin or cisplatin administered either sys-temically or locally and electric pulses delivered by the Cliniporator by means of invasive or non-invasive electrodes. EJC Suppl 4: 14–25, 2006.

[74] Balch CM, Buzaid AC, Soong SJ, et al. Final version of the American Joint Committee on Cancer staging system for cutaneous melanoma. J Clin Oncol 19: 3635–3648, 2001.

[75] Howard JH, Thompson JF, Mozzillo N, et al. Metastasectomy for Distant Metastatic Melanoma: Analysis of Data from the First Multicenter Selective Lymphadenectomy Trial (MSLT-I). Ann Surg Oncol 19:2547-55, 2012.

[76] Roth JA, Silverstein MJ, Morton DL. Metastatic potential of metastases. Surgery 79:669–73, 1976.

[77] Morton DL, Holmes EC, Golub SH. Immunologic aspects of lung cancer. Chest 71:640–3, 1977.

[78] Gulec SA, Faries MB, Lee CC, et al. The role of fluorine-18 deoxyglucose positron emission tomography in the management of patients with metastatic melanoma: im-pact on surgical decision making. Clin Nucl Med 28:961–5, 2003.

Chapter 11

Therapeutic Agents for Advanced Melanoma

Zhao Wang, Wei Li and Duane D. Miller

Additional information is available at the end of the chapter

1. Introduction

Melanoma is an extremely complicated disease, with many gene mutations and alternations in signaling pathways. Because effective treatment for melanoma is lacking, the prognosis for metastatic melanoma patients remains very poor. Over the past 30 years, significant efforts have been made to search for better agents or strategies to fight this deadly disease. Numerous clinical trials at different stages have been carried out. Although most of them have failed, some did show very promising results. New treatment strategies have resulted in paradigm shift in our approach to melanoma therapy. These shining examples may markedly change our philosophy about melanoma treatment.

The year 2011 marked a fruitful year for melanoma research. The FDA approved three drugs for advanced melanoma treatment: ipilimumab (an anti-cytotoxic T lymphocyte antigen-4 monoclonal antibody), vemurafenib (a selective BRAF inhibitor), and pegylated interferon-α2b for adjuvant setting usage [1]. However, there are still significant limitations for melanoma treatment. Ipilimumab only prolonged the survival time for metastatic melanoma patient from an average of 6.5 months to an average of 10 months. This treatment also has been associated with strong immunological adverse effects; severe to fatal autoimmune reactions were seen in 12.9% of patients treated with ipilimumab in a clinical trial that enrolled 676 melanoma patients [2]. Vemurafenib is not effective for melanoma patients with wide type BRAF, and confirmation of BRAFV600E mutation-positive melanoma using an FDA-approved test is required before treatment with vemurafenib. This treatment also only prolonged the median survival time for advanced melanoma patients 2~3 months [1]. More importantly, despite the high initial response rate for patients with BRAFV600E mutation to vemurafenib, virtually all the patients developed primary or acquired resistance to this drug in the end [3]. With the rapidly rising incidents of this disease and the high resistance to current therapeutic agents, developing more effective drugs for melanoma is very important.

In this chapter, we will review available therapeutic agents for advanced melanoma as well as agents that are still under clinical development. We will focus on their mechanism of action, development history, and therapeutic effects. In learning from our efforts in the past, we must continue to challenge the current paradigms of treatment as we forge new paths to more effective treatment options. This will likely involve a multimodal approach to therapy utilizing all of the available tools in our arsenal.

2. Chemotherapy agents

According to the current 7th edition American Joint Committee of Cancer (AJCC) staging system, melanoma can be pathologically classified in the following stages: 0, IA, IB, IIA, IIB, IIC, IIIA, IIIB, IIIC, and IV. Stage 0 is in situ melanoma. Stage I and II are growth phase of localized cutaneous melanoma with increasing thickness. Stage III has regional involvement of lymph node. Stage IV means distant metastasis. Normally stage III and IV melanoma are called metastatic melanoma. Localized melanoma is curable with complete surgical excision in most patients. But currently treatment for metastatic melanoma is still very challenging. Only two chemotherapy drugs in current use have been approved by the Food and Drug Administration (FDA) for metastatic melanoma: dacarbazine (DTIC) and vemurafenib. Other agents that have been tried on melanoma patients are also discussed below.

2.1. Dacarbazine (DTIC)

DTIC is the first FDA approved chemotherapy drug for metastatic melanoma. This drug gained FDA approval in May 1975 as DTIC-Dome for the treatment of metastatic melanoma. It was initially marketed by Bayer. The therapeutic effect of DTIC is believed to be produced through alkylation of DNA. While its anticancer mechanism of action is still not fully understood, DTIC is believed to be first metabolically bioactivated through a series of reactions involving CYP450. Initial demethylation to MTIC [3-methyl-(triazen-1-yl)imidazole-4-carboxamide] is followed by formation of diazomethane, the active moiety of DTIC and a potent methylating agent [4].

DTIC has produced response rates of from 15% to 25% in single-institution trials. But the overall response rate has fallen over the years from 15% to 7% and less than 5% of responses are complete in phase 3 trials. The median response durations to DTIC are 5 to 6 months. Long-term follow-up of patients treated with DTIC alone shows that only <2% can be anticipated to survive for more than 6 years. In recent phase 3 trials that used strict response assessment criteria, the response rates with single-agent DTIC did not exceed 12% [5].

Over the past 30 years after its approval by the FDA, DTIC remains the only currently used cytotoxic drug for the treatment of metastatic melanoma. Despite its low single-agent activity, DTIC has remained the mainstay of many combination chemotherapy regimens and evaluations of resistance-reversing agents. After more than 20 years of research, DTIC is still the standard against which most new chemotherapy agents are compared [6].

As for the dose, it has been demonstrated that 850~1000 mg/m^2 single dose of DTIC is tolerated. This single dose administration appears to deliver clinical improvements similar to those observed with multiple doses that provide the same total dose per cycle. This should be the reference standard for randomized trials comparing new therapies with DTIC [7].

2.2. Temozolomide

Temozolomide (TMZ) is an orally active alkylating agent. It's a prodrug of MTIC and congener of DTIC. It has been available in the US since August 1999 and in other countries since the early 2000s. The therapeutic benefit of temozolomide depends on its ability to alkylate/methylate DNA, which most often occurs at the N-7 or O-6 positions of guanine residues. This methylation damages the DNA and triggers the death of tumor cells. However, some tumor cells are able to repair this type of DNA damage, and therefore diminish the therapeutic efficacy of temozolomide, by expressing an enzyme called O-6-methylguanine-DNA methyltransferase (MGMT) or O-6-alkylguanine-DNA alkyltransferase [8].

The single agent activity of TMZ in metastatic melanoma has been established in several phase 1 and 2 studies [9]. In a randomized trial of 305 patients with advanced melanoma, TMZ showed efficacy at least equivalent to that of DTIC in terms of objective response rate, time to progression, and overall disease-free survival [10]. TMZ was tolerated very well and showed an advantage in terms of improvement in the quality of life. More patients showed improvement or maintenance of physical functioning at Week 12. That trial excluded patients who had brain metastases. Because the trial design was intended to demonstrate the superiority of TMZ over DTIC, rather than equivalence, the FDA did not accept the results of that trial as grounds for approving a melanoma indication for TMZ. But in clinical practice, patients with metastatic melanoma often are treated off-label with TMZ.

TMZ has demonstrated efficacy in the treatment of variety of solid tumors, especially in brain malignancies, which is a manifestation of its far greater ability to penetrate the central nervous system (CNS). Taking into account the high rate of CNS recurrence as a site of failure after cytotoxic chemotherapy, TMZ may represent a viable alternative to DTIC, which is ineffective against melanoma CNS metastases.

2.3. Sorafenib

Sorafenib (BAY43-9006, developed by Bayer Pharmaceuticals, West Haven CT, trade name Nexavar) is an orally administered tyrosine kinase inhibitor. It is a potent inhibitor of the BRAF kinase that is frequently mutated in melanoma, as well as an inhibitor of the Vascular Endothelial Growth Factor (VEGF) receptor and other kinases. It targets the adenosine triphosphate-binding site of the BRAF kinase and inhibits both wild-type and mutant BRAF *in vitro*. Sorafenib was approved by the FDA in December 2005 for use in the treatment of advanced renal cancer. Preclinical studies demonstrated a significant retardation in the growth of human melanoma tumor xenografts with Sorafenib. In a phase 1 study, the maximum tolerated dose of Sorafenib as a single agent was established at 400 mg twice daily, and the most common toxicities were gastrointestinal (mainly diarrhea), dermatologic (skin rash, hand-foot syndrome), and fatigue [11].

But in further phase 2 clinical trials, Sorafenib had shown relatively little activity in metastatic melanoma when using alone. In a phase 2 trial that was conducted in 20 patients with refractory metastatic melanoma, Sorafenib showed modest activity with 1 partial response and 3 patients who achieved stable disease [12]. In another phase 2, randomized, discontinuation trial, no objective responses were achieved, and 19% of patients achieved stable disease [13].

Sorafenib combined with other chemotherapy drugs were also tested clinically. In a phase 1 and 2 study that combined carboplatin and paclitaxel with escalating doses of Sorafenib in 35 patients, a promising response rate of 31% was observed, and another 54% of patients experienced stable disease that lasted longer than 3 months. That study recently was updated to include 105 patients, and the current response rate is 27% [14]. On this basis, 2 phase 3 trials have been launched to assess the efficacy of carboplatin and paclitaxel plus Sorafenib versus placebo in chemotherapy-naive patients and in previously treated patients. In December 2006, Bayer reported the combinations failed to show significant improvement of progression-free survival in melanoma patients [15].

2.4. Vemurafenib

Vemurafenib established a successful model for extracellular chemotherapeutic targeted therapy based on deep understanding cancer biology. It's a paradigm of structured-based drug development. It was first discovered in 2002 that the protein kinase BRAF is mutated in about 70% of malignant melanomas and a significant number of colorectal, ovarian and papillary thyroid cancers, implicating mutated BRAF as a critical promoter of malignancy. Then scientists determined the structure of the BRAF catalytic domain and identified a class of BRAF inhibitors that bind to the active conformation of the protein. Further lead series were developed and crystal structures of complexes combined with molecular modeling studies have resulted in potent selective inhibitors. Vemurafenib is the first one that went into clinical trials and gained FDA approval in August 2011.

Vemurafenib (PLX4032/RG7204) is developed by Plexxikon (now part of the Daiichi Sankyo group and Hoffmann–La Roche) for the treatment of late-stage melanoma. Vemurafenib can induce programmed cell death in melanoma cell lines. It interrupts the BRAF/MEK step on the BRAF/MEK/ERK pathway – if the BRAF has the common V600E mutation [16].

Vemurafenib has very impressive single-agent clinical activity, with unprecedented response rates of about 80% and a clear impact on progression-free survival longer than 6 months. An international randomized open-label trial in patients with previously untreated metastatic or unresectable melanoma with the BRAF[V600E] mutation led to the FDA approval of Vemurafenib for melanoma. This clinical trial enrolled 675 patients. 337 patients were randomly assigned to vemurafenib with 960 mg orally twice daily. 338 patients were randomly assigned to dacarbazine with 1000 mg/m^2 intravenously every three weeks. Treatment end-points are disease progression, unacceptable toxicity, and/or consent withdrawal.

Vemurafenib's efficacy was measured by overall survival (OS), investigator-assessed progression-free survival (PFS) and confirmed investigator-assessed best overall response rate. Overall survival was significantly improved in patients receiving vemurafenib compared with those receiving dacarbazine. The median survival of patients receiving vemurafenib had not been reached and was 7.9 months for those receiving dacarbazine. Progression-free survival (PFS) was also significantly improved in patients receiving vemurafenib. The median PFS was 5.3 months for patients receiving vemurafenib and 1.6 months for patients receiving dacarbazine. 48.4% for patients who received vemurafenib showed complete or partial response while only 5.5% patients who received dacarbazine showed complete or partial response [17].

Arthralgia, rash, photosensitivity, fatigue, alopecia, pruritis, and skin papilloma were observed in at least 30% of patients treated with vemurafenib. Cutaneous squamous cell carcinomas were detected in approximately 24% of patients. Other adverse reactions reported in patients treated with vemurafenib included hypersensitivity, Stevens-Johnson syndrome, toxic epidermal necrolysis, uveitis, QT prolongation, and liver enzyme laboratory abnormalities [18].

2.5. Other single chemotherapy agents

Cisplatin and carboplatin have shown modest activity as single agents in patients with metastatic melanoma. Cisplatin as single-agent therapy induced a 15% response rate with a short median duration of 3 months [19]. A response rate of 19% has been reported in 26 chemotherapy-naive patients with metastatic melanoma who received carboplatin. In those patients, there were 5 partial responses, and thrombocytopenia was the dose-limiting toxicity [20]. *In vitro* studies suggested that oxaliplatin may be more active than cisplatin or carboplatin. But a small phase 2 trial in 10 patients who had received and failed prior chemotherapy produced no objective responses [21].

The nitrosoureas (carmustine, lomustine, and semustine) induce objective responses in 13~18% patients. They can cross the blood-brain barrier. But at conventional doses, little or no activity was observed against melanoma brain metastases [22]. Another drawback of the nitrosureas is they induce prolonged myelosuppression. Despite these, they have been included frequently in multi-agent chemotherapy combinations, presumably for their ability to penetrate into the CNS and lack of viable alternatives for metastatic melanoma.

The vinca alkaloids (vindesine and vinblastine) have produced responses in approximately 14% of patients [23]. The taxanes have produced responses in 16~17% patients [24]. All of these response rate data were obtained from phase 2 trials. None of those drugs have been evaluated as single agents in phase 3 trials. Based on the experience with DTIC, it is likely that the phase 3 trial objective response rates would be less than the rates reported from phase 2 trials. All of these drugs are rarely used currently as single-agent therapy in metastatic melanoma, but they frequently have been incorporated into combination chemotherapy and biochemotherapy regimens.

2.6. Chemotherapy drug combinations

Theoretically drug combination should be based on laboratory or clinical evidence of syner-gistic effect. But since single-agent chemotherapy regimens only provided modest activity against metastatic melanoma and lack of viable alternatives, many combination regimens have been evaluated in clinical trials. Initially two-agent combinations were tested in which DTIC was combined with a nitrosourea, vinca alkaloid, or platinum compound. In most of these trials, only 10~20% response rates were observed. There was little evidence to suggest superiority of these combinations compared with DTIC treatment alone [25-27].

In order to improve response rates, more aggressive multi-drug combinations using 3 or 4 different drugs were also tested clinically. Two most widely studied combinations are cis-platin, vinblastine, and DTIC (CVD) and the Dartmouth regimen. The latter is a 4-drug com-bination consisting of cisplatin, DTIC, carmustine, and tamoxifen (also called CDBT). Both combinations showed improved response rates that ranged from 30% to 50% in single-insti-tution phase 2 studies [28, 29]. But in further randomized phase 3 trials which involved more patients, they all showed much lower efficiency: In a randomized trial comparing CVD with single-agent DTIC that involved approximately 150 patients, the CVD arm pro-duced a 19% response rate compared with 14% for the DTIC arm, and there was no differen-ces in either response duration or survival. In another randomized phase 3 trial, the CDBT combination was compared with single-agent DTIC. That cooperative group trial involved 240 patients, and the response rate was 10% for the DTIC regimen compared with 19% for the CDBT regimen (P=0.09). The median survival was 7 months, with no significant differ-ence between the 2 treatment arms [6].

The main reason for such discrepancies between the results from single-institution studies and those from large, multicenter, cooperative trials probably is selection bias. Differences in performance status, percentages of patients with visceral involvement, and number of meta-static sites easily could account for some of the observed differences. In fact, all of those fac-tors are known to have an impact on both response rate and survival [30].

Overall, controlled trials have produced no compelling evidence to support the value of combination chemotherapy, with or without tamoxifen, in patients with metastatic melano-ma. Toxicity was substantially greater for the combination regimen, with bone marrow sup-pression, nausea, emesis, and fatigue significantly more frequent with CDBT than with DTIC [6]. So it is difficult to justify the use of either CVD or CDBT instead of single-agent DTIC or TMZ for the treatment of most patients with metastatic melanoma.

3. Immunotherapy agents

3.1. Interleukin-s (IL-2)

In 1998, the FDA approved intermittent high-dose bolus IL-2 based on its ability to mediate durable complete response in metastatic melanoma patients [31]. IL-2 is a type of cytokine immune system signaling molecule, which is a leukocytotrophic hormone that is instrumental in the body's natural response to microbial infection and in discriminating between for-eign (non-self) and self. It's a glycosylated 15,500 dalton single protein molecule. IL-2 mediates its effects by binding to IL-2 receptors, which are expressed by lymphocytes, the cells that are responsible for immunity. It is one of the only two FDA approved agents for the treatment of metastatic melanoma. Although the overall response rate is only about 15% and less than 5% of patients achieve complete remission with IL-2, its performance on mela-noma is better than DTIC.

One of the major immunologic effects of IL-2 upon the immune system is to expand the total number of T-lymphocytes (CD4+ and CD8+) and to prevent lymphocyte apoptosis. Another key role of IL-2 is to provide the appropriate cytokine milieu necessary to over-come tumor-induced immune tolerance. But the exact molecular and genetic mechanisms involved in this complex interaction between the tumor and the host immune response is still largely unknown [32].

There is currently a wide spectrum of dosing schedules and regimens for IL-2 therapy, with the current standard used by most oncologists being 600,000 to 720,000 IU/kg/dose, given at 8 h intervals. Although the optimal dosing schedule resulting in the best clinical response is currently unknown, previous data would suggest that the higher dose regi-mens as well as the number of total doses received correlates best with clinical response. Thus, several groups have begun to look at alternative dosing strategies to achieve an in-creased drug tolerance and tolerability profile, such as the continuous infusion of IL-2 (18 mIU/m^2/day) over an extended period of 72 h [33]. But the multiorgan toxicity of many IL-2 regimens limits its use. In addition, the tumor-killing cytotoxic T cells and natural killer cells, which are the presumed target cells for IL-2, are frequently inefficient in the tumor environment, partly due to suppressive and apoptosis-inducing signals from tumor-infiltrating mononuclear phagocytes [34].

3.2. Interferon α

Interferons (IFNs) are proteins made and released by the cells of most vertebrates in re-sponse to the presence of pathogens or tumor cells. They allow communication between cells to trigger the protective defenses of the immune system that eradicate pathogens or tu-mors. IFNs belong to the large class of glycoproteins known as cytokines. They are named after their ability to "interfere" with viral replication within host cells. IFNs have other func-tions: they activate immune cells, such as natural killer cells and macrophages; they increase recognition of infection or tumor cells by up-regulating antigen presentation to T lympho-cytes; and they increase the ability of uninfected host cells to resist new infection by virus.

Based on the type of receptors through which they signal, human interferons have been clas-sified into three major types. The type I interferons present in human are IFN-α, IFN-β and IFN-ω [35]. High-dose IFN therapy using IFN-α was the first form of medical therapy to be approved by the FDA for use in high-risk melanoma in the adjuvant setting. Adjuvant nor-mally means using IFN- α weeks after the surgical excision of the melanoma tumor. Com-mon treatment scheme is IFN-α2b at 20 million units (MU)/m^2/day intravenous injection 5 days a week for 4 weeks, then 10 MU/m^2/day subcutaneous injection 3 days a week for the next 48 weeks for a full year's. But IFN-α2b can also be used one month before definitive surgical lymphadenectomy. This is called 'neoadjuvant' treatment [36].

The first randomized comparison of high-dose IFN versus observation found the median re-lapse-free survival was 1.72 years in the high-dose IFN arm versus 0.98 year in the observa-tion arm (P=0.0023) and the median overall survival was 3.82 versus 2.78 years (P=0.0237) respectively [37]. But in a later pooled analysis of more patients in more clinical trials, the relapse-free survival benefit was maintained but no overall survival benefit was seen [38].

The exact mechanism of IFN IFN-α's anti-tumor efficacy is still unknown. But it was found that the STAT1/STAT3 expression ratios rose in association with IFN treatment. The clinical effects of IFN-α2b in human melanoma are also found to be inversely related to STAT3 ex-pression (41). Induction of apoptosis has been shown to be important *in vitro*, if not *in vivo*. IFN-α can induce apoptosis in transformed cell lines as well as primary tumor cells [39].

High-dose IFN is the standard of care for high-risk melanoma patients in the adjuvant set-ting. However, it is associated with significant toxicity. The incidence and severity of these adverse events is clearly dose-related. Consequently, there has been a great deal of interest in intermediate- and low-dose regimens administered through subcutaneous injection. However, none of the trials using intermediate or low dosing so far have been able to dem-onstrate any reliable benefit in terms of relapse-free survival or overall survival [40].

3.3. Pegylated interferon-α2b

Pegylated interferon-α2b gained its approval from the FDA in March 2011 in the adjuvant setting for melanoma patients with lymph-node-positive disease (stage III) after lymph-node dissection. The approval was based on a randomized controlled phase-III trial in 1256 stage-III melanoma patients. This trial compared treatment with pegylated interferon- α2b for up to 5 years with observation. The results revealed a significant and sustained impact on relapse free survival (RFS) in the intention-to-treat (ITT) population. This trial also showed that interferon-α2b treatment didn't significantly improve distant metastasis-free survival (DMFS) or overall survival (OS) [41]. Pegylated interferon-α2b also showed much better effect in patients with sentinel-node-positive disease (stage III-N1: microscopic in-volvement only) compared with patients with palpable nodal disease (stage III-N2). It also significantly improved DMFS in sentinel-node-positive patients in contrast to a marginal ef-fect in patients with palpable nodes. The authors identified tumor stage as a predictive fac-tor in trials. One very important finding from clinical trials was that ulceration of the primary melanoma indicated a distinct biology that was clearly IFN sensitive in contrast to the non-ulcerated type of melanoma.

3.4. Anti-CTLA4 antibodies: Ipilimumab and tremelimumab

Cytotoxic T-Lymphocyte Antigen 4 (CTLA4) also known as CD152 (Cluster of differentia-tion 152) is a member of the immunoglobulin super family, which is expressed on the sur-face of Helper T cells and transmits an inhibitory signal to T cells that eventually shuts off the activated state. The rationale for involving this in treatment of metastatic melanoma is to block the negative signal sending by CTLA4 by using anti-CTLA4 antibodies, thus reduce the sensitivity of activated T cells to negative regulatory signals and enhance the immune response of the host to tumor cells.

As of October 2007 there are two fully human monoclonal anti-CTLA4 antibodies in advanced clinical trials, one from Medarex, Inc. (Princeton, NJ) and Bristol-Myers Squibb (New York), called ipilimumab (MDX-010), and one from Pfizer (New York), called tremelimumab (formerly ticilimumab, CP-675,206) [42]. These antibodies were produced using different types of mice with engineered immune systems, and are thus fully human, with long half-lives of 2– 4 weeks.

Ipilimumab (MDX-010) is an IgG1 monoclonal antibody. Preclinical and early clinical studies of patients with metastatic melanoma show that ipilimumab promotes antitumor activity as monotherapy and in combination with treatments such as chemotherapy, vaccines, or cytokines. The initial success with these antibodies has encouraged the rapid development of new agonistic and antagonistic antibodies that alter immune regulation, such as anti-PD-1, anti-4-1BB, anti-CD40, and anti-OX-40. On December 10, 2007, Bristol-Myers Squibb and Medarex released the results of three studies on ipilimumab [42]. The three studies tested 487 patients with metastatic melanoma. Short-term tumor progression prior to delayed regression has been observed in ipilimumab-treated patients, and objective responses may be of prolonged duration. In some patients clinical improvement manifests as stable disease, which may also extend for months or years. One of the three studies failed to meet its primary goal of shrinking tumors in at least 10% of the study's 155 patients. Overall the medication produced weaker-than-anticipated efficacy on melanoma patients.

In the meantime, the side effect profile was high in the ipilimumab treated group, with the generation of autoimmune-like effects, such as diarrhea, dermatitis and effects upon the thyroid and pituitary glands. Several patients also experienced vitiligo, indicative of anti-melanocyte autoimmunity. However, the majority of the side effects were noted to be transient (except the vitiligo), improving or disappearing after the completion of therapy. Early clinical data suggest a correlation between these side effects and response to ipilimumab treatment and most likely reflect the drug mechanism of action and corresponding effects on the immune system [42].

In 2011, the first-line pivotal trial data for ipilimumab was released. The median survival of patients treated with ipilimumab at a dose of 10 mg/kg in combination with dacarbazine was 11.2 months. Patients treated with dacarbazine alone showed a median survival of 9.1 months. The improvement in the median survival was 2.1 months. The estimated survival rates in the two groups of, respectively, 47.3% and 36.3% at 1 year, 28.5% and 17.9% at 2 years, and 20.8% and 12.2% at 3 years. These results are not better than those observed with the 3 mg/kg dose in second-line treatment. One possible reason is that a significant and unexpectedly high rate of hepatitis in the dacarbazine + ipilimumab arm did take a significant percentage of patients off treatment before the third or especially the fourth dose of ipilimumab could be administered, thus limiting both the number of administrations of dacarbazine as well as of ipilimumab in the combination arm. Other immune-related adverse events were not increased compared to those with the 3 mg/kg dose experience. The overall interpretation therefore is that dacarbazine did not help, but may rather have mitigated the results in the dacarbazine plus ipilimumab arm. Based on all the data available, the large cumulative phase-II experience, and the two phase-III trials, the FDA approved treatment of melanoma with ipilimumab alone at the 3mg/kg dose [43].

Tremelimumab is an IgG2 monoclonal antibody produced by Pfizer. It blocks the binding of the antigen-presenting cell ligands B7.1 and B7.2 to CTLA-4, resulting in inhibition of B7-CTLA-4-mediated down-regulation of T-cell activation. Subsequently, B7.1 or B7.2 may interact with another T-cell surface receptor protein, CD28, resulting in a B7-CD28-mediated T-cell activation unopposed by B7-CTLA-4-mediated inhibition. Tremelimumab is thought to stimulate patients' immune systems to attack their tumors. It has been shown to induce durable tumor responses in patients with metastatic melanoma in phase 1 and phase 2 clinical studies [44].

On April 2, 2008, Pfizer announced that it has discontinued a phase 3 clinical trial for patients with metastatic melanoma after the review of interim data showed that the trial would not demonstrate superiority to standard chemotherapy [45]. Studies for other tumors are planned as of October 2009, namely for prostate cancer and bladder cancer.

3.5. Anti-integrin antibody: Etaracizumab

Etaracizumab (also known as etaratuzumab, MEDI-522, trade name Abegrin) is an IgG1 humanized monoclonal antibody directed against the $\alpha V\beta 3$ integrin. $\alpha V\beta 3$ is essential for endothelial cell proliferation, maturation, and survival. When it is blocked, proliferating endothelial cells undergo apoptosis and regress. In addition, $\alpha V\beta 3$ is highly expressed in melanomas and is associated with tumor growth and invasion. In preclinical studies using $\alpha V\beta 3$ antagonists, inhibition of melanoma tumor growth independent of its antiangiogenic effects was reported [46]. Etaracizumab has been investigated in 3 phase 1, dose-escalation studies in patients with refractory melanoma. In the phase 2 trial, 57 patients received etaracizumab alone, and 55 patients received etaracizumab plus DTIC. Etaracizumab with or without DTIC generally was well tolerated and was active in patients with metastatic melanoma. The median survival was 12.6 months for the group that received etaracizumab with DTIC and 9.4 months for the group that received etaracizumab without DTIC [47]. These results encouraged people to further test this antibody in more clinical trials.

Early 2010, a study by the Etaracizumab Melanoma Study Group was reported. In this study, 112 patients were randomized to receive etaracizumab alone or etaracizumab plus DTIC. None of the patients in the etaracizumab alone study arm and 12.7% of patients in the etaracizumab plus DTIC study arm achieved an objective response. Stable disease occurred in 45.6% of patients in the etaracizumab alone study arm and 40.0% of patients in the etaracizumab plus DTIC study arm. Despite a modest increase in survival, 12.6 months in the etaracizumab alone arm, versus 9.4 months in the etaracizumab plus DTIC arm, the researchers concluded that the survival results in both treatment arms of this study were considered unlikely to result in clinically meaningful improvement over DTIC alone [48]. At the present time, clinical development of etaracizumab has been interrupted.

3.6. Vaccines based on tumor cells: Canvaxin, melacine, and MVax

The basic idea is to use tumor cell-based vaccine to stimulate and activate the host immune system to recognize, contain and eliminate cancer cells. This effect may be based on the following two pathways: direct migration of the tumor cells to the draining lymph node basin after injection, or uptake of apoptotic or necrotic tumor cells by host dendritic cells located within the skin [49].

The most extensively studied tumor cell-based vaccine is a polyvalent, antigen-rich whole cell vaccine called Canvaxin (CancerVax Corp., Carlsbad, CA). It is comprised of three melanoma cell lines that contain over 20 immunogenic melanoma tumor antigens, given intradermally every two weeks for 3 to 5 doses, followed by monthly injections for the remainder of the first year. However, several small, single-institution phase 1 and 2 clinical trials of Canvaxin have not yielded a striking clinical benefit in most patients when administered with BCG as an immunoadjuvant [50]. But the rare complete responder to Canvaxin therapy has prompted the initiation of two multicenter phase 3 randomized trials of Canvaxin therapy in 1998. In these trials, patients who have undergone complete resection of regional (stage III) or distant (stage IV) metastatic melanoma receive postoperative adjuvant immunotherapy with Canvaxin plus Bacillus of Calmette and Guerin (BCG) or BCG alone. In April 2005, CancerVax announced the discontinuation of their phase 3 clinical trial of Canvaxin in patients with Stage IV melanoma based upon the clinical funding that it was unlikely that the trial would provide significant evidence of a survival benefit for Canvaxin-treated patients versus those receiving placebo. On October 3, 2005, CancerVax announced the discontinuation of another phase 3 clinical trial of Canvaxin in patients with Stage III melanoma base on a similar reason [51].

The second tumor cell-based vaccine that has been well studied since 1988 is Melacine. It is an allogeneic melanoma cell lysate combined with an immunologic adjuvant which is composed of a mixture of detoxified endotoxin, cell wall cytoskeleton and monophosphoryl lipid A. Early phase 1 and 2 clinical trials in 1987 and 1988 revealed some promising results, with one complete and three partial responses seen in 25 patients treated with Melacine. These results prompted the completion of seven open-label phase 2 trials involving 139 patients with stage III/IV melanoma and a multicenter phase 3 clinical trial of Melacine versus the Dartmouth regimen. The objective response rates for all of the above studies have been between 5 and 10%. Based largely upon these former results and the clinical results of other phase 3 trials, a phase 3 observation controlled trial of Melacine in melanoma patients was conducted. But the results revealed no evidence of a benefit from Melacine in patients with melanoma [52].

One very promising autologous cell vaccine is MVax which is now in active phase 3 clinical trial sponsored by AVAX Technologies, Inc. This vaccine is derived from autologous tumor cells that have been irradiated and then modified with the hapten dinitrophenyl (DNP) [53]. In February 2004 the Journal of Clinical Oncology published an article by Dr. David Berd on the treatment of 214 Stage IIIb and IIIc melanoma patients that showed a five-year survival rate of 44%. Comparison to published results of similar patients treated with surgery alone showed five-year survival figures of 22%. In stage IV patients MVax has demonstrated significant response rates as a monotherapy and in published reports MVax plus adjuvant IL-2 have reported response rate of 35% (13% Complete Response, 22% Partial Response). This compares to published response rates in low dose IL-2 of 3% [54].

In October 2006, AVAX obtained a Special Protocol Assessment (SPA) agreement with the FDA for its phase 3 protocol. The SPA allows for the start of the phase 3 registration clinical trial for MVax for the treatment of patients with metastatic melanoma. In addition, the SPA addressed AVAX's ability to use a surrogate endpoint as a basis for accelerated approval. Based on this SPA, a phase 3 trial for stage IV melanoma was started on May 2007. AVAX plans to enroll up to 387 patients who will be assigned in a double-blind fashion at a 2:1 ratio to MVax or placebo vaccine. The MVax arm will consist of an initial dose of MVax followed by cyclophosphamide and then six weekly doses of MVax administered with BCG. Following vaccine administration patients will receive a specific schedule of low dose IL-2. Patients assigned to the control group will receive a treatment identical to the MVax group, except that a placebo vaccine will replace MVax. The primary endpoints of the study are best overall anti-tumor response rate and the percentage of patients surviving at least 2 years. Secondary endpoints of the study will include overall survival time, response duration, percentage complete and partial responses, progression free survival and treatment related adverse events [55].

3.7. Vaccines based on peptides: MDX-1379, astuprotimut-R, and others

The identification of tumor antigens that are present on the surface of melanoma cells is the basis for developing cancer vaccines that utilize peptide based immunotherapy. There are several melanoma differentiation antigens known involved in the synthesis of melanin and recognized by melanoma-reactive T cells, for example, gp100, MART-1/Melan-A, tyrosinase, TRP-1 and TRP-2, NY-ESO-1and the melanoma-associated antigen (MAGE) *etc*. One big advantage of peptide based-vaccination is that it has few toxic side effects or adverse reactions. Data suggests that most tumor cell lines established from fine needle aspiration biopsies of patients with metastatic melanoma exhibit a relatively homogeneous co-expression of MART-1 and tyrosinase, with a much more heterogeneous expression of other tumor antigens, such as gp100, NY-ESO 1 and the MAGE antigens [56].

Rosenberg and his colleagues developed a with a peptide based-vaccine using modified immunodominant peptide of the gp100 antigen, g209-2M. They used this agent vaccinated stage IV melanoma patients subcutaneously every three weeks. Following two immunizations, 10 of 11 (91%) of patients showed a consistently high level of immunization against the native g209~217 peptide, but not against the control peptide g280~288. This study also demonstrated that the majority of patients immunized with the g209-2M peptide in incomplete Freund's adjuvant (IFA) consistently developed high levels of circulating immune precursors reactive against the native g209~217 peptide. Clinically, one of nine patients who received the g209~217 peptide in IFA experienced an objective cancer regression that lasted 4 months. Three of the eleven patients exhibited mixed responses with complete or partial regression of several lesions. However, all patients eventually developed progressive disease [57].

MDX-1379 vaccine consists of two gp100 melanoma peptides. These peptides are part of a protein normally found on melanocytes, or pigmented skin cells, and on melanoma cells. These melanoma peptides are recognized by cytotoxic T cells in melanoma patients that are positive for HLA-A2, a human immune system compatibility antigen that is expressed in approximately half of the melanoma population. Phase II data show limited evidence of MDX-1379's clinical activity although there is strong proof-of-concept for therapeutic vaccines based on gp100 in melanoma. Medarex is currently conducting a phase 3 clinical trial with ipilimumab and MDX-1379 combination therapy in stage III and IV melanoma at multiple sites within the United States. Preliminary data showed MDX-1379 plus ipilimumab induced a modest percentage of durable response in stage IV melanoma. But autoimmune events could make the risk/benefit ratio for MDX-1379 plus ipilimumab unfavorable [58].

Astuprotimut-R (also called recombinant MAGE-A3 antigen-specific cancer immunotherapeutic GSK1203486A) is a cancer vaccine consisting of a recombinant form of human melanoma antigen A3 (MAGE-A3) combined with a proprietary adjuvant with potential immunostimulatory and antineoplastic activities. Upon administration, astuprotimut-R may stimulate a cytotoxic T-lymphocyte response against tumor cells expressing the MAGE-A3 antigen, resulting in tumor cell death. MAGE-A3, a tumor-associated antigen (TAA) originally discovered in melanoma cells, is expressed by various tumor types including melanoma, non-small cell lung cancer, head and neck cancer, bladder cancer, with no expression in normal cells. MAGE-A3 protein has been in-licensed by GlaxoSmithKline (GSK) from the Ludwig Institute for Cancer Research. The proprietary immunostimulating adjuvant in this agent is composed of a specific combination of immunostimulating compounds selected to increase the anti-tumor immune response to MAGE-A3. Using this vaccine as intramuscular administration together with GSK's two proprietary adjuvant systems, AS15 or AS02B, they have developed a treatment regimen for cancer patients called Antigen-Specific Cancer Immunotherapeutic (ASCI).

In 2008, GSK reported a randomized, open-label phase 2 study designed to evaluate Astuprotimut-R. A total of 72 patients with measurable metastatic MAGE-A3-positive cutaneous melanoma (unresectable or in transit stage III or stage IV M1a) were randomized to receive immunization with MAGE-A3 protein combined with either AS15 or AS02B as first-line metastatic treatment. Patients were to receive a maximum of 24 immunizations over four years. Clinical activity is assessed by the Response Evaluation Criteria In Solid Tumors (RECIST) criteria, the international standards for evaluation of solid tumors. Complete response (CR) and partial response (PR) i.e., disappearance or significant reduction of tumor, were reported in 4 patients in the AS15 group (3 CR and 1 PR) with two of these ongoing for more than two years; in the AS02B arm, 1 patient showed a partial response which lasted for 6 months. The safety profile was similar in both groups with the majority of reported adverse events being mild or moderate local or systemic reactions [59]. Currently this agent still is under phase 2 clinical development for progressive metastatic cutaneous melanoma.

Because melanoma tumors are heterogeneous in their antigenic profile, it is very difficult to make vaccines that can elicit cytotoxic T-cell responses universally in all the host immune systems. Rosenberg's group analyzed 28 different peptide-based vaccines utilized in stage

IV melanoma patients. A total of 381 patients were treated with 370 patients showing no response, 9 patients showing a partial response and 2 patients with a complete response, for an overall objective response rate of only 2.9%. This suggested the lack of effectiveness with this single peptide based vaccination approach [60].

Next logical step is to make vaccines with multiple peptides to overcome tumor cell antigenic heterogeneity. A recent randomized phase 2 trial was performed in 26 patients with metastatic melanoma, vaccinating with four melanoma peptides. Although a high level of specific T-cell responses were noted (in 42% of the peripheral blood, 80% of sentinel lymph nodes), only three patients had a clinical response [61].

Here is the biggest issue in this area, actually many peptide based-vaccinations have resulted in a significant increase in the number of lymphocyte precursors reactive against a variety of tumor differentiation antigens by immunization with native or modified peptides. However, such immunological responses to peptide-based therapy have not translated into meaningful clinical responses for the vast majority of patients. To date, there is no study that has clearly shown a direct correlation between an immunologic response to therapy (immune cell activation) and a clinical response (regression of established tumor).

3.8. Vaccines based on dendritic cells

In the normal human epidermis and dermis, dendritic cells (DC) are present as relatively immature antigen presenting cells, exhibiting relatively low levels of class II major histocompatibility complex (MHC) molecules and co-stimulatory molecules. But these immature DC are quite capable of capturing various soluble protein antigens, such as apoptotic and necrotic tumor cells and then cross-presenting such tumor-associated antigens to cytotoxic CD8+ T cells. When relatively immature DC in the skin is triggered to enter afferent lymphatic channels, this migrating pathway also initiates a phenotypic conversion that has profound immunological consequences [30]. When the DC arrives in the lymph node, it is characterized by an abundant levels of class II MHC antigens, as well as high surface levels of costimulatory molecules, such as CD40, CD54, CD80, CD83, and CD86. The matured DC is then capable of forming stable MHC class II-peptide complexes available to activate antigen specific CD4+ T cells [62].

To make the dendritic cell-based vaccine, the monocyte-derived, autologous DC can be pulsed *in vitro* with either whole irradiated, autologous tumor cells or tumor cell lysate. Once the tumor cells are "fed" to the DC *in vitro*, the apoptotic or necrotic cells are then processed and tumor-specific peptide antigens are then transported to the surface in both an MHC class I- and II-restricted fashion. Both immature and mature DC can be administered to patients as vaccine safely with few adverse side effects. The administration of DC via various routes of vaccination (intradermal, intranodal and intravenous) is also feasible. The first published clinical trial of DC vaccination was in 1995 and has since been followed by 98 additional clinical trials describing more than 1,000 DC-based vaccines performed in 15 different countries. Twenty-eight trials focused on patients with various advanced stages of melanoma. The safety profile was again noted to be quite remarkable, however, despite the treatment of over 1,000 patients with DC-based vaccines, the record of effectiveness have been disappointing [63].

One very successful DC-based trial for patients with advanced, metastatic melanoma was reported by Nestle *et al*. He used plastic adherent monocytes matured with a xenogeneic-based 10% fetal calf serum, subsequently pulsed with either tumor cell lysate or multiple HLA-matched peptides injected intranodally. This trial involved 16 patients who were immunized on an outpatient basis. Overall, 5 of 16 patients experienced an objective response, 2 complete and 3 partial responses. The side effects were noted to be minimal in all cases, with the development of vitiligo in a few patients. One dramatic feature of this treatment was the durability of the clinical responses, with the 2 complete responders remaining free of disease for over 15 months [64].

One phase 3 clinical trial about using DC-based vaccine to treat metastatic melanoma was report by Schadendorf and colleagues recently [65]. The trial was a prospective, randomized trial that analyzed the therapeutic effects of an autologous peptide-pulsed DC-based vaccine in patients with stage IV melanoma compared to standard chemotherapy with DTIC alone. The results revealed that the overall response in the vaccine group was 3.8% compared to 5.5% in the DTIC group, with no statistically significant differences noted in response, toxicity, overall and progression-free survival between the two groups. The median time to progression was 2.8 months versus 3.2 months respectively and the median survival was 11 months for the DTIC arm but only 9 months for the vaccine arm [65].

Although disappointed by many trials, several new avenues of DC-based immunotherapy are actively being pursued and in various stages of development, focusing on different ways to enhance the therapeutic efficacy of DC in combination with various immunoadjuvants and other anticancer agents.

3.9. Individual therapy based on activated T-cells

One very promising approach to treat metastatic melanoma is to use fully activated anti-tumor T-cells as warhead. This regimen involves the adoptive autologous transfer of highly selective tumor-reactive T-cells directed against over-expressed self-derived differentiation antigens after lymphodepleting chemotherapy. Rosenberg group reported in 2004 a clinical trial using this method. Cancer regression in patients with refractory metastatic melanoma with large, vascularized tumors was noted in a remarkable 18 of 35 patients (51% response rate), including four patients with a complete regression of all metastatic disease. Such results may stem from the ability to infuse a large number of fully activated tumor infiltrating lymphocytes with anti-tumor activity into a host that is depleted of regulatory T-cells [66].

4. Gene therapy agents

The recent developments in the field of gene transfer have advanced the use of gene therapy as a novel strategy against a variety of human malignancies. Because of its unique set of characteristics, melanoma represents a suitable target for gene therapy. Several strategies have been used by gene therapy to treat melanoma. First is to target melanoma cells to introduce "suicide" genes. Second is to transfer tumor suppressor genes. Third is to inactivate aberrant oncogene expression. Fourth is to introduce genes encoding immunologically relevant molecules. Last is to target the host's immune cells to redirect immune responses against melanoma. Clinical trials have shown the feasibility and safety of gene therapy against malignant melanoma. Although no major successes have been reported, the positive results observed in some patients support the potential for gene therapy in the management of this disease. To make gene therapy as an effective modality of treatment for malignant melanoma, better vector technology as well as increased understanding of the "bystander effect" triggered by gene transfer approaches are needed [67].

The gene therapy in our discussion is to introduce oligonucleotide or DNA sequence into host body thus to stimulate immune response to tumor cells. So it is also called DNA vaccination. This approach has been shown to induce long-lasting immunity against infectious agents and protection from tumor outgrowth in several animal models [68]. Likewise, intramuscular injections of DNA (composed of naked DNA expression plasmids) into humans have also resulted in the development of an immunologic response [69]. It is hypothesized that one mechanism of tumor antigen expression may involve the DNA introducing the appropriate genes into dendritic cells for subsequent processing and presentation to the host immune system. One of the obvious advantages of DNA vaccinations is that they can be administered to patients regardless of HLA-phenotype and without identifying immunogenic epitopes.

4.1. Anti-BCL2 antisense oligonucleotide genasense

Genasense (Oblimersan sodium developed by Genta Inc. which is a biopharmaceutical company based in Berkeley Heights, New Jersey) is a phosphorothioate antisense oligonucleotide directed against the first six codons of the Bcl-2 messenger RNA. Binding of the drug to the mRNA recruits RNAse H, resulting in cleavage of the mRNA. As a result, further translation is halted and intracellular protein concentrations of Bcl-2 decrease with time. Melanoma cell lines having Bcl-2 overexpression have been shown to enhance activity of metastasis-related proteinases, *in vitro* cell invasion, and *in vivo* tumor growth [70]. Many *in vitro* studies have demonstrated increased sensitivity of melanoma cells to chemotherapy when combined with antisense Bcl-2 therapy [71]. Genasense is the first oncology drug of its kind to directly target the biochemical pathway (known as apoptosis) whereby cancer cells are ultimately killed by chemotherapy. Genasense is believed to inhibit the production of Bcl-2, a protein that is believed to be a fundamental cause of resistance to anticancer therapy. By inhibiting Bcl-2, Genasense may greatly improve the activity of anticancer therapy.

Encouraged by previous data, numerous clinical trials were started to evaluate the addition of oblimersan to chemotherapy in various solid tumors, including melanoma. Updated analysis from a randomized phase 3 trial, comparing DTIC combined with oblimersan, with DTIC alone in 771 patients with Stage IV or unresectable Stage III melanoma who had not previously received chemotherapy has shown a response rate of 12.4% in the former compared with 6.8% in the latter group (P=0.007) [72]. Median progression-free survival for the oblimersan group was 2.4 months as compared with 1.6 months for the DTIC group, with a relative risk reduction of 27% (P=0.0003). The median survival was increased from 7.8 months in the DTIC arm to 9 months in the oblimersan arm with a P value of 0.077, which became significant when the patients with normal baseline LDH were analyzed. In terms of toxicity, no new or unexpected adverse events were observed in this study, which had not been seen with DTIC alone.

However, in May 2004, a new drug application (NDA) based on 6-months of minimum follow-up data from this trial failed to receive an affirmative vote for approval by an advisory committee to the FDA. Genta subsequently withdrew that application, and the Company has not yet made a decision regarding re-filing the U.S. application [73].

4.2. DNA Plasmid-lipid complex allovectin-7

Allovectin-7 is a bicistronic plasmid formulated with a cationic lipid system containing the DNA sequences encoding HLA-B7 and beta-2 microglobulin, which together form a MHC1 antigen. Injection of Allovectin-7 directly into tumors is designed to stimulate an immune response against both local and distant metastatic tumors. Allovectin-7 is a novel gene therapy approach for cancer with a unique mechanism of action that is fundamentally different from currently approved treatments. The following three mechanisms were believed to play roles in this agent's efficacy. Mechanism one, in HLA-B7 negative patients, a vigorous allogeneic immune response may be initiated against the foreign MHC class I antigen. Mechanism two, in all patients, ß2 microglobulin may reconstitute normal class I antigen presentation and/or increase tumor antigen presentation to the immune system. Mechanism three, in some patients, an innate pro-inflammatory response may occur that induces tumor responses following intralesional injection of the DNA/lipid complex. The final outcome of all these mechanisms is to initially cause recognition of the tumor at the local site to allow a then sensitized immune response to recognize un-injected tumors at distant metastatic sites [74].

In 2001, Dr. Richards and his colleagues began a high-dose, 2 mg, phase 2 trial evaluating the Allovectin-7 immunotherapeutic alone for patients with stage III or stage IV melanoma, who have few other treatment options. The high-dose phase 2 trial completed enrollment in 2003. The data showed that the trial had a total of 15 responders among the 127 patients receiving the high dose (11.8%), with four of the patients having complete responses and 11 having partial responses. The Kaplan-Meier estimated median duration of response was 13.8 months. The Kaplan-Meier median survival was 18 months. The safety profile was excellent with no reported Grade 3 or Grade 4 adverse events associated with Allovectin-7 [75].

Allovectin-7 has been granted orphan drug designation for the treatment of invasive and metastatic melanoma by the FDA's Office of Orphan Products Development. Orphan drug designation provides U.S. marketing exclusivity for seven years if marketing approval is received from the FDA

Vical is conducting the AIMM (Allovectin-7 Immunotherapeutic for Metastatic Melanoma) trial, a phase 3 pivotal trial of Allovectin-7 as first-line therapy in approximately 375 patients with Stage III or IV recurrent metastatic melanoma in accordance with a SPA agreement completed with the FDA. The trial is being conducted at approximately 60 clinical sites worldwide. They designed the trial to include patients most likely to benefit from our treatment, and specifically excluded patients with brain or liver metastases, patients previously treated with chemotherapy, and patients with elevated lactate dehydrogenase (LDH) levels.

In January 2010 Vical announced that the company has completed enrollment of the planned 375 subjects in its multinational phase 3 trial of Allovectin-7 in patients with metastatic melanoma. Allovectin-7®'s safety profile is excellent with no drug-related serious adverse events reported to date in the phase 3 trial [74].

4.3. Herpes simplex virus based oncoVEX

OncoVEX (GM-CSF) is an enhanced potency, immuneenhanced oncolytic herpes simplex virus type 1 (HSV-1). It is deleted for infected-cell protein gene 34.5 (ICP34.5), providing tumor selective replication, and ICP47 gene which otherwise blocks antigen presentation. In addition, ICP47 deletion increases unique short region protein 11 (US11) gene expression thereby enhancing virus growth and replication in tumor cells. The coding sequence for human granulocyte-macrophage colony-stimulating factor (GM-CSF) is inserted, replacing ICP34.5, to enhance the immune response to tumor antigens released following virus replication.

OncoVEX is developed by BioVex (Woburn, MA). It is a first-in-class oncolytic, or cancer destroying virus, that works by replicating and spreading within solid tumors (leaving healthy cells unaffected), thereby causing cancer cell death and stimulating the immune system to destroy un-injected metastatic deposits. Both modes of action have been clearly validated in the clinic, where multiple patients with metastatic disease progressing at enrollment have been declared disease free.

BioVex recently concluded a 50-patient phase 2 trial for OncoVEX (GM-CSF) as a standalone therapy in patients with Stage IIIc and Stage IV melanoma. The trial was designed to measure overall objective response, which is defined as a complete response, where disease is completely eliminated, or partial response, where there is a >50% reduction in disease burden. 74% of patients who entered the study were progressing after having failed prior therapy. 13 objective systemic responses (26% objective response rate) were achieved including eight CRs, seven of which remain free of disease. 12 responses have so far continued for more than 6 months (ranging from 6 to more than 29 months). Responses were observed in patients with all stages of disease, including the complete resolution of un-injected visceral deposits. Adverse effects were primarily limited to transient flu-like symptoms [76].

In April 2009, BioVex Inc. announced that its OPTiM (OncoVEX Pivotal Trial in Melanoma) phase 3 study with OncoVEX (GM-CSF) in previously treated patients with Stage III and Stage IV melanoma had initiated. The study has commenced recruiting patients in the U.S. and with sites in the United Kingdom, Germany and Australia. The OPTiM trial is a multinational, open label, randomized study designed to assess the efficacy and safety of treat-ment with OncoVEX (GM-CSF) as compared to subcutaneously administered GM-CSF in patients with unresectable stage III (b-c) and stage IV (M1a-c) disease. Patients will have re-ceived at least one prior therapy for active disease which includes any type of therapy in-cluding investigational drugs. A total of 360 patients will be enrolled (240 to the OncoVEX (GM-CSF) arm and 120 to the control arm). The study design was agreed with the FDA un-der the special protocol assessment process [77].

5. Possible reasons for extremely high resistance of metastatic melanoma

Despite an epic number of clinical trials to test a wide variety of anticancer strategies, the average survival rate for patients with metastatic melanoma remains unimproved during the past 30 years (41). Though constant clinical trials effort, although some approaches showed promising intermediate results, still no agent has been granted FDA approval for the treatment of metastatic melanoma. There are several reasons that may account for the extremely high resistance of metastatic melanoma to current treatment modalities.

5.1. Reasons for chemotherapy resistance

Melanoma cells are quite resistant to most chemotherapy reagents. This is associated with the specific feature of melanoma cells. In nature, these cells have low levels of spontaneous apoptosis *in vivo* compared with other tumor cell types, and they are relatively resistant to drug-induced apoptosis *in vitro* [78]. The natural role of melanocytes is to protect inner or-gans from UV light, a potent DNA damaging agent. Therefore, it is not surprising that mela-noma cells may have special DNA damage repair systems and enhanced survival properties [79]. Moreover, recent studies showed that, during melanoma progression, it acquired com-plex genetic alterations that led to hyperactivation of efflux pumps, detoxification enzymes, and a multifactorial alteration of survival and apoptotic pathways. All these have been pro-posed to mediate the multi-drug resistant phenotype of melanoma [80].

5.2. Barriers for successful immunotherapy

The major barrier is immunosuppressive effects activated by tumors. Tumor cell can escape immune rejection and induce immunosuppression through the following five major paths. Firstly, tumor cells may lose or down-regulate either the melanoma associated antigens or MHC molecules. Secondly, tumor cells may produce a plethora of immunosuppressive fac-tors such as interleukin-10, VEGF and transforming growth factor. These factors create an inherently unfavorable microenvironment that limits the host immune response, in addition to tolerating the T-cell response to established tumor. Third possible reason is intrinsic inef-ficiency of DC whereby the appropriate co-stimulatory molecules are not being presented on the cell surface. Fourth possible reason is tumor-related alterations in T-cell signaling and a skewing of the immune response from a Th1 (immunoactivating) to a Th2 response (im-munotolerant). Lastly, the concept of tumor cell escape and immune tolerance is an exceedingly complex process. We need to further understand these mechanisms before we can have successful immunotherapy to melanoma [32].

Specifically for cancer vaccines, there are some further barriers. First is the characterization of vaccines potency and toxicity. This is especially important in the transition from phase 2 to phase 3 trials. To select a meaningful and validated end point for trials is a big challenge most of the time. Second barrier is selection of the maximum tolerated dose of cancer vaccine, particularly compared with traditional anticancer agents. Cancer vaccines are typically not very toxic. So the optimum dose often has to be based on the immune response of patients. But if the patients have previously been heavily treated with other anticancer agents, this can lead to a compromised immune system that makes it difficult to detect an evoked immune response. The third barrier is appropriate trial design and statistical data process. This is also a key part and can substantially affect final trial outcome [53].

6. Future directions

With the rapidly rising incidence and the high resistance to current therapeutic agents, developing more effective drugs for metastatic melanoma is urgently needed. But before we can thoroughly understand all the major molecular pathological changes associated with melanoma malignancy, it is very difficult to reach a cure for it.

Melanoma is an extremely complicated disease, with many gene mutation and signaling pathway changes. Elevated signaling pathway in melanoma including mitogen-activated protein kinase (MAPK) pathway, phosphatidylinositol 3 kinase (PI3K)-AKT pathway, Wnt-Frizzled-β-catenin pathway, JAK/Stat pathway and α-MSH-MC1R or microphthalmia-associated transcription factor (MITF) pathway. The first two are crucial pathway accounting for melanoma malignance. Gene mutation that are involved in melanoma include the following oncogenes: BRAF, N-ras, akt3; tumor suppressors: CDKN2A, PTEN, p53, APAF-1, p16, p15, p19; others: Cyclin D1, MITF etc [81].

The binding of growth factors to their respective receptors leads to activation of RAS proteins. Ras will then activate Raf. Raf activate mitogen-activated protein kinase (MEK), which then act on extracellular-related kinase (ERK). Phosporylated ERK kinases (ERK-P) translocate to the nucleus and activate transcription factors, which promote cell cycle progression and proliferation. The PI3K-AKT pathway mediates cell survival signaling via growth factors. Phosphatase and tensin homolog (PTEN) inhibits growth factor signaling by inactivating phosphatidylinositol triphosphate (PIP3) generated by PI3K. Activated PI3K converts the plasma membrane lipid phosphatidylinositol 4,5-bisphosphonate to PIP3, which acts as a second messenger leading to the phosphorylation AKT and subsequent up-regulation of cell cycle, growth, and survival proteins. AKT can also up-regulate mTOR (mammalian target of rapamycin), S6K, and NFκb leading to cell growth and inhibition of apoptosis.

Knowing the huge complexity of melanoma, it's easy to understand why so many random trials of single agents or combinational treatment have failed. So targeted therapy in a systemic way based on the understanding about melanoma molecular pathology seems to be a reasonable way to fight this disease.

Individualized T-cell-based therapy is a very promising approach. Combined with other suitable tumor killing agents, it could improve the patient survival rate and time. Unfortunately, the selective tumor-reactive T-cells isolated from a patient can only be used for this same patient. Thus the cost associated with this treatment method is very high. Such an expensive treatment may not be available to all the patients in the near future.

In learning from our efforts in the past, we must continue to challenge the current paradigms of treatment as we forge new paths to more effective treatment options. This will likely involve a multimodal approach to therapy utilizing all of the available tools in our arsenal. Several agents given in unique combinations may then synergize with standard chemotherapeutic regimens resulting in prolonged clinical responses and long term survival. Take Sorafenib as an example, its failure maybe largely due to the fact that it only blocks the RAF-MEK-ERK signaling pathway. Melanoma cells can still survive by compensatory up-regulation in other survival pathways such as the PI3K-AKT pathway. Melanoma can also develop drug resistance with time by over-expressing MDR genes. Ideally, if we can use drugs to synergistically block all the major survival pathways in melanoma cells and then educate our immune system to fight the tumor cells, we will have a much better chance to conquer this deadly disease.

Author details

Zhao Wang, Wei Li* and Duane D. Miller

*Address all correspondence to: wli@uthsc.edu

Department of Pharmaceutical Sciences, University of Tennessee Health Science Center, Memphis, USA

References

[1] Eggermont, A.M. and C. Robert, *New drugs in melanoma: It's a whole new world*. Eur J Cancer, 2011. 47(47): p. 2150-2157.

[2] Kahler, K.C. and A. Hauschild, *Treatment and side effect management of CTLA-4 antibody therapy in metastatic melanoma*. J Dtsch Dermatol Ges, 2011. 9(4): p. 277-86.

[3] Roukos, D.H., *PLX4032 and melanoma: resistance, expectations and uncertainty*. Expert Rev Anticancer Ther, 2011. 11(3): p. 325-8.

[4] Williams, D.A. and T.L. Lemke, *Foye's Principles of Medicinal Chemistry*. Fifth Edition ed2002, Philadelphia, PA: Lippincott Williams & Wilkins.

[5]   Falkson, C.I., et al., *Phase III trial of dacarbazine versus dacarbazine with interferon al-pha-2b versus dacarbazine with tamoxifen versus dacarbazine with interferon alpha-2b and tamoxifen in patients with metastatic malignant melanoma: an Eastern Cooperative Oncology Group study.* J Clin Oncol, 1998. 16(5): p. 1743-51.

[6]   Chapman, P.B., et al., *Phase III multicenter randomized trial of the Dartmouth regimen versus dacarbazine in patients with metastatic melanoma.* J Clin Oncol, 1999. 17(9): p. 2745-51.

[7]   Eggermont, A.M. and J.M. Kirkwood, *Re-evaluating the role of dacarbazine in metastatic melanoma: what have we learned in 30 years?* Eur J Cancer, 2004. 40(12): p. 1825-36.

[8]   Jacinto, F.V. and M. Esteller, *MGMT hypermethylation: a prognostic foe, a predictive friend.* DNA Repair (Amst), 2007. 6(8): p. 1155-60.

[9]   Newlands, E.S., et al., *Phase I trial of temozolomide (CCRG 81045: M&B 39831: NSC 362856).* Br J Cancer, 1992. 65(2): p. 287-91.

[10] Middleton, M.R., et al., *Randomized phase III study of temozolomide versus dacarbazine in the treatment of patients with advanced metastatic malignant melanoma.* J Clin Oncol, 2000. 18(1): p. 158-66.

[11] Strumberg, D., et al., *Phase I clinical and pharmacokinetic study of the Novel Raf kinase and vascular endothelial growth factor receptor inhibitor BAY 43-9006 in patients with advanced refractory solid tumors.* J Clin Oncol, 2005. 23(5): p. 965-72.

[12] Ahmad T, M.R., Pyle L, James M, Schwartz B, Gore M, Eisen T., *BAY 43-9006 in patients with advanced melanoma: The Royal Marsden experience.* Journal of Clinical Oncology 2004 ASCO Annual Meeting Proceedings., 2004. 22(14s).

[13] Eisen, T., et al., *Sorafenib in advanced melanoma: a Phase II randomised discontinuation trial analysis.* Br J Cancer, 2006. 95(5): p. 581-6.

[14] Flaherty KT, B.M., Schucter L, et al, *Phase I/II trial of BAY 43-9006, carboplatin (C) and paclitaxel (P) demonstrates preliminary antitumor activity in the expansion cohort of patients with metastatic melanoma.* Journal of Clinical Oncology 2004 ASCO Annual Meeting Proceedings., 2004. 22(14s): p. 7507.

[15] Herlyn, M., *recent development in melanoma research (review on literature).* 2007.

[16] Sala, E., et al., *BRAF silencing by short hairpin RNA or chemical blockade by PLX4032 leads to different responses in melanoma and thyroid carcinoma cells.* Mol Cancer Res, 2008. 6(5): p. 751-9.

[17] Chapman, P.B., et al., *Improved survival with vemurafenib in melanoma with BRAF V600E mutation.* N Engl J Med, 2011. 364(26): p. 2507-16.

[18] Young, K., A. Minchom, and J. Larkin, *BRIM-1, -2 and -3 trials: improved survival with vemurafenib in metastatic melanoma patients with a BRAF(V600E) mutation.* Future Oncol, 2012. 8(5): p. 499-507.

[19] Atkins, M.B., *The treatment of metastatic melanoma with chemotherapy and biologics*. Curr Opin Oncol, 1997. 9(2): p. 205-13.

[20] Evans, L.M., E.S. Casper, and R. Rosenbluth, *Phase II trial of carboplatin in advanced malignant melanoma*. Cancer Treat Rep, 1987. 71(2): p. 171-2.

[21] Gogas, H.J., J.M. Kirkwood, and V.K. Sondak, *Chemotherapy for metastatic melanoma: time for a change?* Cancer, 2007. 109(3): p. 455-64.

[22] Boaziz, C., et al., *[Brain metastases of malignant melanomas]*. Bull Cancer, 1991. 78(4): p. 347-53.

[23] Quagliana, J.M., et al., *Vindesine in patients with metastatic malignant melanoma: a Southwest Oncology Group study*. J Clin Oncol, 1984. 2(4): p. 316-9.

[24] Bedikian, A.Y., et al., *Phase II trial of docetaxel in patients with advanced cutaneous malignant melanoma previously untreated with chemotherapy*. J Clin Oncol, 1995. 13(12): p. 2895-9.

[25] Avril, M.F., et al., *Combination chemotherapy of dacarbazine and fotemustine in disseminated malignant melanoma. Experience of the French Study Group*. Cancer Chemother Pharmacol, 1990. 27(2): p. 81-4.

[26] Fletcher, W.S., et al., *Evaluation of cis-platinum and DTIC combination chemotherapy in disseminated melanoma. A Southwest Oncology Group Study*. Am J Clin Oncol, 1988. 11(5): p. 589-93.

[27] Vorobiof, D.A., R. Sarli, and G. Falkson, *Combination chemotherapy with dacarbazine and vindesine in the treatment of metastatic malignant melanoma*. Cancer Treat Rep, 1986. 70(7): p. 927-8.

[28] Legha, S.S., et al., *A prospective evaluation of a triple-drug regimen containing cisplatin, vinblastine, and dacarbazine (CVD) for metastatic melanoma*. Cancer, 1989. 64(10): p. 2024-9.

[29] Del Prete, S.A., et al., *Combination chemotherapy with cisplatin, carmustine, dacarbazine, and tamoxifen in metastatic melanoma*. Cancer Treat Rep, 1984. 68(11): p. 1403-5.

[30] Flaherty, L.E., et al., *Comparison of patient characteristics and outcome between a single-institution phase II trial and a cooperative-group phase II trial with identical eligibility in metastatic melanoma*. Am J Clin Oncol, 1997. 20(6): p. 600-4.

[31] Smith, F.O., et al., *Treatment of metastatic melanoma using interleukin-2 alone or in conjunction with vaccines*. Clin Cancer Res, 2008. 14(17): p. 5610-8.

[32] Riker, A.I., et al., *Immunotherapy of melanoma: a critical review of current concepts and future strategies*. Expert Opin Biol Ther, 2007. 7(3): p. 345-58.

[33] Quan, W., Jr., et al., *Repeated cycles with 72-hour continuous infusion interleukin-2 in kidney cancer and melanoma*. Cancer Biother Radiopharm, 2004. 19(3): p. 350-4.

[34] Kiessling, R., et al., *Tumor-induced immune dysfunction.* Cancer Immunol Immunother, 1999. 48(7): p. 353-62.

[35] Liu, Y.J., *IPC: professional type 1 interferon-producing cells and plasmacytoid dendritic cell precursors.* Annu Rev Immunol, 2005. 23: p. 275-306.

[36] Moschos, S.J., et al., *Neoadjuvant treatment of regional stage IIIB melanoma with high-dose interferon alfa-2b induces objective tumor regression in association with modulation of tumor infiltrating host cellular immune responses.* J Clin Oncol, 2006. 24(19): p. 3164-71.

[37] Kirkwood, J.M., et al., *Interferon alfa-2b adjuvant therapy of high-risk resected cutaneous melanoma: the Eastern Cooperative Oncology Group Trial EST 1684.* J Clin Oncol, 1996. 14(1): p. 7-17.

[38] Kirkwood, J.M., et al., *High-dose interferon alfa-2b does not diminish antibody response to GM2 vaccination in patients with resected melanoma: results of the Multicenter Eastern Co-operative Oncology Group Phase II Trial E2696.* J Clin Oncol, 2001. 19(5): p. 1430-6.

[39] Sangfelt, O., et al., *Induction of apoptosis and inhibition of cell growth are independent responses to interferon-alpha in hematopoietic cell lines.* Cell Growth Differ, 1997. 8(3): p. 343-52.

[40] Kirkwood, J.M., et al., *Mechanisms and management of toxicities associated with high-dose interferon alfa-2b therapy.* J Clin Oncol, 2002. 20(17): p. 3703-18.

[41] Eggermont, A.M., et al., *Adjuvant therapy with pegylated interferon alfa-2b versus observation alone in resected stage III melanoma: final results of EORTC 18991, a randomised phase III trial.* Lancet, 2008. 372(9633): p. 117-26.

[42] Weber, J., *Review: anti-CTLA-4 antibody ipilimumab: case studies of clinical response and immune-related adverse events.* Oncologist, 2007. 12(7): p. 864-72.

[43] Robert, C., et al., *Ipilimumab plus dacarbazine for previously untreated metastatic melanoma.* N Engl J Med, 2011. 364(26): p. 2517-26.

[44] Reuben, J.M., et al., *Biologic and immunomodulatory events after CTLA-4 blockade with ti-cilimumab in patients with advanced malignant melanoma.* Cancer, 2006. 106(11): p. 2437-44.

[45] Johnston, R.L., et al., *Cytotoxic T-lymphocyte-associated antigen 4 antibody-induced colitis and its management with infliximab.* Dig Dis Sci, 2009. 54(11): p. 2538-40.

[46] Mitjans, F., et al., *In vivo therapy of malignant melanoma by means of antagonists of alphav integrins.* Int J Cancer, 2000. 87(5): p. 716-23.

[47] Hersey, P., et al., *A phase II, randomized, open-label study evaluating the antitumor activity of MEDI-522, a humanized monoclonal antibody directed against the human metastatic melanoma (MM),* in *Proc Am Soc Clin Oncol*2005. p. 711s..

[48] Hersey, P., et al., *A randomized phase 2 study of etaracizumab, a monoclonal antibody against integrin alpha(v)beta(3), +/- dacarbazine in patients with stage IV metastatic melanoma.* Cancer.

[49] Ward, S., et al., *Immunotherapeutic potential of whole tumour cells.* Cancer Immunol Immunother, 2002. 51(7): p. 351-7.

[50] Hsueh, E.C. and D.L. Morton, *Antigen-based immunotherapy of melanoma: Canvaxin therapeutic polyvalent cancer vaccine.* Semin Cancer Biol, 2003. 13(6): p. 401-7.

[51] *CancerVax Announces Results of Phase 3 Clinical Trials of Canvaxin(TM) in Patients With Stage III and Stage IV Melanoma.* Market Wire, 2006.

[52] Sondak, V.K., et al., *Adjuvant immunotherapy of resected, intermediate-thickness, node-negative melanoma with an allogeneic tumor vaccine: overall results of a randomized trial of the Southwest Oncology Group.* J Clin Oncol, 2002. 20(8): p. 2058-66.

[53] *Rethinking therapeutic cancer vaccines.* Nat Rev Drug Discov, 2009. 8(9): p. 685-6.

[54] Berd, D., et al., *Immunopharmacologic analysis of an autologous, hapten-modified human melanoma vaccine.* J Clin Oncol, 2004. 22(3): p. 403-15.

[55] Avax Technologies, I., *Harnessing the patient's immune system for the treatment of cancer.* Avax fact sheet, 2007.

[56] Riker, A.I., et al., *Development and characterization of melanoma cell lines established by fine-needle aspiration biopsy: advances in the monitoring of patients with metastatic melanoma.* Cancer Detect Prev, 1999. 23(5): p. 387-96.

[57] Rosenberg, S.A., et al., *Immunologic and therapeutic evaluation of a synthetic peptide vaccine for the treatment of patients with metastatic melanoma.* Nat Med, 1998. 4(3): p. 321-7.

[58] Report, D., *Pipeline Insight: Therapeutic Cancer Vaccines - Prospect of first approval set to reinvigorate interest from major companies.* PipelineReview, 2009.

[59] Kruit W, S.S., Dreno B, et al, *Immunization with recombinant MAGE-A3 protein combined with adjuvant systems AS15 or AS02B in patients with unresectable and progressive metastatic cutaneous melanoma: a randomized open-label phase II study of the EORTC Melanoma Group.* J Clin Oncol, 2008. 26: p. abstr 9065.

[60] Rosenberg, S.A., J.C. Yang, and N.P. Restifo, *Cancer immunotherapy: moving beyond current vaccines.* Nat Med, 2004. 10(9): p. 909-15.

[61] Slingluff, C.L., Jr., et al., *Clinical and immunologic results of a randomized phase II trial of vaccination using four melanoma peptides either administered in granulocyte-macrophage colony-stimulating factor in adjuvant or pulsed on dendritic cells.* J Clin Oncol, 2003. 21(21): p. 4016-26.

[62] Albert, M.L., B. Sauter, and N. Bhardwaj, *Dendritic cells acquire antigen from apoptotic cells and induce class I-restricted CTLs.* Nature, 1998. 392(6671): p. 86-9.

[63] Ridgway, D., *The first 1000 dendritic cell vaccinees.* Cancer Invest, 2003. 21(6): p. 873-86.

[64] Nestle, F.O., et al., *Vaccination of melanoma patients with peptide- or tumor lysate-pulsed dendritic cells.* Nat Med, 1998. 4(3): p. 328-32.

[65] Schadendorf D, N.F., Broecker EB, Enk A, Grabbe S, Ugurel S, Edler L, Schuler G, De-COG-DC Study Group., *Dacarbacine (DTIC) versus vaccination with autologous peptide-pulsed dendritic cells (DC) as first-line treatment of patients with metastatic melanoma: Results of a prospective-randomized phase III study.* Journal of Clinical Oncology, ASCO Annual Meeting Proceedings, 2004. 22(14s): p. 7508.

[66] Rosenberg, S.A. and M.E. Dudley, *Cancer regression in patients with metastatic melanoma after the transfer of autologous antitumor lymphocytes.* Proc Natl Acad Sci U S A, 2004. 101 Suppl 2: p. 14639-45.

[67] Sotomayor, M.G., et al., *Advances in gene therapy for malignant melanoma.* Cancer Control, 2002. 9(1): p. 39-48.

[68] Piechocki, M.P., S.A. Pilon, and W.Z. Wei, *Complementary antitumor immunity induced by plasmid DNA encoding secreted and cytoplasmic human ErbB-2.* J Immunol, 2001. 167(6): p. 3367-74.

[69] Ulmer, J.B., et al., *Heterologous protection against influenza by injection of DNA encoding a viral protein.* Science, 1993. 259(5102): p. 1745-9.

[70] Trisciuoglio, D., et al., *Bcl-2 overexpression in melanoma cells increases tumor progression-associated properties and in vivo tumor growth.* J Cell Physiol, 2005. 205(3): p. 414-21.

[71] Jansen, B., et al., *Chemosensitisation of malignant melanoma by BCL2 antisense therapy.* Lancet, 2000. 356(9243): p. 1728-33.

[72] Millward MJ, B.A., Conry RM, Gore ME, Pehamberger HE, Sterry W, Pavlick AC, De Conti RC, and I.L. Gordon D, *Randomized multinational phase 3 trial of dacarbazine (DTIC) with or without Bcl-2 antisense (oblimersen sodium) in patients (pts) with advanced malignant melanoma (MM): Analysis of long-term survival.* Journal of Clinical Oncology, (Post-Meeting Edition), 2004. 22(14S (July 15 Supplement)).

[73] Genta, A.a., *FDA Advisory Committee Reviews Genasense(reg) For Use in Advanced Melanoma.* Medical News Today, 2004.

[74] Vical, *Vical Completes Enrollment in Allovectin-7(r) Phase 3 Trial for Metastatic Melanoma.* Globe Newswire, 2010.

[75] J. M. Richards, A.B., R. Gonzalez, M. B. Atkins, E. Whitman, J. Lutzky, M. A. Morse, T. Amatruda, E. Galanis, J. Thompson Vical Clinical Research Operations Team *High-dose Allovectin-7 in patients with advanced metastatic melanoma: final phase 2 data and design of phase 3 registration trial* Journal of Clinical Oncology 2005 ASCO Annual Meeting Proceedings., 2005. 23(16s): p. 7543.

[76] Nemunaitis., N.N.S.H.K.T.A.M.N.T.R.G.D.R.G.J.G.E.W.K.H.R.C.J., *Updated Results of a Phase II Clinical Trial with a Second Generation, Enhanced Potency, Immune-enhanced,*

Oncolytic Herpesvirus in Unresectable Metastatic Melanoma. American Society of Clinical Oncology, 2009. annual meeting: p. poster.

[77]   biovex, *BioVex Commences OncoVEX (GM-CSF) Phase 3 Trial In Metastatic Melanoma.* Medical News Today, 2009.

[78]   Gray-Schopfer, V., C. Wellbrock, and R. Marais, *Melanoma biology and new targeted therapy.* Nature, 2007. 445(7130): p. 851-7.

[79]   Dothager, R.S., et al., *Synthesis and identification of small molecules that potently induce apoptosis in melanoma cells through G1 cell cycle arrest.* J Am Chem Soc, 2005. 127(24): p. 8686-96.

[80]   Fernandez, Y., et al., *Differential regulation of noxa in normal melanocytes and melanoma cells by proteasome inhibition: therapeutic implications.* Cancer Res, 2005. 65(14): p. 6294-304.

[81]   Smalley, K.S. and M. Herlyn, *Targeting intracellular signaling pathways as a novel strategy in melanoma therapeutics.* Ann N Y Acad Sci, 2005. 1059: p. 16-25.

Chapter 12

Update in Ocular Melanoma

Victoria de los Ángeles Bustuoabad,
Lucia Speroni and Arturo Irarrázabal

Additional information is available at the end of the chapter

1. Introduction

1.1. Ocular anatomy

In order to understand the pathophysiology of this condition we will describe the *uvea* anatomy.

The Iris is a contractile diaphragm that controls the degree of retinal illumination, it has a central aperture, the pupil, located slightly nasally. It consists of the following layers from anterior to posterior:

1. Stroma: a thin avascular layer with fibroblasts and melanocytes. It is heavily pigmented in persons with brown eyes less pigmented in green and hazel irises and least in blue. Posteriorly, the stroma contains the sphincter pupillae muscle (parasympathetic, miosis).

2. Pigment epithelium: consists of 2 layers of cells: -anterior layer, which intermingles with the dilator pupillae muscle (sympathetic, mydriasis) -posterior layer, which is continuous with the pigment epithelium of the ciliary body and RPE of the retina, all having the same embryologic origin.

The cilliary body is one of the three parts of the uvea and extends for 6 mm from the end of the retina (ora serrata) till the scleral spur. Its epithelial portion (adjacent to vitreous) consists of a posterior portion (pars plana) and an anterior portion (pars plicata). The latter has 60-70 folds called the ciliary processes which secrete the aqueous humor into the posterior chamber. Its uveal portion contains the ciliary muscle which has 3 parts, all under parasympathetic innervation: longitudinal (outermost), radial and circular.

The choroid is a dark brown vascular sheet, 0.25mm thick, lying between the sclera and the retina. The outer vascular bed has large vessels (layer of Haller) and the inner bed consists of an extensive network of fenestrated vessels, the choriocapillaris which is the major blood supply to the outer layers of the retina and to the whole macula The inner layers, up to the middle of the Pigmented Epithelium are supplied by the central retinal artery.

1.2. Difference between ocular melanoma and cutaneous melanoma

Ocular and cutaneous melanomas show several differences despite they both derive from melanocytes. Both malignancies show a high tendency to metastasize though they display different preferential sites. Skin melanomas spread to distant skin sites, lung, liver, central nervous system and bone. However uveal melanoma, the most frequently diagnosed of the ocular melanomas, gives rise to metastases almost exclusively in the liver which is affected in 90% of the cases.

Interestingly, both malignancies display similar chromosomal aberrations as well as a similar gene expression profile [1]. The similarity in this aspect, despite the difference in tumor behaviour, serves as a proof of the role of the microenvironment in tumor development.

With respect to the early diagnosis, in the skin melanoma the suspected diagnosis and the subsequent clinical follow-up are based on the ABCDE rule.On the other hand, in the diagnosis of ocular melanoma the most relevant information comes from the ophthalmoscopy and the ultrasonography. Finally, consulting times for patients and prognosis are different for both types of melanoma.

2. Objectives

In this chapter we will focus in the clinical management of ocular melanoma from the diagnosis to the treatment.

3. Immunopathology

The eye is an immunologically privileged site; from an evolutionary point of view this condition helps to control or eliminate pathogens while generating the least inflammatory damage to the ocular tissues. However, the counterpart of this phenomenon is that it favors the escape of the tumor cells from the controls of the immune system, facilitating the growth of the uveal melanoma and its metastatic dissemination. Experiments in mice it have shown that cytotoxic cell activity in the ocular tissue might be modulated by two mechanisms:

1.   By direct interference of the specific effector function of CD8 + lymphocytes.

2.   Indirectly affected by stimulation of macrophages [2].

The inhibition of macrophage action was expressed by an insufficient production of nitric oxide in the ocular tissue, which is known to modulate the tumoricidal activity of cytotoxic T lymphocytes [3]. It has also been shown that tumor rejection in mice by the CD8 + CTL is mediated by TNF-α [4].

The study of the mechanisms that facilitate the growth of an immunogenic tumor in the anterior chamber, demonstrated an influx of CD8 + CTL infiltrating the tumor. This phenomenon was preceded by intratumoral accumulation of CD11 + myeloid cells B, which exert a powerful immunosuppressive activity on the CTL, facilitating tumor escape from the immune system. Regulatory T cells, myeloid suppressor cells and stroma cells could also reduce the delayed type hypersensitivity reaction to induce apoptosis of CD8 + and NK cells [5]

4. Demographic and epidemiological data

The *racial* background of the patient is an important factor. Whites have been shown to be eight times more likely to develop choroidal melanoma than African-Americans. This trend is also observed in skin melanoma, whites are six times. More likely to develop this malignancy than African-Americans [6-7]. The individuals with light iris are at increased risk of developing uveal melanoma. This is a finding that implicates *sunlight exposure* as an important environmental risk factor. The protective effect of melanin may be particularly important in the iris as it is the only part of the uveal tract positioned in front of the lens, which serves as an effective ultraviolet filter.

The median *age* at diagnosis is about 55-65 years and the incidence decreases after 70 years of age. With regards to incidence depending on *sex*, there is a slight predominance of males [8].

In a study involving 4500 patients with uveal melanoma, only 0.6% of the cases had a family history of this disease [9]. Thus *heredity* does not seem to be a significant determinant of uveal melanoma. With respect to *occupational and chemical exposures*, the only specific occupational exposure that has been linked to uveal melanoma is welding. Ocular melanomas have been induced in laboratory animals after administration of *radium, methylcholanthrene, N-2fluorenylacetamide, ethionine and nickel subsulfide.*

5. Diagnosis of ocular melanoma

Accuracy in the early diagnosis of ocular melanoma is crucial to improve the prognosis. Currently the diagnosis of ocular melanoma is based on both the clinical experience of the specialists and on the use of modern diagnostic techniques.

The rate of misdiagnosis for eyes enucleated for choroidal melanoma was 20 % until the 1970's but it has decreased to 1% since then. [10-16]

5.1. Clinical

The most common symptoms include *visual loss, photopsias and visual field defects*. None of these symptoms are specific of choroidal melanoma. Pain is very atypical in ocular melanoma, except in those cases that present massive extraocular extension, inflammation or neovascular glaucoma.

Indirect Ophthalmoscopy through a well-dilated pupil is the most important examination in the diagnosis of choroidal melanoma. The classic image is a pigmented, dome-shaped or collar button-shaped tumor in a minority of cases and an associated exudative retinal detachment, orange tumor pigmentation (Lipofuscin) and sentinel vessels (prominent episcleral vessels especially in those involving ciliary body). Scleral transillumination has been advocated by Reese. [17]

The lesions most commonly mistaken for choroidal melanoma are choroidal nevus (49%), periphereal exudative hemorrhagic chorioretinopathy (8%), congenital hypertrophy of the retinal pigment epithelium (6%), hemorrhagic detachment of the retina or pigment epithelium (5%), circumscribed choroidal hemangioma (8%) and age related macular degeneration (4%) [18]

5.2. Complementary studies

Ultrasonography: The most important ancillary test in the evaluation of a patient with intraocular mass lesions is the combination of both A-mode and B-mode ultrasonography (see Box 1). For tumors larger than 3 mm in thickness, a combination of both scans in skilled hands can diagnose choroidal melanomas with greater than 95% accuracy [19].

A-mode:

1. medium to low internal echoes with smooth attenuation.

2. vascular pulsations within the tumor

B-mode: 3 classic futures

1. Low to medium reflectivity within the melanoma.

2. Choroidal excavation.

3. Shadowing in the orbit.

Box 1. Ultrasonography

Fluorescein angiography: Early hyperfluorescence with late leakage and multifocal punctate hyperfluorescence. This study is of major importance in order to distinguish lesions that simulate choroidal melanoma.

Other studies like Optical Coherence Tomography and Indocyanine Green angiography may be useful in the diagnosis of this pathology. Magnetic resonance imaging, nuclear magnetic resonance spectography, color Doppler ultrasonography, electrophysiologic testing and inmmunologic testing do not offer reliable results. [20-26]

6. Current medical management of patients with Ocular Melanoma

a.   Cytogenetic: Personalized Targeted Therapy

Currently much effort is directed toward understanding uveal melanoma genetics and genomics [27], hoping that this knowledge will contribute to the development of effective molecular therapies

Inhibitors of B.Raf and MEK kinases hold promise for treatment of cutaneous melanomas harboring BRAF mutations. BRAF are rare in ocular melanomas, but somatic mutations in the G protein alfa subunits G alfa q and G alfa 11 (encoded by *Gnaq* and *Gna11*, respectively) occur, in a mutually exclusive pattern, in 80% of uveal melanomas. The impact of the B-Raf inhibitor PLX4720 and the MEK inhibitor AZD6244, the AKT inhibitor MK2206 and the PKC inhibitors bisindolylmaleimide I (GF109203X) has been assessed [28].

A randomized phase II study compared MEK inhibition (AZD6244) to temozomide in advanced uveal melanoma. MEK inhibition seems to be a rationale therapeutic strategy in uveal melanoma, using Gnaq/11 as a potential predictor of sensitivity [29].

b.   Surgery: Resection/Enucleation

Enucleation is indicated when the tumor size exceeds 16 mm of base and 10 mm of height, is diffuse and with bad prognosis; however it is very important to emphasize that there is no scientific evidence of increased survival after enucleation. Also, enucleation does not prevent metastases.

A novel minimally invasive surgical technique for resection of selected cases of small iris tumours has been described. This technique avoids the potential morbidity associated with a large corneoescleral incision allowing for rapid visual recovery [30].

Radiotherapy, *Brachytherapy* (BT: I125, 103 Pd, 131 Cs, Ru) and Proton Beam Radiotherapy (PBRT)

The most commonly employed form of radiotherapy has been the application of an episcleral radioactive plaque and the most frequently employed isotopes include *60 Co (Cobalt), 106 Ru (Ruthenium), 192 Ir (Iridium) and 125 I (Iodine)* [31-32].

It is extremely important to highlight the conservative treatment of melanoma, proposed by *Irarrazabal A. et al* using brachytherapy. This procedure has shown positive results in preserving the eye, without increase in mortality. Moreover useful vision was retained in more than half of the treated patients [33].

In a study comparing patients treated with *Ruthenium* brachytherapy with patients undergoing simultaneous thermotherapy or BT alone, combined treatment provided higher local control, eye globes preservation, better recurrence-free survival rates, lower rates of metastases and prolonged survival than treatment with BT alone.

I125 episcleral brachytherapy in uveal melanoma is effective in tumor control, allowing preservation of the eye and useful visual function for the majority of patients [34].

It has been suggested that length of remaining life after diagnosis of uveal melanoma is similar following enucleation (removal of the eye) to local eye-conserving radiotherapy. The multidisciplinary COMS Group emphasized that there were no differences in survival outcomes and a small difference in quality-of-life outcomes between patients in the brachytherapy arm and those in the enucleation arm [35].

Radiation treatment was found to reduce the tumor in 94% of the cases. Mean tumor thickness decreased from 3.7 to 2.5 and 2.1 after 3 and 5 years respectively. Recurrence occured in 6% of the treated patients. Although this therapy is associated with complications like radiation optic neuropathy in 81% and vitreous bleeding in 30% of cases, it is a promising treatment given that enucleation was necessary in only 3% of patients and metastasis developed in 15% during follow up. Even though the visual acuity decreases considerably after optic disc irradiation with proton beam therapy, the rates of tumor control and eye retention are favourable.

The second most frequent method of radiotherapy is the use of heavy ions such as *Proton Beam Radiotherapy* [36]. In a comparison of the efficacy of PBRT and Ruthenium-106 notched plaque radiotherapy with or without TTT for the treatment of juxtapapillary choroidal melanoma, it was found that the tumors were successfully treated using either proton beam or notched plaque combined with adjuvant TTT [37].However, vision is often sacrificed. On the other hand, Notched plaque alone is not as efficient in reducing the tumor but results in improved visual outcome [37].

Proton beam irradiation of uveal melanoma has great advantages over brachytherapy because of the homogenous dose delivered to the tumor and the possibility of sparing normal tissue close to the tumor. Complications such as retinal detachment, maculopathy, papillopathy, cataract, glaucoma, vitreous hemorrhage and dryness are described. The severest complication that usually leads to secondary enucleation is neovascular glaucoma and it is encountered after irradiation of large to extra-large tumors. It is hypothesized that the residual tumor scar may produce proinflammatory cytokines and Vascular endothelial growth factor- VEGF (toxic tumor syndrome) leading to intraocular inflammation and neovascular glaucoma. Additional treatments after proton beam such as transpupillary thermotherapy, endoresection of the tumor scar or intravitreal injections of anti-VEGF may reduce the rate of these complications [38].

c.   Monoclonal Antibodies

Current systemic treatments for metastatic uveal melanoma have not improved overall survival. The fully human anti-cytotoxic T-lymphocyte antigen-4 (CTLA-4) monoclonal antibody, *ipilimumab*, improved overall survival of patients with advanced cutaneous melanoma in a phase 3 trial. However, uveal melanoma patients were excluded from this study. A sub-analysis, performed by the ipilimumab-ocular melanoma expanded access program (I-OMEAP) study group, aimed at assessing the activity and safety of ipilimumab in patients with uveal melanoma in a setting similar to daily clinical practice. The results indicated that uveal melanoma is a potential target for ipilimumab treatment and that it should be further investigated in clinical trials [39].

The *R24 monoclonal antibody*, that recognizes the disialoganglioside GD3 expressed on the surface of malignant melanoma cells, could mediate destruction of these cells. A combination of R24 with a low dose of IL-2 was found to promote destruction of cultured melanoma cells and it can be safely administered to patients with metastatic melanoma [40].

d.   Transpupillary Thermotherapy (TTT):

Choroidal melanomas should be diagnosed and treated at the very early stage as the initial spread of metastases is thought to occur during the proliferative stage of tumor development.

TTT is recomended for the management of posterior choroidal nevi suspected for malignant transformation or small choroidal melanomas that are less than 2-5 mm in thickness [41]. TTT might be the treatment of choice for selected, very small melanomas. However, studies with long follow-up and large number of patients are needed to evaluate its effectiveness.

Choroidal melanomas treated with TTT as stand-alone procedure need a close monitoring since these tumors developed a significant rate of local recurrences and ocular side-effects in the long run.

e.   Antiangiogenic drugs (Bevacizumab)

Anti-angiogenic therapy is based on the assumption that a tumor cannot grow beyond the limits of diffusion (about 1-2 mm) of oxygen and nutrients from capillaries, unless angiogenesis takes place. VEGF plays a key role in angiogenesis, regulating vasopermeability and the proliferation and migration of endothelial cells. VEGF levels are significantly elevated in uveal melanoma patients with metastatic disease compared to patients without metastases. Anti-angiogenic therapy, such as bevacizumab, is currently used for the treatment of metastases of several malignancies. [43].

Bevacizumab may be used as an adjuvant agent when used following plaque brachytherapy in the treatment of choroidal melanoma. The combination of this treatments was assessed in an interventional case series of 100 patients treated from 2006-2008 for choroidal melanoma and the results were satisfactory. Melanoma specific mortality was 0% at 9 months after treatment. Mean visual acuity for combined treatment at 6 months was 20/30 [42]

The *bevacizumab - radiotherapy combination* could be a promising clinical approach for the management of human uveal melanoma, since it may allow the use of lower doses of radiotherapy without compromising the antitumor effect [44].

f.   Chemotherapy

There is no current evidence that chemotherapy has a significant role in the primary management of uveal melanoma. Such treatment may prolong survival for a few months but it is unlikely that it will be curative.

Uveal melanoma metastases develop in 6.5-35% of patients, most commonly to the liver. Metastatic uveal melanoma survival is poor, with 5-7 months of median survival. A retrospective study including 58 patients with uveal melanoma metastases showed that the median overall survival (OS) for all the patients was 10.83 months. Patients who had undergone chemotherapy presented 10.83 months of median OS whereas the patients who did not undergo this treatment had an OS of 8.033 months. Patients with metastatic uveal melanoma should be included in clinical trials evaluating other options with newer agents [45].

g.   Others (Adjuvant therapy with interferon, Imatinilo Mesylate, Paclitaxeldocosahexaenoico Acid, Factionated Radiosurgery Cyberknife, aflibercept, vaccine).

7. Medical prognosis: Mortality (Hepatic metastasis), loss of the eye, loss of vision

These three variables will affect directly the patient survival:

Variable	Importance for prognosis
A Size (Base more than 16 mm and altura more than 10 mm).	+
B Cell Type (Epithelloid Cells)	++
C Genetic Type (GEP: Gene Expression Profile)	+++

Prognosis: GEP (Gene Expression Profile) In a prospective evaluation involving 514 uveal melanoma patients [46], the gene expression profile prognostic assay helped in classifying the primary tumor into two prognostic subgroups:

Class I (60% of the cases)

Low metastatic risk :

IA (87%) almost without metastasis (0.8% of the patients).

IB (13%) few metastasis (10.8%) + disomy cr3 few metastasis.

Class II (40% of the cases)

High metastatic risk: metastasis (29.8%) + monosomy or pseudodisomy cr3 metastasis is not sure, + Trisomy cr6: 80 % of patients will show metastasis 4 years after diagnosis.

This classification might be helpful for the prognosis in three aspects: in the screening targeted to metastasis, in the earlier diagnosis of the metastasis and for an earlier preventing treatment of the metastasis in high risk cases. In this regard, it is important to highlight that there is no scientific evidence about increased survival due to metastasis treatment [47].

8. Uveal melanoma TNM staging and survival: Implications in patient management and prognosis

Damato, B; Eleuteri, A [48] support the idea that Kaplan-Meier survival curves based only in tumour size and extend do not provide a true indication of prognosis. This is because the survival prognosis in uveal melanoma correlates not only with clinical stage but also with histologic grade, genetic type and competing causes of death. They propose an online predictor tool using the following data:

8.1. Parameters

Age

Sex

Large ultrasound diameter

Cilliary body involvement

Extraocular extension

Years since treatment

Epithelloid Cells

Closed PAS+ ve loops

Mitotic rate/40

Monosomy 3

Regional Lymph nodes

Distant metastasis

First scan (years)

Threshold for next scan (number)

8.2. TNM Stage

C.

Survival

Controls

Subjects

Difference

Relative

9. Conclusion

The uveal melanoma, which arises from melanocytes residing in the stroma, is the most common primary intraocular tumour in adults. More than 90% involve the choroid, the remainder being confined to the ciliary body and iris.

The most common symptoms in uveal melanoma include visual loss, photopsias and visual field defects but none of these symptoms are specific of this malignancy. Diagnosis is based on slit-lamp biomicroscopy and/or ophthalmoscopy, with ultrasonography, autofluorescence photography. Although each day we count with more variety and helpful complementary studies, suspicious lesions should be closely monitored. Uveal melanomas are diverse in their clinical features and behaviour. Despite ocular treatment almost 50% of patients with primary uveal melanoma will develop distance metastasis [50]. The metastatic disease occurs almost exclusively in patients whose tumour show chromosome 3 loss and/or class 2 gene expression profile. When the tumour shows such lethal genetic changes, the survival time depends on the anatomical stage and the histological grade of the malignancy.

Prognostication has improved as a result of progress in multivariate analysis including all the major risk factors.

Screening for metastases is more sensitive as a consequence of the advances in liver scanning with magnetic resonance imaging and other methods. More patients with metastases are living longer, benefiting from therapies such as: partial hepatectomy; radiofrequency ablation; ipilumumab immunotherapy; selective internal radiotherapy; intra-hepatic chemotherapy, possibly with isolated liver perfusion; and systemic chemotherapy [48].

Conservation of the eye with useful vision has improved thanks to the advances in brachytherapy, proton beam radiotherapy, transpupillary thermotherapy. The current trend is to try to preserve the affected eye by all means, as there is no scientific evidence that shows that removing the affected eye will improve survival.. This is a great difference in the treatment of ocular vs cutaneous melanoma. The specialists must take into consideration the need to protect the eye with melanoma and preserve as much vision as possible as the other eye may be affected by another pathology in the future with the consequent loss of vision.

On the basis of the currently available information it appears that patients treated with radiotherapy have a survival rate at least as good, if not better than those treated with enucleation [36].

Several drugs, such as bortezomib, celecoxib, dacarbazine, anti-angiogenic agents (such as bevacizumab, sorafenib and sunitinib), temsirolimus, mitogen-activated protein kinase kinase (MEK) inhibitors, ipilimumab and AEB071 are candidate drugs, and studies are underway to determine the therapeutic effects of these drugs in uveal melanoma [51].

Currently, the aim is to improve the detection of uveal melanoma so as to maximize the opportunities for conserving the eye and vision, as well as preventing metastatic spread. Patient management has been enhanced by the formation of multidisciplinary teams in specialized ocular oncology centers all over the world.

Acknowledgements

This publication was supported by grants from Raymos S.A.C.I. laboratory.

Author details

Victoria de los Ángeles Bustuoabad[1], Lucia Speroni[2] and Arturo Irarrázabal[3]

1 German Hospital, Buenos Aires, Argentina

2 Department of Anatomy and Cellular Biology, Tufts University, Boston, USA

3 Consultores Oftalmológicos Institute, Montevideo, Buenos Aires, Argentina

References

[1] Van den Bosch T, Kilic E, Paridaens D, de Klein A. Genetics of uveal melanoma and cutaneous melanoma: two of a kind? Dermatol Res Pract. 2010;2010:360136.

[2] Vicetti Miguel RD, Cherpes TL, Watson LJ, Mc Kenna KC: CTL induction of tumoricidal nitric oxide production by intratumoral macrophages is critical for tumor elimination. J Immunol 2010, 185:6706-18.

[3] Dace DS, Chen PW, Niederkorn JY: CD8+ Tcells circumvent privilege in the eye and mediate intraocular tumor rejection by aTNF-alfa dependent mechanism. J Immunol, 2007, 178:6115-22

[4] McKenna KC, Kapp JA: Accumulation of immunosuppressive CD11B+ myeloid cells correlates with the failure to prevent tumor grouth in the anterior chamber of the eye. J Immunol, 2006, 177:1599-608.

[5] Poggi A, Zocchi MR: Mechanisms of tumor escape: role of tumor microenviroment inducing apoptosis of cytolytic effector cells. Arch. Immunol The Exp (Warsz) 2006, 54:323-33.

[6]   Margo CE, Mc Lean IW: Malignant melanoma of the choroid and ciliary body in black patiens. Arch Ophthalmol 1984; 102:77-79.

[7]   Graham BJ, Duane TD: Meetings, conferences, symposia: report of ocular melanoma task force. Am J Ophthalmol 1981; 90:728-733.

[8]   Gragoudas ES: First 1000 patients with uveal melanoma treated by proton beam irradiation. Presented at the second International Meeting in the Diagnosis and Treatment of Intraocular Tumors in Nyon, Switzerland, November, 1987.

[9]   Singh AD, Shields CL, De Potter P, Shields JA, Trock B, Cater J, Pastore D. Familial uveal melanoma. Clinical observations on 56 patients. Arch Ophthalmol.1996 Apr; 114(4):392-9.

[10] Ferry AP: Lesions mistaken for malignant melanoma of the posterior uvea: a clinicopathologic analysis of 100 cases with ophthalmoscopically vivible lesions. Arch, Ophthalmol 1964; 72:463-469.

[11] Shields JA, Zimmerman LE: Lesions simulating malignant melanoma of the posterior uvea. Arch Ophthalmol 1973; 89:466-471.

[12] Zimmerman LE: Bedell Lecture. Problems in the diagnosis of malignant melanoma of the choroid and ciliary body. Am J Phthalmol 1973; 75:917-929.

[13] Chang M, Zimmerman LE. Mc Lean IW: The persisting pseudomelanoma problem. Arch Ophthalmol 1984, 102:726-727.

[14] Shields JA, Augsburger JJ, Brown GC, Stephens RF: The Differential diagnosis of posterior uveal melanoma. Ophthalmology 1980; 87:518-522.

[15] Shields JA, Mashayekhi A, Ra S, Shields CL: Pseudomelanomas of the posterior uveal tract. Retina 2005; 25:767-771.

[16] Char DH, Stone RD, Irvine AR, et al: Diagnostic modalities in choroidal melanoma. Am J Ophthalmol 1980; 89:223-230.

[17] Reese AB: Tumors of the eye 3rd edn. Hagerstown, MD: Harper & Row; 1976:174-262.

[18] Shields JA, Mashayekhi A, Ra S, Shields CL: Pseudomelanomas of the posterior uveal tract. Retina 2005; 25:767-771

[19] Char DH, Stone RD, Irvine AR, et al: Diagnostic modalities in choroidal melanoma. Am J Ophthalmol 1980; 89:223-230.

[20] Char DH: Inhibition of leukocyte migration with melanoma-associated antigens in choroidal tumors. Invest Ophthalmol Vis Sci 1977; 16:176-179.

[21] Brownstein S, Phillips TM, Lewis MG: Specificity of tumor-associated antibodies in serum of patients with uveal melanoma. Can J Ophthalmol 1978; 13:190-193.

[22] Felberg NT, Donoso LA, Federman JL: Tumor-associated antibodies in the serum of patients with ocular melanoma. Ophthalmology 1980; 87:529-533.

[23] Felberg NT, Pro-Landazuri JM, Shields JA, Federman JL: Tumor-associated antibodies in the serum of patients with ocular melanoma. Arch Ophthalmol 1979; 97:256-259.

[24] Donoso LA, Felberg NT, Edelberg K, et al: Metastasic uveal melanoma: an ocular melanoma-associated antigen in the serum of patients with metastatic deasease.

[25] Meyer F, Naron d, Zonix S: The role of carcinoembryonic antigen in surveillance of patients with choroidal melanoma: a prospectibe study. Ann Ophthalmol 1987; 19:24-25.

[26] Bomanji J, Hungerford JL, Granowska M, Britton Ke: Radioimmunoscintigraphy of ocular melanoma with 99m Tc labeled cutaneous melanoma antibody fragments. Br J Ophthalmol 1987; 71:651-658.

[27] Leyvraz S, Keilholz U: Ocular Melanoma: whats new? Curr Opin Oncol. 2012 Mar; 24(2):162-9.

[28] Vasiliki Poulaki, Sue Anne Chew, Bin He, Nicholas Mitsiades. Personalized Targeted Therapy harboring GNAq and GNA 11 Mutations. Inhibition of genes (Mek, B-Raf, Akt, PkC). Uveal Melanoma. XVth Biannual Meeting ISOO International Society of Ocular Oncology, 2011, Nov 14-17.

[29] Carvajal R, Wolchok JD, Chapman PB, Dickson M, Bluth M, Ambrosini G, Marr B, Heinemann M, Fusco A, Nalysnyk, Martin N, Doyle A, Bastian B, Abramson D, Schwartz G: Rationale, study design and accrual status of a randomized phase II study of AZD6244, a MEK inhibitor, vs temozomide in advanced uveal melanoma. XVth Biannual Meeting ISOO International Society of Ocular Oncology, 2011, Nov 14-17.

[30] Singh A: Resection of iris tumours: Internal approach. XVth Biannual Meeting ISOO International Society of Ocular Oncology, 2011, Nov 14-17.

[31] Shields JA, Augsburger JJ, Brady LW, Day JL: Cobalt plaque therapy of posterior uveal melanomas. Ophthalmology 99:1201-1207, 1982.

[32] Shields JA: Diagnosis and Management of Intraocular Tumours. St. Louis, the CV Mosby Co, 1983.

[33] Irarrázabal A, Cazon P: Results of melanoma brachytherapy in Argentina. XVth Biannual Meeting ISOO (International Society of Ocular Oncology), 2011, Nov 14-17.

[34] García-Álvarez C, Saornil MA, López-Lara F, Almaraz A, Muñoz MF, Frutos-Baraja J, Muiños Y: Episcleral brachytherapy for uveal melanoma: analysis of 136 cases. Clin Transl Oncol. 2012 May;14(5):350-5.

[35] Hawkins BS: Collaborative ocular melanoma study randomized trial of I-125 brachytherapy. Clin Trials. 2011 Oct;8(5):661-73.

[36] Gragoudas ES, Goiten M, Verhey L, Munzenreider J, Suit HD, Kohler A: Proton Beam irradiation, an alternative to Enucleation for intraocular melanoma. Ophthalmology 87:571-581, 1980.

[37] Tsimpida M, Hungerford J, Cohen V: Treatment of juxtapapillary choroidal melanoma. XVth Biannual Meeting ISOO International Society of Ocular Oncology, 2011, Nov 14-17.

[38] Damato B: Progress in the management of patients with uveal melanoma. Eye (Lond). 2012 Jun 29. The 2012 Ashton Lecture. [Epub ahead of print]

[39] Danielli R, Ridolfi R, Chiarion-Sileni V, Queirolo P, Testori A, Plummer R, Boitano M, Calabró L, Rossi CD, Giacomo AM, Ferrucci Pf, Ridolfi L, Altomonte M, Miracco C, Balestrazzi A, Maio M: Ipilimumab in pretreated patients with metastatic uveal melanoma.: safety and clinical efficacy. Cancer Immunol Immunother, 2012 Jan; 61(!): 41-8. Epub 2011 Aug 11.

[40] Soiffer RJ, Chapman PB, Murray C, Williams L, Unger P, Collins H, Houghton AN, Ritz J: Administration of R24 monoclonal antibody and low-dose interleukin 2 for malignant melanoma. Clin Cancer Res, 1997 Jan; 3(1):17-24.

[41] Mordechai R, Moroz I, Moisseiev J, Vishnevskia-Dai V: Our experience with transpupillary thermo therapy for suspected or small choroidal melanomas. XVth Biannual Meeting ISOO International Society of Ocular Oncology, 2011, Nov 14-17.

[42] Houston SK, Murray T, Markoe A, Pina Y, Decataur C: Intravitreal bevacizumab as an adjuvant agent when used immediately after treatment with plaque brachytherapy. XVth Biannual Meeting ISOO International Society of Ocular Oncology, 2011, Nov 14-17.

[43] el Filali M, van der Velden PA, Luyten GP, Jager MJ: Anti-angiogenic therapy in uveal melanoma. Dev Ophthalmol. 2012;49:117-36. Epub 2011 Oct 21.

[44] Sudaka A, Susini A, Lo Nigro C, Fischel JL, Toussan N, Formento P, Tonissi F, Lattanzio L, Russi E, Etienne-Grimaldi MC, Merlano M, Milano G: Combination of bevacizumab and irradiation on uveal melanoma: an in vitro and in vivo preclinical study. Invest New Drugs. 2012 Jun 20. [Epub ahead of print]

[45] Pons F, Plana M, Caminal JM, Pera J, Fernandes I, Perez J, Garcia-Del-Muro X, Marcoval J, Penin R, Fabra A, Piulats JM: Metastatic uveal melanoma: is there a role for conventional chemotherapy? - A single center study based on 58 patients. Melanoma Res. 2011 Jun;21(3):217-22.

[46] Harbour JW, Onken M, Worley L, Augsburger J, Correa Z, Devron HC, Nudleman E, Aaberg TJr, Altaweel MM, Bardenstein D, Finger P, Gallie B, Harocopos GJ, Hovland PG, McGowan H, Milman T, Mruthyunjaya P, Simpson ER, Smith M, Wilson D, Wirostko WJ: Prospective evaluation of a gene expression profile prognostic assay for uveal melanoma in 514 patients. XVth Biannual Meeting ISOO International Society of Ocular Oncology, 2011, Nov 14-17.

[47] Augsburger JJ, Correa ZM, Shaikh AH: Quality of evidence about effectiveness of treatments for metastatic uveal melanoma, Trans Am Ophthalmol Soc, 2008; 106:128-35; discussion 135-7.

[48] Damato B, Eleuteri A, Taktak AF, Coupland SE: Estimating prognosis for survival after treatment of choroidal melanoma. Prog Rtin Eye Res, 2011 Sep; 30(5):285-95. Epub 2011 May 30.

[49] Eye (Lond). 2012 Jun 29. doi: 10.1038/eye.2012.126. [Epub ahead of print]

[50] Spagnolo F, Caltabiano G, Queirolo P: Uveal Melanoma. Cancer Treat Rev 2012 Aug; 38(5):549-53. Epub 2012 Jan 24.

[51] Velho TR, Kapiteijn E, Jager MJ: New therapeutic agents in uveal melanoma. Anticancer Res. 2012 Jul;32(7):2591-8.

Permissions

The contributors of this book come from diverse backgrounds, making this book a truly international effort. This book will bring forth new frontiers with its revolutionizing research information and detailed analysis of the nascent developments around the world.

We would like to thank Guy Huynh Thien Duc, for lending his expertise to make the book truly unique. He has played a crucial role in the development of this book. Without his invaluable contribution this book wouldn't have been possible. He has made vital efforts to compile up to date information on the varied aspects of this subject to make this book a valuable addition to the collection of many professionals and students.

This book was conceptualized with the vision of imparting up-to-date information and advanced data in this field. To ensure the same, a matchless editorial board was set up. Every individual on the board went through rigorous rounds of assessment to prove their worth. After which they invested a large part of their time researching and compiling the most relevant data for our readers. Conferences and sessions were held from time to time between the editorial board and the contributing authors to present the data in the most comprehensible form. The editorial team has worked tirelessly to provide valuable and valid information to help people across the globe.

Every chapter published in this book has been scrutinized by our experts. Their significance has been extensively debated. The topics covered herein carry significant findings which will fuel the growth of the discipline. They may even be implemented as practical applications or may be referred to as a beginning point for another development. Chapters in this book were first published by InTech; hereby published with permission under the Creative Commons Attribution License or equivalent.

The editorial board has been involved in producing this book since its inception. They have spent rigorous hours researching and exploring the diverse topics which have resulted in the successful publishing of this book. They have passed on their knowledge of decades through this book. To expedite this challenging task, the publisher supported the team at every step. A small team of assistant editors was also appointed to further simplify the editing procedure and attain best results for the readers.

Our editorial team has been hand-picked from every corner of the world. Their multi-ethnicity adds dynamic inputs to the discussions which result in innovative outcomes. These outcomes are then further discussed with the researchers and contributors who give their valuable feedback and opinion regarding the same. The feedback is then collaborated with the researches and they are edited in a comprehensive manner to aid the understanding of the subject.

Apart from the editorial board, the designing team has also invested a significant amount of their time in understanding the subject and creating the most relevant covers. They scrutinized every image to scout for the most suitable representation of the subject and create an appropriate cover for the book.

The publishing team has been involved in this book since its early stages. They were actively engaged in every process, be it collecting the data, connecting with the contributors or procuring relevant information. The team has been an ardent support to the editorial, designing and production team. Their endless efforts to recruit the best for this project, has resulted in the accomplishment of this book. They are a veteran in the field of academics and their pool of knowledge is as vast as their experience in printing. Their expertise and guidance has proved useful at every step. Their uncompromising quality standards have made this book an exceptional effort. Their encouragement from time to time has been an inspiration for everyone.

The publisher and the editorial board hope that this book will prove to be a valuable piece of knowledge for researchers, students, practitioners and scholars across the globe.

List of Contributors

Sherif S. Morgan, Joanne M. Jeter, Evan M. Hersh and Lee D. Cranmer
Section of Hematology and Oncology, Melanoma/Sarcoma Program, University of Arizona Cancer Center, University of Arizona, USA

Sun K. Yi
Department of Radiation Oncology, College of Medicine, University of Arizona, USA

Paul J. Speicher, Douglas S. Tyler and Paul J. Mosca
Division of Surgical Oncology, Department of Surgery, Duke University Medical Center, Durham, USA

Andrea Zangari
Pediatric Surgery Department San Camillo Hospital, Roma, Italy

Federico Zangari, Mercedes Romano, Elisabetta Cerigioni and Martino Ascanio
Pediatric Surgery Department, University Hospital of Ancona, Italy

Maria Giovanna Grella and Anna Chiara Contini
Catholic University of the Sacred Heart, Roma, Italy

Jennifer Makalowski and Hinrich Abken
Center for Molecular Medicine Cologne (CMMC), University of Cologne, Cologne, Germany
Dept. I Internal Medicine, University Hospital Cologne, Cologne, Germany

Z. Al-Hilli, D. Evoy, J.G. Geraghty, E.W. McDermott and R.S. Prichard
St. Vincent's University Hospital, Elm Park, Dublin, Ireland

Luis Sanchez del-Campo, Maria F. Montenegro, Magali Saez-Ayala, María Piedad Fernández-Pérez and Jose Neptuno Rodriguez-Lopez
Department of Biochemistry & Molecular Biology A, University of Murcia, Spain

Juan Cabezas-Herrera
Research Unit of Clinical Analusis Service, University Hospital Virgen de la Arrixaca, Spain

Jonathan Castillo Arias
Pharmacological Biochemistry Laboratory, Institute of Biochemistry, Faculty of Sciences, Universidad Austral de Chile, Valdivia, Chile

Miriam Galvonas Jasiulionis
Pharmacology Department, Universidade Federal de São Paulo, São Paulo, Brazil

Yasuhiro Nakamura and Fujio Otsuka
Department of Dermatology, Faculty of Medicine, University of Tsukuba, Tsukuba, Japan

Yoshitaka Kai and Sakuhei Fujiwara
Department of Dermatology, Faculty of Medicine, Oita University, Oita, Japan

Mario Santinami, Roberto Patuzzo, Roberta Ruggeri, Gianpiero Castelli, Andrea Maurichi, Giulia Baffa and Carlotta Tinti
Melanoma Sarcoma Unit Fondazione Istituto Tumori Milano, Italy
Dermatology Unit Ospedale Umberto I Siracusa, Italy

Zhao Wang, Wei Li and Duane D. Miller
Department of Pharmaceutical Sciences, University of Tennessee Health Science Center, Memphis, USA

Victoria de los Ángeles Bustuoabad
German Hospital, Buenos Aires, Argentina

Lucia Speroni
Department of Anatomy and Cellular Biology, Tufts University, Boston, USA

Arturo Irarrázabal
Consultores Oftalmológicos Institute, Montevideo, Buenos Aires, Argentina

www.ingramcontent.com/pod-product-compliance
Lightning Source LLC
Chambersburg PA
CBHW070730190326
41458CB00004B/1108